This book

Outcome Measures in Orthopaedics and Orthopaedic Trauma

Outcome Measures in Orthopaedics and Orthopaedic Trauma

2nd Edition

Edited by

Paul B. Pynsent
Research and Teaching Centre, Royal Orthopaedic Hospital,
Birmingham, UK

Jeremy C. T. Fairbank
Nuffield Orthopaedic Centre, Oxford, UK

Andrew J. Carr
University of Oxford, Nuffield Orthopaedic Centre, Oxford, UK

A member of the Hodder Headline Group
LONDON

First published as *Outcome Measures in Orthopaedics* in 1992, and as *Outcome Measures in Trauma* in 1994 by Butterworth-Heinemann, Linacre House, Jordan Hill, Oxford, OX2 8DP.

This edition published in Great Britain in 2004 by Arnold, a member of the Hodder Headline Group, 338 Euston Road, London NW1 3BH

http://www.arnoldpublishers.com

First published 1992; 1994
Second edition 2004

Distributed in the United States of America by Oxford University Press Inc., 198 Madison Avenue, New York, NY10016 Oxford is a registered trademark of Oxford University Press

British Library Cataloguing in Publication Data
A catalogue record for this book is available from the British Library

Library of Congress Cataloging-in-Publication Data
A catalog record for this book is available from the Library of Congress

ISBN   0 340 80707 5

1 2 3 4 5 6 7 8 9 10

Commissioning Editor: Serena Bureau
Development Editor: Layla Vandenbergh
Project Editor: Zelah Pengilley
Production Controller: Deborah Smith
Cover Design: Stewart Larking
Indexer: Laurence Errington

Typeset in 10/13 Sabon by Charon Tec Pvt. Ltd, Chennai, India
Printed and bound in the UK by Butler & Tanner Ltd.

What do you think about this book? Or any other Arnold title?
Please send your comments to **feedback.arnold@hodder.co.uk**

Contents

Contributors

Roger M. Atkins, MA, FRCS, DM Oxon
Consultant Orthopaedic Surgeon, Bristol Royal
Infirmary and Avon Orthopaedic Centre,
Bristol Royal Infirmary, Bristol, UK

Peter P. Belward, MCSP, SRP
Clinical Specialist Hand Therapist,
Southampton General Hospital,
Southampton, UK

Harry Brownlow, BSc, MBChB, MD, FRCS (Ortho)
Consultant Orthopaedic Surgeon,
Royal Berkshire Hospital,
Reading, UK

Andrew J. Carr, ChM, FRCS
Nuffield Professor of Orthopaedic Surgery,
Nuffield Department of Orthopaedic Surgery,
Nuffield Orthopaedic Centre, Oxford, UK

Philip J. Chapman-Sheath, BSc, FRCS (Tr & Orth)
Consultant Orthopaedic Surgeon,
Southampton General Hospital,
Southampton, UK

Jonathan C. Clasper, DPhil, DM FIMC FRCSEd (Orth)
DMCC
Consultant Orthopaedic Surgeon,
Frimley Park Hospital, Surrey, UK

Julian P. Cooper, BSc, FRCS (Tr & Orth)
Consultant Orthopaedic Trauma Surgeon,
South Birmingham Trauma Unit,
Selly Oak Hospital, University Hospital
Birmingham NHS Trust, Birmingham, UK

Edel Daly, DPhil
Research Officer, Unit of Health Care
Epidemiology, Department of Public Health,
Oxford University, Oxford, UK

T. R. C. Davis, BSc, FRCS
University Hospital, Queens Medical Centre,
Nottingham, UK

Joseph J. Dias, MD, FRCS(Ed), FRCS
Consultant Orthopaedic and Hand Surgeon,
Glenfield Hospital, Groby Road, Leicester, UK

D. M. Eastwood, MB, FRCS
Consultant Orthopaedic Surgeon, The Royal
National Orthopaedic Hospital and the
Royal Free Hospital, London, UK

Lars B. Engesæter, MD, PhD
Orthopaedic Surgeon, Department of Orthopaedic
Surgery, Haukeland University Hospital,
Bergen, Norway

Birgitte Espehaug, MSc, PhD
Statistician, The Norwegian Arthroplasty
Register, Department of Orthopaedic Surgery,
Haukeland University Hospital, Bergen, Norway

Jeremy C. T. Fairbank, MD, FRCS
Consultant Orthopaedic Surgeon, Nuffield
Orthopaedic Centre, Oxford, UK

Raymond Fitzpatrick, BA, MSc, PhD
Professor of Public Health and Primary Care,
Department of Public Health, University of
Oxford, Institute of Health Sciences,
Oxford, UK

Simon P. Frostick, MA, DM, FRCS
Department of Musculoskeletal Science,
Royal Liverpool University Hospital,
Liverpool, UK

Ove Furnes, MD, PhD
Orthopaedic Surgeon and Head of the
Norwegian Arthroplasty Register, Department of
Orthopaedic Surgery, Haukeland University
Hospital, Bergen, Norway

Andrew Garratt, BA, MSc, PhD
Research Lecturer, Unit of Health Care
Epidemiology, Department of Public Health,
Oxford University, Oxford, UK

Michael J. Goldacre, BM, BCh, FFPHM
Professor of Public Health, Unit of Health Care
Epidemiology, Department of Public Health, Oxford
University, Oxford, UK

Alastair Gray, PhD
Director, Health Economics Research Centre,
Department of Public Health, University of
Oxford, Institute of Health Sciences, Oxford, UK

Amir W. Hanna, MS, PhD, FRCS
Clinical Lecturer Orthopaedics and Trauma,
Dundee University, Tayside University Hospitals,
Dundee, UK

Paul Harvie, BSc, MBChB, MRCS
Girdlestone Scholar in Orthopaedic Surgery,
Nuffield Department of Orthopaedic Surgery,
University of Oxford, Oxford, UK

Leif I. Havelin, MD, PhD
Orthopaedic Surgeon, Head of the Department of
Orthopaedic Surgery, Haukeland University
Hospital, Bergen, Norway

Mark L. Herron, FRCS (Tr & Orth)
The Royal Orthopaedic Hospital,
Birmingham, UK

Raman V. Kalyan, D Ortho, Dip N B Ortho Surg
Spine Fellow, Department of Trauma and
Orthopaedics Surgery, Queen's University of
Belfast, Musgrave Park Hospital, Belfast, UK

Stein A. Lie, PhD, MSc
Research Fellow, Section for Epidemiology and
Medical Statistics, Department of Public Health

and Primary Health Care, University of Bergen,
Bergen, Norway

Nikos Maniadakis, PhD, MSc
General Manager, General University Hospital of
Patras, Rion Patras, Greece

David R. Marsh, MD, FRCS
Professor of Trauma and Orthopaedics,
Queens University, Belfast
Musculoskeletal Education and Research Unit,
Musgrave Park Hospital, Belfast, UK

Alastair Mason, FRCP, FFPHM
Epidemiologist, Cobblers Close, Gotherington, UK

Henry J. McQuay
Pain Research, Nuffield Department of
Anaesthetics, University of Oxford,
The Churchill Oxford Radcliffe Hospital,
Oxford, UK

Badri Narayan, MS, MCh (Orth),
FRCS (Tr & Orth)
Consultant Orthopaedic Surgeon, Royal Liverpool
and Broadgreen University Hospitals NHS Trust,
Liverpool, UK

Martyn J. Parker, MD, FRCS
Orthopaedic Research Fellow, Peterborough
District Hospital, Peterborough, UK

Andrew Pearson, FRCS (Trt & Orth)
Specialist Registrar, The Royal Orthopaedic
Hospital, Birmingham, UK

Paul B. Pynsent, PhD
Director, Research and Teaching Centre,
Royal Orthopaedic Hospital, Birmingham, UK

Alasdair J. A. Santini, FRCS (Orth)
Royal Liverpool Hospital, Liverpool, UK

Michael M. Stephens, MSc (Bioeng), FRCSI
Consultant Orthopaedic Surgeon, Cappagh
National Orthopaedic, Mater Misericordae and
University Children's Hospitals,
Dublin, Ireland

T. N. Theologis, FRCS
Consultant Orthopaedic Surgeon, Nuffield
Orthopaedic Centre, Oxford, UK

Stein E. Vollset, MD, DrPH
Section for Epidemiology and Medical Statistics,
Department of Public Health and Primary Health
Care, University of Bergen, Bergen, Norway

David Warwick, MD, BM, DIME, FRCS, FRCS (Orth)
Consultant Hand Surgeon, Southampton
University Hospitals, Southampton, UK

Keith M. Willett, FRCS
Consultant Orthopaedic Trauma Surgeon, Trauma
Service, John Radcliffe Hospital, Oxford, UK

Preface

'Outcome' is defined by *The Oxford English Dictionary* as 'a visible or practical result'. Outcome measures play an important rôle in medical practice. They should provide the basis for both clinical audit and research. The principal object of this book is to provide references to sources of instruments and techniques used for outcome measurement in orthopaedics and trauma and to advise on the optimum choice of instrument. It will become clear to any student of this topic that it is not an easy subject and there remain many areas without adequate outcome measures.

The text is aimed at medical staff in orthopaedic units, trauma centres and accident and emergency departments. The book may also be of value to physiotherapists, metrologists, research nurses and others involved in clinical research into orthopaedics and trauma. There is a medico-legal dimension to this topic. Outcome measures are vital to the setting of standards of care and their measurement, as well as in the assessment of disease or injury severity. This is of relevance to both lawyers and clinicians in this area, who will find in this book a reference to the most appropriate outcome measures for their purpose. The setting of standards of care and the assessment of the quality of care is also of concern to doctors in public health medicine, purchasers and government. It is important for the clinician to maintain an interest in this field, not least to ensure that managers are receiving accurate and relevant clinical information about his or her activities.

The British Paediatric Association Outcome Measures Working Group (British Paediatric Association 1992) has presented a number of definitions:

- A *Health Status Measurement* is a direct measure of some aspect of health in which improvement is sought, whether or not its relationship to any intervention, social or environmental circumstance is understood. An example is infant mortality rate.

- An *Outcome Measurement* is a sub-type of health status measurement where changes in the measure are known (or at least believed) to be largely attributable to a health service intervention. An example, in the field of paediatrics is life expectancy for people with cystic fibrosis.

- An *Implied Outcome Measurement* is an indirect indicator of health that can be used as a valid proxy for an outcome measurement. Examples are immunization coverage, and coverage of a screening programme of proven effectiveness. In our view, the health status measurement may also be described as 'functional status measurement' and a 'quality of life measure'. These measurements can be made without necessarily seeking improvement.

The Editors of this book have all had a longstanding interest in outcome measures. Each has contributed both to the original development of outcome instruments and to studies to establish their validity, reliability and responsiveness. We have collaborated to produce collections of outcome measures for orthopaedics (Pynsent *et al.* 1993) and for trauma (Pynsent *et al.* 1994) in separate texts, and also in a text on methodology (Pynsent *et al.* 1997). We have also collected classification systems in trauma (Pynsent *et al.* 1999).

In this book, we have combined orthopaedic and trauma outcome measures in a single volume. In our original texts we used a conference based on the Dahlem model to review draft chapters (Dixon 1987) but on this occasion we have asked authors to collect, classify and – where possible – to tabulate outcome measures. We also asked them to rank outcome measures according to a formula laid out below. This has not always been achieved but we believe that the results will be of value to both clinical research and audit. There may be some circumstances where instruments can be used to evaluate individual patients as an aid to clinical assessment and decision making.

OUTCOME INSTRUMENTS

Where possible, instruments (questionnaires or other outcome systems) have been either actually included as an appendix or carefully referenced. A summary of instruments (questionnaires or other outcome systems) has been tabulated in Table 1.

SCORING OUTCOME INSTRUMENTS

Instruments have been scored according to Table 2.

Where a paper has been published showing poor validity, reliability or responsiveness results, it has been included in the summary table, but with an asterisk beside it and comments in the chapter text. These papers have not been added into the score. In the event of a score tie, then if one is self-reporting (i.e. completed by the patient) then it wins. If they are both self-reporting then the one with the fewest questions wins – otherwise it is a tie.

In general, many of the outcome measures in clinical practice are based on scoring systems, though most of these systems are poorly validated. Newcomers to the field will experience difficulties not only in finding the available instruments but also in making an informed choice as to the most appropriate for their purpose. This book is designed to help in making such a choice. We have tried to be descriptive as well as proscriptive. Often, there are differences between the requirements of outcome measures for audit as opposed to clinical research. In most cases there is a pay-off between the demands of speed, efficiency and acceptability to both doctor and patient and the demands of precision and specificity. In our opinion, some instruments are so complex that they have become impossible to use. Where possible, it should be indicated where apparently clear-cut measures of outcome (for example, the union of a fractured tibia) may be

Table 1

Instrument name (reference)	What it measures	Validation	Reliability	Responsiveness	Usage	Score

Table 2

	No	Yes (by author)	Independent (by another author)
Validated	0	1	2
Reliability tested	0	1	2
Responsiveness tested	0	1	2
Usage published[†]	0	Scores from 1 for each publication, to a maximum of 4	

[†] This should exclude any publications that have scored in the three previous categories.

vulnerable to confounding factors, such as clinical judgement, age or intercurrent illness. An instrument should be quick, simple to use, reliable, specific to the question being investigated, cost-effective, and applicable. In most cases this ideal instrument does not exist, although many measures have come into general use without meeting these criteria.

In this book we have tried to indicate areas where there are deficiencies in the currently available instruments and these may represent avenues for future research. We would expect that the pragmatic reader should be content with the best available instrument but, if dissatisfied, an innovator should be stimulated to develop new systems for the future. Streiner and Norman (2003) provide invaluable advice on how this may be achieved. An area that has not been addressed is the question of who should carry out the measurements in research. It is sometimes possible to have a research nurse or an independent observer to fulfil this important task but in practice it is usually the surgeon who is obliged to perform the measurements. Whoever performs this task will introduce their own biases. A North American view on general outcome measures can be found in Spilker (1990) but these should be only used in the United Kingdom with some circumspection.

Outcome measures may be broadly distinguished into those used to measure the doctor's assessment, and those used to measure the patient's own assessment of their problem. In most cases it is appropriate to record both types of outcome. The latter are widely used by health economists, managers and politicians. As these two approaches are likely to be measuring different factors, it is our opinion that they should normally be presented as separate outcomes. The problems and advantages of these two groups of measurement should be addressed in the text. The more we have investigated this field, the more we have become convinced of the value of patient-based measures. In the past, these have been dismissed as being too unreliable for serious consideration by clinical investigators but, in fact, these assessments tend to follow closely the main indication for the original intervention.

We have found the World Health Organization's (World Health Organization 1986) definitions of impairment, disability and handicap of considerable value. *Impairment* is a demonstrable anatomical loss or damage, such as the loss of range of movement of a joint. *Disability* is the functional limitation caused by an impairment, which interferes with something a patient wishes to or must achieve. *Handicap* depends on the environment. For example, a patient confined to a wheelchair may be fully mobile on the level, yet be completely immobilized by a flight of stairs.

The measurement of complications is not, strictly speaking, an outcome measure. However, complications are commonly the major component of review in clinical audit, as it is currently practised in the UK. They may be of importance in clinical trials and are routinely reported in most retrospective reviews of a condition and its treatment.

REFERENCES

British Paediatric Association (1992): *Outcome Measurements for Child Health*. British Paediatric Association, London.

Dixon, B. (1987): Scientifically speaking. *Br Med J* **294**, 1424.

Pynsent, P. B., Fairbank, J. C. T., and Carr, A. J. (1993): *Outcome Measures in Orthopaedics*. Butterworth-Heinemann, Oxford.

Pynsent, P. B., Fairbank, J. C. T., and Carr, A. J. (1994): *Outcome Measures in Trauma*. Butterworth-Heinemann, Oxford.

Pynsent, P. B., Fairbank, J. C. T., and Carr, A. J. (1997): *Assessment Methodologies in Orthopaedics*. Butterworth-Heinemann, Oxford.

Pynsent, P. B., Fairbank, J. C. T., and Carr, A. J. (1999): *Classification of Musculoskeletal Trauma*. Butterworth-Heinemann, Oxford.

Spilker, B. (1990): *Quality of Life Assessments in Clinical Trials*. Raven Press, New York.

Streiner, D. L., and Norman, G. R. (2003): *Health Measurement Scales: A practical guide to their development and use*. 3rd edition. Oxford Medical Publications, Oxford.

World Health Organization (1986): *International Classification of Impairments, Disabilities and Handicaps*. World Health Organization, Geneva.

Acknowledgements

The editors are indebted to Ann Weaver at the Research and Teaching Centre, The Royal Orthopaedic Hospital for help in preparation of the manuscripts including reorganizing all the references for our reference-management software. In addition her help with the proof corrections was invaluable.

We should also like to thank Zelah Pengilley, the publisher's Project Editor, for her unerring support. We are most grateful to Bill Down, the copy-editor, and Marian Haimes, the proof-reader, for their meticulous work.

1
Choosing an outcome measure
Paul B. Pynsent

INTRODUCTION

Many instruments have been designed to measure some aspect of health. They are commonly used to measure changes over time, either as a result of treatment or natural history, such instruments are termed outcome measures. Today, most orthopaedic surgeons are being asked to document the outcome of their practice with very little guidance on how to accomplish this. The methods range from regularly auditing complications (usually short-term perioperative complications) to implementing some form of measuring instrument given to all patients. Often, the surgeon would be happy to implement an outcome measure but is unable to decide or find advice on what this measure should be. These motivated practitioners often end up merely applying a fashionable generic health status measure, for example SF-36 (Tarlov *et al.* 1989; Ware 1993), that will usually get the blessing of the local health authority. However, although general measures may be suitable for comparisons of health, a measure more specific to a condition will normally be more appropriate. Unfortunately, such a measure may be difficult to find partly because of the wide range of conditions faced by orthopaedic surgeons. For example, in addition to pain and functional problems, much of orthopaedics is concerned with the correction of deformity. Measuring deformity is very difficult,

and few have attempted to define it (Theologis and Fairbank 1997, see also Chapter 11). In trauma, it is difficult to assess the pre-trauma status of the patient. Both in elective surgery and in trauma, the outcome may take many years to be established.

Most outcome instruments do not stand alone, in the sense that a disorder must be classified to ensure that any comparative results are for the same condition and severity. For example, it may be that an instrument designed to measure disability due to low back pain in primary care is more sensitive to changes of low disability than one designed for use in a hospital setting (Fairbank and Pynsent 2000). This article leads the reader through the essential requirements for choosing an outcome measure.

WHAT IS A GOOD OUTCOME INSTRUMENT?

Two essential requirements of an outcome instrument are that it measures what it is supposed to and that this measure is made with the minimum of error. The former is called 'validity' and the latter 'reliability'. These terms cause confusion but can be visualized by borrowing a target analogy used by Good and Card to explain precision and accuracy (Good and Card 1971). In Fig. 1.1 the 'bull's eye' represents the true outcome to be measured

A shortened version of this chapter first appeared in the *Journal of Bone and Joint Surgery*: Pynsent, P. B. (2001): Choosing an outcome measure. *J Bone Joint Surg* **83-B**, 792–4.

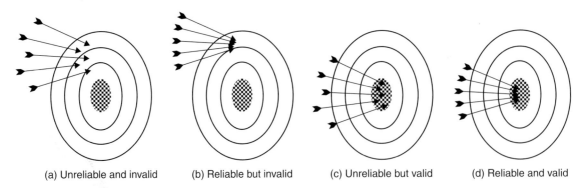

(a) Unreliable and invalid   (b) Reliable but invalid   (c) Unreliable but valid   (d) Reliable and valid

Figure 1.1 A target analogy for reliability and validity. The 'bull's eye' represents the true outcome to be measured, and each arrow represents a single application of the outcome instrument.

(e.g. disability), each arrow represents a single application of the outcome instrument. It can be seen, for example, that it is possible to have a very reliable instrument that does not measure what it purports to (Fig. 1.1b), the arrows are tightly packed but are not hitting the bull's eye. Note that there are measures in common use that fit Fig. 1.1a rather well – for example, the assessment of scoliosis using the Cobb angle (Cobb 1948). This does not measure what it is supposed to – that is, a three-dimensional deformity – and what it does measure is unreliable (Carman *et al.* 1990; Morrissy *et al.* 1990). Spinal surgeons may not agree with this point of view (see Chapter 14). The goal is the situation shown in Fig. 1.1d.

The measurement of reliability and validity is not straightforward. Most of the studies in this area have been carried out by psychologists in the application of questionnaires. Hence, the term 'psychometrics' is now used for the study of the properties of outcome instruments.

The remainder of this discussion will be a brief resume of the methodology of establishing validity and reliability, so that a prospective user of an instrument can check that these metrics have been attained. The text also shows that designing a new instrument is a complex task not to be undertaken lightly. Instrument design is explained in detail by Streiner and Norman (1995). McDowell and Newell (1996) discuss the methodology and also review many instruments, showing how validity and reliability have been attained. The design pathway for such an instrument is summarized in Fig. 1.2.

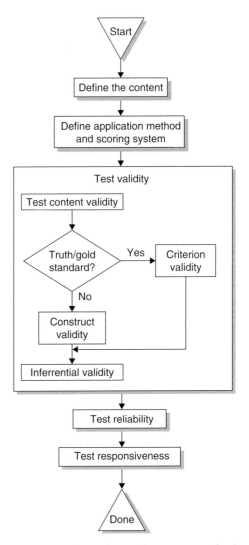

Figure 1.2 A flow diagram showing the requirements for the design of an outcome measure.

INSTRUMENT CONTENT

The items measured for outcome may be based on signs, symptoms, complications and investigations. Any of these items may be intermixed, for example the Harris Hip Score (Harris 1969) uses both symptoms and signs to produce a final score. The resultant measure is reported either as a statistic, values or categories for each dimension measured or an overall score (also termed an index).

After establishing that the validity and reliability have been demonstrated, the choice of an instrument should be a measure that is practical to implement. Measures that comprise solely self-reported symptoms are much easier to use than those requiring a clinical component such as X-ray, operative or range of movement data. The inclusion of such data should be carefully weighed against ease of implementation and the concomitant compliance both of the user and colleagues. Incomplete data collection renders useless results.

In the past, the belief was that the patient's view was of no value in measurement. Thus, the so-called 'subjective' tests were dismissed in favour of 'objective' data. (In this context, subjective means pertaining to a perceived condition within the patient's own consciousness, objective is a condition of the mind or body as perceived by another.) In fact, it is now clear that well-designed self-reported questionnaires are very good at determining health traits. Furthermore, many clinical signs have never been tested for reliability. It might come as a surprise that the physicians' icon – the stethoscope – is unreliable, even in the hands of a specialist chest physician (Spiteri *et al.* 1988). Range of motion features in many scoring systems (e.g. the Harris Hip Score (Harris 1969), Constant Shoulder Assessment (Constant and Murley 1987)), even though both inter- and intra-rater reliability are very low (O'Doherty 1997). These points should encourage the reader to follow the route of self-reported questionnaires when this is possible. It is also worth noting that when the instrument is available in computerized form (Pynsent and Fairbank 1989; Hanna *et al.* 1999), data can be entered directly into a database.

Written questionnaires will usually be constructed from simple binary (yes/no) and graded questions. The graded or scaled questions are normally based on visual analogue scales (VASs), Likert scales or some form of adjectival question. The advantages and disadvantages of these are discussed at length by Streiner and Norman (1995; see Chapter 4). Guyatt *et al.* (1987) compared Likert scales to VASs and showed no difference in their sensitivities to change, although patients found VAS questions more difficult to understand. In the present author's own experience, VASs confuse patients and delude surgeons into believing that they have continuous data. Redundant items should not be included in an instrument. Redundancy may not always be obvious – two items may ask the same question in a different way, or an item may be asking a question about a different trait from that being measured. This heterogeneity may be identified by correlating the questions of an instrument with each other. There are various ways of doing this, but Cronbach's α (Cronbach 1951) is the most generally applicable. Results for homogeneity should have been published for an instrument, and α should lie between 0.7 and 0.9.

Good content will produce a reliable and valid instrument.

VALIDITY

Unfortunately, there is no one statistic that will tell the reader the validity of an instrument. Any published inferential statistics about a measure may add validity to that measure. Validation has two aspects. First, have results of content and criterion or construct validity been published? Second – and more importantly – do the published results using the instrument confirm that it does allow inferences to be made about the trait it purports to measure?

Content validity examines the ability of the instrument to measure all aspects of the condition for which it was designed so that it is applicable to all patients with that condition. One problem with increasing the content is that the reliability tends to decrease;

however, validity at the expense of some reliability is the rule.

Criterion validity establishes if the instrument agrees with the 'truth'. Methods of measuring agreement are discussed below.

When no truth or 'gold standard' exists, then construct validity should be established. This occurs, for example, in the measurement of non-specific low back pain or anterior knee pain, where clearly the patient believes that pain is present but no physical signs or investigations can be used to confirm either its presence or its severity. There is no easy way to test construct validity; the best approach is to ensure that the inferences made with the measure in published data are substantiated over time. Indeed, the current view of the psychometricians is that the most important aspect of the verification of validity is by inferences derived from use of the measure.

RELIABILITY

The application of a totally reliable instrument would produce the same result each time when used under exactly the same conditions. In reality, the results would differ due to error. Thus:

$$\text{Measurement} = \text{True value} + \text{Error}$$

There will be several sources of this error, from the rater, from the instrument itself, random error and error from the patient. These errors or variances may not be separated in any one particular experiment to measure reliability. Some of the issues specifically relating to reliability in orthopaedics have been reviewed by Wright and Feinstein (1992). Measures of reliability and, to some extent, validity are concerned mainly with the comparison of data. They define variances including inter-rater, intra-rater and between methods and the words agreement, concordance, repeatability or reproducibility are often used. A short review of the statistics of agreement is considered in the next section.

Let us return to the statement that reliability is about separating errors from the true value. This is classical teaching of the subject, as there is of course

not a 'true value'. The modern view on measuring reliability is to adopt the 'generalizability theory' originally developed by Cronbach in the early 1960s. This uses analysis of variance methods to investigate the sources of error as separate entities. The approach develops methods for finding and reducing the main components of error. The text of Feldt and Brennan (1989) is recommended for a statistical account of reliability with many useful references to both 'classical' and 'generalizability theory'.

Agreement

An intra-class correlation coefficient (ICC) should be used for continuous data to measure agreement between or within methods or raters. There are other measures available but the ICC is appropriate and the most commonly used. There is not only one ICC, just as in analyses of variance, the mean squared differences are used as sample variances to calculate an ICC. Hence, the method of calculating of an ICC will depend on the design of an experiment.

Results published showing agreement using Pearson's product moment correlation coefficient should be treated with caution. The latter overestimated the agreement, and is unable to distinguish data when there is a systematic error. For example, if a mercury thermometer was compared with a digital thermometer and the mercury device measured exactly the same as the digital equipment but 2° lower, then Pearson's coefficient would be 1, suggesting 100 per cent agreement. It is always worth plotting the results to find systematic biases when comparing data. The best way to plot the data is by placing the mean of points on the x-axis and the difference (if the comparison is between two) on the y-axis. This method used by Oldham (1968) has been extended by Altman and Bland (1983) for normally distributed data, to include lines at two standard deviations (SD) above and below the mean line; these were termed the limits of agreement. This graphical technique should be viewed as complementary to the ICC (Lee 1992).

If binary results are to be compared, then the kappa statistic should be used. This uses the proportion of agreement but also adjusts for the chance agreement. For ordinate data kappa has been extended to a weighted kappa where the amount of disagreement is weighted. If the correct weighting is applied, then the weighted kappa statistic – and indeed kappa itself – can be compared directly to an ICC value. Lee *et al.* (1989) suggest three measures of the agreement between two methods for these methods to be interchangeable:

1. The lower limit of the 95 per cent confidence interval for the ICC should be ≤0.75.

2. There should be no systematic bias.

3. The two means should not be statistically significantly different.

Diagnostic tests

If the instrument is being assessed for its reliability as a clinical test, then sensitivity, specificity should be used. These are derived from the proportions of a 2 × 2 table. The reader unfamiliar with these terms is referred to any standard medical statistics book (e.g. Armitage and Berry 1987).

Test-retest

The idea here is to apply an instrument, to re-apply it after a short time (5 to 14 days), and then to compare the results for agreement using an ICC or kappa. However, as pointed out by Kramer and Feinstein (1981), there is often learning bias in the retest, and there are also situations where retesting is not possible. These authors suggest methods that use inter-item correlations such as Cronbach's α to be a good measure of test-retest reliability.

SENSITIVITY TO CHANGE

This section deals with the ability of an instrument to detect changes with time; this is also termed 'responsiveness'. Some measures may not need this property – for example, if death or peri-operative complications are used as a outcome. However, in many situations a measure is required that is sensitive to changes that occur over time due to the natural history of the condition or medical intervention. The major issue here is to ensure that the instrument can detect a clinically important change, even if this is quite small. This latter point has two implications. First, that a clinically important change can be defined; the present author's experience is that many outcome measures are in use today without the users having any idea of what is the smallest clinically important change. Second, this change must be considered when designing an experiment so that power calculations are made accordingly; clearly, if a small change must be detected and the instrument is only moderately reliable, then large numbers of patients would be required. The effect size is usually quoted as a measure of sensitivity to change for instruments whose sample means are reasonably normally distributed:

$$\text{Effect size index} = \frac{\text{Mean at time 1} - \text{Mean at time 2}}{\text{SD at time 1}}$$

This is a commonly used definition (Kazis *et al.* 1989), although the assumption is that the SDs of both samples are the same. This index is dimensionless, and its value gives the number of SDs apart of the two means. Cohen (1977) mentions values of 0.2, 0.5 and 0.8 as small, medium and large effect sizes, respectively. Thus, for two normal curves, at an effect size of 0.2, only 14.7 per cent of their areas will not overlap, whereas at 0.8 some 47.4 per cent of the curves' areas will not overlap (Cohen 1977; pp. 24–7). Cohen also considers definitions for proportions and nominal variables. The situation for ordinal data is more difficult, and requires conversion to binary data or transforming and using the definitions for continuous data.

SUMMARY

The aim of this chapter has been to draw the reader's attention to the methodology required to establish an outcome measure as a valid and reliable instrument to be implemented within a practice. Checks should be made in the original paper or subsequently that the steps shown in Fig. 1.2 have been established. Is the instrument to be applied to a sample from a similar population that it was designed for? Remember, for example, that English words in North America may have different intonations to the UK population. A hip score may be valid for an elective total hip replacement (THR), but invalid for a THR following trauma to the proximal femur.

For a chosen outcome measure, if a scoring system has been specified, then use it. Inventing a new system will make the results incomparable, and also greatly detract from the value of the efforts made to collect the data. Ensure that the instructions for missing items and incorrectly ticked boxes are adhered to.

Do not modify the instrument unless the user is prepared to go through the validation and reliability tests again. These hurdles are high and should not be undertaken lightly. As an example, some consequences of modifying the Oswestry Disability Questionnaire are highlighted by Fairbank and Pynsent (2000).

An outcome measure should be easy to administer, and regular feedback of aggregated results encourages staff compliance.

REFERENCES

Altman, D. G., and Bland, J. M. (1983): Measurement in medicine: an analysis of method comparison studies. *The Statistician* **32**, 307–17.

Armitage, P., and Berry, G. (1987): *Statistical Methods in Medical Research* (Chapter 16). Blackwell Scientific, Oxford.

Carman, D. L., Browne, R. H., and Birch, J. G. (1990): Measurement of scoliosis and kyphosis radiographs, intraobserver and interobserver variation. *J Bone Joint Surg* **72-A**, 328–33.

Cobb, J. R. (1948): An outline for the study of scoliosis. *Am Acad Orthop Surg Instructional Course Lectures* **5**, 261–75.

Cohen, J. (1977): *Statistical Power Analysis for the Behavioral Sciences*. Academic Press, New York, pp. 24–7.

Constant, C. R., and Murley, A. H. G. (1987): A clinical method of functional assessment of the shoulder. *Clin Orthop* **214**, 160–4.

Cronbach, L. (1951): Coefficient alpha and the internal structure of tests. *Psychometrica* **16**, 297–334.

Fairbank, J. C. T., and Pynsent, P. B. (2000): The Oswestry Disability Questionnaire. *Spine* **25**, 2940–53.

Feldt, L. S., and Brennan, R. L. (1989): Reliability, In: Linn, R. L. (ed.), *Educational Measurement*. Macmillan, New York, pp. 105–46.

Good, I. J., and Card, W. I. (1971): The diagnostic process with special reference to errors. *Methods Inform Med* **10**, 176–88.

Guyatt, G. H., Townsend, M., Berman, L. B., and Keller, J. L. (1987): A comparison of Likert and Visual Analogue Scales for measuring change in function. *J Chron Dis* **40**, 1129–33.

Hanna, A. W., Pynsent, P. B., Learmonth, D. J., and Tubbs, O. N. (1999): A comparison of a new computer-based interview for knee disorders with conventional history taking. *The Knee* **6**, 245–56.

Harris, J. E. (1969): Traumatic arthritis of the hip after dislocation in acetabular fractures: treatment by mould arthroplasty. *J Bone Joint Surg* **51-A**, 737–55.

Kazis, L. E., Anderson, J. J., and Meenan, R. F. (1989): Effect sizes for interpreting changes in health status. *Medical Care* **27**, S178–89.

Kramer, M. S., and Feinstein, A. R. (1981): Clinical biostatistics LIV. The biostatistics of concordance. *Clin Pharmacol Ther* **29**, 111–23.

Lee, J. (1992): Evaluating agreement between two methods for measuring the same quantity: a response. *Comput Biol Med* **22**, 369–71.

Lee, J., Koh, D., and Ong, C. N. (1989): Statistical evaluation of agreement between two methods for measuring a quantitative variable. *Comput Biol Med* **19**, 61–70.

McDowell, I., and Newell, C. (1996): *Measuring Health: A guide to rating scales and questionnaires*. Oxford University Press, New York.

Morrissy, R. T., Goldsmith, G. S., Hall, E. C., Kehl, D., and Cowie, G. H. (1990): Measurement of the Cobb Angle on radiographs of patients who have scoliosis: evaluation of intrinsic error. *J Bone Joint Surg* **72-A**, 320–7.

O'Doherty, D. P. (1997): Measuring joint range of motion and laxity. In: Pynsent, P.B., Fairbank, J. C. T., and Carr, A. J. (eds), *Orthopaedic Methodology*. Heinemann-Butterworth, Oxford, pp. 120–30.

Oldham, P. D. (1968): *Measurement in Medicine*. English Universities Press, London.

Pynsent, P. B. (2001): Choosing an outcome measure. *J Bone Joint Surg* **83-B**, 792–4.

Pynsent, P. B., and Fairbank, J. C. T. (1989): A computer interview system for patients with back pain. *J Biomed Eng* **11**, 25–9.

Spiteri, M. A., Cook, D. G., and Clarke, S. W. (1988): Reliability of eliciting physical signs in examination of the chest. *Lancet* **ii**, 873–5.

Streiner, D. L., and Norman, G. R. (1995): *Health Measurement Scales. A practical guide to their development and use.* Oxford University Press, New York.

Tarlov, A. R., Ware, J. E., Greenfield, S., Nelson, E. C., Perrin, E., and Zubkoff, M. (1989): The Medical Outcomes Study: an application of methods for monitoring the results of medical care. *JAMA* **262**, 925–30.

Theologis, T. N., and Fairbank, J. C. T. (1997): Deformity and cosmesis of the spine. In: Pynsent, P. B., Fairbank, J. C. T., and Carr, A. J. (eds), *Orthopaedic Methodology*. Heinemann-Butterworth, Oxford, pp. 199–214.

Ware, J. E. (1993): Measuring patients' views: the optimum outcome measure. SF-36: a valid, reliable assessment of health from the patient's point of view. *Br Med J* **306**, 1429–30.

Wright, J. G., and Feinstein, A. R. (1992): Improving the reliability of orthopaedic measurements. *J Bone Joint Surg* **74-B**, 287–91.

2

A systematic approach to developing comparative health outcome indicators

Alastair Mason, Andrew Garratt, Edel Daly and Michael J. Goldacre

COMPARATIVE HEALTH OUTCOME INDICATORS

Although interest has been expressed in using comparative health outcomes in management of the health service for some years, it is only during the past decade that a systematic national approach to their development has taken place (Department of Health 1993, 2001; McColl and Gulliford, 1993; Public Health Development Unit NHS Executive 1998; NHS Executive 1999a, b). In this chapter, we focus on a project which was commissioned by the Department of Health in the late 1990s in order to develop 'ideal' indicators of health outcome for ten clinical conditions, one of which was fractured proximal femur (Fairbank *et al.* 1999).

Health outcomes can be defined as changes in health, health-related status or risk factors affecting health, or lack of change when change is expected. Such a broad definition may include data about all the factors shown in Table 2.1. In the national work, an indicator has been defined as an aggregated statistical measure describing a group of patients or a whole population, compiled from measures or assessments made on the people concerned.

Throughout the development work it has been emphasized that indicators do not necessarily provide answers as to whether care is good or bad or better in one place than another. Well-chosen indicators will provide pointers to circumstances that may be worth further investigation; no more, despite politicians' current enthusiasm for league tables.

Table 2.1: Factors that could be used as health outcomes

- Environmental factors in the general population such as air pollution
- Environmental factors relating to the individual such as smoking
- Knowledge, attitudes, behaviour in the general or specific populations
- Patients' symptoms, function, health status and well-being
- Patients' clinical state
- Patients' pathological and physiological state
- Events occurring to patients such as:
  1. end-points of earlier occurrence of disease
  2. interventions such as GP contact, admission, death

Indicators may be derived from a number of data sources. Data about environmental factors are obtained from population surveys. Patients are the source for knowledge, attitudes, health status and other related factors, and the data may be obtained either opportunistically or collected in a planned survey. Clinical information is recorded by health professionals and events' data are available from administrative systems.

Indicators may be used for a variety of purposes. Clinicians have for many years compiled indicators for audit and research purposes and, more recently, national comparable audits have been organized for conditions such as stroke (Rudd *et al.* 1999).

Those involved in the strategic and operational development of health services have always required comparative indicators to inform their decision making.

However, uses are now dominating the drive to develop health outcome indicators. The performance assessment framework (NHS Executive 1999b) contains a range of health outcome indicators for comparing both health authorities and NHS trusts. Associated with this, policy documents such as 'Our Healthier Nation' (Secretary of State for Health 1998) contain outcome targets, derived from the research literature or set by political decisions. Third, the Department of Health is now promoting the development of national standards of quality and promoting the development of clinical governance (Department of Health 2000). Fourth, professionals are increasingly in the vanguard of innovation in quality assessment and audit.

SYSTEMATIC APPROACH

In the work on fractured proximal femur commissioned by the Department of Health, ideal indicators were defined as to what should be known, and what realistically could be known, about the condition being addressed. Thus, the work was not constrained by existing data sets and could take into account known information developments such as the introduction of the new NHS number.

The overall aim was to recommend a comprehensive menu of indicators with a standard approach taken for all the conditions addressed. The work was overseen for each condition by a broadly based multidisciplinary working group that included clinicians, managers and representatives of patients' and research interests.

The initial task was to choose a list of candidate indicators – measures that were considered worthy of being worked up in detail. To do this, a number of checklists were developed including a comprehensive health model. Researchers from the NHS Centre for Reviews and Dissemination at the University of York and the Clearing House on Health Outcomes at the University of Leeds were also available to carry

Table 2.2: Factors considered in developing candidate indicator list

---

Reduce risk of fracture
- prevent accidents, particularly in elderly persons
- prevent osteoporosis

Reduce risk of death
- effective operation

Reduce risk of complications (types of complication)
- general (pneumonia, pressure sores, pulmonary embolism)
- intra-capsular (reoperation with arthroplasty, mechanical failure of fixation)
- extra-capsular (failure of fixation, reoperation with device extraction)

Reduce risk of complications (specific interventions)
- thromboprophylaxis
- reduction in delay before operation

Restore function and well-being
- multidisciplinary rehabilitation

---

out literature reviews to assist the working group's deliberations.

The development of a comprehensive health outcome model was crucial to the success of the systematic approach. The main aims of intervention were identified and under each of these headings factors that might be considered for the candidate indicator list were identified. Those relevant to fractured proximal femur are shown in Table 2.2.

In working up the list of candidate indicators it was considered important to include indicators with different characteristics. The four factors taken into account were measurement perspective, specificity, timeframe, and outcome relationship.

Measurement perspective was classified as being from the patients', the clinicians' or population viewpoint. Thus, for fractured proximal femur a measure of quality of life might be more appropriate from the patients' perspective, while clinicians may be more concerned about post-operative complications. The population perspective includes measures such as mortality rates.

The specificity of an indicator relates to whether it is either specific or generic. For example, pre-operative thromboprophylaxis is specific to fractured femur while the measurement of mobility is much less so, and will be influenced by a number of conditions. Condition-specific indicators have the advantage that their relative insensitivity to other conditions increases their sensitivity to the condition of interest. Generic measures provide outcomes relevant to a wide range of conditions.

With respect to timeframe, indicators may be either cross-sectional, recorded at a single point of time for an individual; or longitudinal, a measure of progression over time. At present, with limited ability to link data, most indicators are cross-sectional.

The outcome relationship relates to whether the indicator is a direct indicator of health outcome or an indirect, proxy one. There is now adequate evidence that some care processes are so closely related to the production of benefits that the successful completion of the intervention may be used as a proxy for the actual outcome.

The full list of candidate indicators chosen by the group is shown in Table 2.3, while their characteristics and the means by which data can be derived are shown in Table 2.4.

After considerable deliberation it was agreed not to include on the list indirect indicators relating to the prevention of osteoporosis and rehabilitation after surgery. It was considered that in both cases there was not yet sufficient evidence of a specific effective intervention that could be used as a proxy indicator. Apart from this, candidate indicators were identified for all the factors noted in Table 2.2.

A full technical specification was then worked up for each candidate indicator by staff of CASPE Research of London. The working group completed their task by considering the specification for each candidate indicator and giving it a recommendation relating to whether it should be generally implemented as a routine or whether studied by periodic sample surveys; and whether further work or further information developments were required before it could be implemented.

Since the publication of the Report, further work on indicator development has been carried out by

Table 2.3: Candidate health outcome indicators for fractured proximal femur (FPF)

Related to reduction of risk of fracture

1A. Hospitalized incidence of FPF

1B. *Hospitalized incidence of second (contralateral) FPF*

2. *Rate of A&E attendance for fractured distal radius*

Related to reduction of risk of death

3. Population-based mortality rates for patients admitted with FPF

4. Case fatality rates for patients admitted with FPF

Related to reduction of risk of complications

5. *Thromboprophylaxis rates for patients admitted with FPF*

6. *Percentage of patients with FPF with pre-operative stay more than 2 days*

7. *Incidence rates of pressure sores in patients admitted with FPF*

8. *Ipsilateral hip surgery rates in patients admitted for FPF within 120 days*

9. Emergency re-admission rates for FPF within 30 days of discharge

Related to restoration of function and well-being

10. Summary of a measure of post-operative pain in patients after operation for FPF

11. Summary of a measure of return to pre-FPF level of social integration

12. *Summary of a measure of return to pre-FPF level of activities of daily living*

13. Summary of a measure of return to pre-FPF level of mobility

14. Summary of a measure of attainment of patient specified outcome goals

15. Percentage of patients returning to pre-FPF accommodation

---

Indicators in *italics* are not considered as yet to be generally implementable.

NCHOD staff. Pilot studies to collect the requisite data and derive some of the recommended indicators have been mounted. Specific projects have been undertaken addressing the main issues involved in

Table 2.4: Characteristics of candidate indicators

Indicator	Perspective	Specificity	Timeframe	Relationship	Data
Related to reduction of risk of fracture					
1A	Population	Generic	Cross-section	Direct	Routine
1B	Population	Specific	Cross-section	Direct	Routine
2	Population	Specific	Cross-section	Indirect	Survey
Related to reduction of risk of death					
3	Population	Generic	Cross-section	Direct	Routine
4	Clinical	Generic	Cross-section	Direct	Routine
Related to reduction of risk of complications					
5	Clinical	Specific	Cross-section	Indirect	Survey
6	Clinical	Specific	Cross-section	Indirect	Routine
7	Clinical	Specific	Cross-section	Direct	Routine
8	Clinical	Specific	Cross-section	Direct	Routine
9	Clinical	Generic	Cross-section	Direct	Routine
Related to restoration of function and well-being					
10	Patient	Specific	Cross-section	Direct	Survey
11	Patient	Generic	Longitudinal	Direct	Survey
12	Patient	Generic	Longitudinal	Direct	Survey
13	Patient	Specific	Longitudinal	Direct	Survey
14	Patient	Generic	Cross-section	Direct	Survey
15	Patient	Specific	Cross-section	Direct	Survey

using comparative mortality, admission, case fatality and re-admission rates.

The implementation recommendations for the indicators made by the working group have been reviewed in the light of this further work, and in some cases they have been revised to take into account this additional information.

CANDIDATE INDICATORS NOT YET GENERALLY IMPLEMENTABLE

Seven of the 16 candidate indicators are not yet generally implementable, and these are shown in italic text in Table 2.3.

Two of the indicators, potentially available from routine systems, require coding of the side on which the operation was done. The hospitalized incidence of a second fracture (indicator 1B) was suggested in order to obtain a measure of the success of preventive measures in the group at high risk having had an initial fracture. The rate of ipsilateral hip surgery within 120 days of discharge (indicator 8) would have been a good measure of complications following initial surgery.

Although codes exist for recording whether the operation was on the left or right hip, these are too poorly completed to recommend now for routine implementation of these indicators. They both also require the linkage of separate hospital episodes. However, it would be possible to mount special surveys to obtain the data from which to derive these two indicators for an individual hospital.

It was considered that the rate of distal radius fractures (indicator 2) might reflect the risk of falls and the prevalence of reduced bone density. The value of this marker needs further assessment. Its routine compilation requires accurate diagnostic coding in accident and emergency information systems and as this is not yet common the requisite data can only be collected by special survey. Given the doubts about its usefulness and the difficulty of data collection, this indicator is not yet recommended for implementation.

A literature review was commissioned by the working group to assist in the decision of whether thromboprophylaxis (indicator 5) was so effective in reducing deep vein thrombosis (DVT) and pulmonary thrombosis that it could be used as a proxy health outcome. Thromboprophylaxis was found to be effective but the best method of delivery was not clear, and it was felt that further work was required on assessing the balance of benefits and risks of pharmacological and non-pharmacological methods of DVT prevention.

The literature review has been updated, and since publication of the Report two major studies have been completed. A Cochrane Collaborative review (Handoll *et al.* 2000) examined the effect of heparin, low molecular-weight heparin and physical methods for the prevention of DVT and pulmonary embolism following surgery for hip fracture. The multi-centre pulmonary embolism prevention trial (Pulmonary Embolism Prevention Trial Collaborative Group 2000) investigated the prevention of DVT with low-dose aspirin started pre-operatively and continued for 35 days among patients undergoing hip surgery for hip fracture randomized to aspirin or placebo.

The studies showed that both pharmacological and mechanical thromboprophylactic methods reduced the incidence of DVT following hip fracture, but any noteworthy overall clinical benefit has not been conclusively established. The effectiveness evidence is still not strong enough to develop a proxy health outcome indicator related to thrombolysis.

A literature review was also commissioned by the working group to assess whether a short time to operation (indicator 6) was a proxy for good outcomes after surgery. The Audit Commission (1995) had identified hospital delays in accident and emergency departments as a cause for concern. As well as discomfort, prolonged periods of immobility on trolleys may increase the risk of pressure sores. Delays of several days before an operation may predispose to complications of immobility such as pneumonia and pulmonary embolism. However, against the need for speedy intervention, many patients with co-morbidities may need time to be stabilized before surgery.

The literature review showed that there was insufficient evidence to support the use of time to operation as a health outcome indicator. The studies analysed were poor and mainly concerned with mortality and clinical complications. Their design was not rigorous enough to attribute differences in outcome to the time between admission and operation. Patients experiencing delays frequently had concomitant illness that would have influenced their survival.

The literature review has been updated, and no new evidence supporting the use of time to operation as a proxy indicator of outcome has been found. In particular, the analysis of hospital episode statistics by Hamilton and Bramley-Harker (1999) shows no relationship between wait time for surgery and outcomes such as in-patient mortality, post-surgical length of stay and discharge destination.

Using Oxford Record Linkage Study (ORLS) data, NCHOD has compared hospital rankings for case fatality with those for pre-operative stay, and no relationship was found between a short time to operation and lower 30-, 90- and 365-day case fatality rates (Mason 2000). Although length of pre-operative stay should not be used as a proxy outcome indicator, it may be an appropriate indicator of the quality of the process of care.

In the Report, the incidence of pressure sores (indicator 7) was recommended for general implementation. However, testing this indicator in stroke patients suggests that it is much less useful than initially thought. The Royal College of Physicians' stroke audit (Mant 2000) has shown major differences in definition and recording between hospitals and a low incidence overall, suggesting that it is an insensitive indicator at NHS trust level.

It is unclear whether hospitals that report a relatively high occurrence of pressure sores are providing poorer care or have a better surveillance system and/or lower reporting thresholds. Rather than worrying about comparative rates, clinicians would do better by treating the occurrence of each pressure sore as a sentinel event to be fully investigated.

Indicator 12 requires activities of daily living to be measured by the Barthel Index (Mahoney and Barthel 1965) before the incident and 120 days after discharge. There are major difficulties in obtaining a pre-fracture and post-fracture score and linking them, and any longitudinal indicator of this nature must be presented with a count of those lost to follow-up. Much of the information given by Barthel can be obtained by simpler measures such as indicators 11 and 13–15.

CANDIDATE INDICATORS TO BE DERIVED FROM ROUTINE SYSTEMS

Four of the candidate indicators can be derived from routine systems now that the NHS number has been implemented. Two of them (indicators 1A and 3) can be used to compare populations, and two (indicators 4 and 9) to compare hospitals or NHS trusts. Extensive work has been carried out by NCHOD since the publication of the Report to determine the best ways of compiling these indicators and to refine the definitions included in the indicator specifications. The main issues that have been addressed are shown in Table 2.5.

The definition of an admission is crucial to all admission-based indicators. The admission forms the numerator for the calculation of admission rates and also the denominator for the calculation of adverse event rates following admission. Routine NHS statistics are currently based on the 'building block' of 'finished consultant episodes' (the time a patient spends in the care of each consultant). If a patient is transferred between consultants within the hospital admission, a new 'consultant episode' is generated. The 'continuous in-patient spell' is the time spent

Table 2.5: Issues relevant to compiling indicators derived from linked data

Related to initial admission (all indicators)
- finished consultant episodes or continuous in-patient spells
- event- or person-based rates
- emergency, elective or all admissions
- diagnostic codes to be included
- principal diagnosis only or anywhere on the clinical record

Related to death (indicators 3 and 4)
- location of death, in hospital or anywhere
- time interval from start of initial admission to death
- diagnostic coding, underlying cause or anywhere on certificate
- diagnostic coding, condition-specific or all causes

Related to re-admission (indicator 9)
- exclusion of initial admissions ending in death accounting for transfers between hospitals
- finished consultant episodes or continuous in-patient spells
- emergency or all re-admissions
- diagnostic coding, condition-specific or all causes
- time interval from end of initial admission and start of re-admission

General points (all indicators)
- age/sex and other standardization
- statistical power, adequate numbers to show differences
- accuracy and completeness of data
- methodology used for linking records and its accuracy

from admission to discharge from hospital and this, rather than the consultant episode, is generally the right measure for these indicators.

A trickier issue arises when a patient has more than one admission for fractured proximal femur. The admissions may relate to the same fracture or to successive fractures. If they relate to two different fractures, the investigator needs to decide whether the count of admissions should be a count of 'fractures' or of 'people who experienced fracture'. Data from ORLS show an annual ratio of about 106 admissions for fractured proximal femur per 100 people admitted with the condition.

Another issue concerns diagnostic coding. The current Tenth Revision of the International Classification of Diseases has codes for fracture of specified parts of the femur (e.g. S72.0 for fracture of neck of femur, S72.1 for pertrochanteric fracture, and so on), with a code S72.9 for 'fracture of femur, part unspecified'. A decision is needed on whether to include patients with the latter code. A common, albeit arbitrary, decision is to include such patients if over the age of 65 years.

The code for fractured proximal femur, when present, is generally recorded in the position for the principal diagnosis. When it is recorded in another position, the investigator must decide whether to include such patients. Recording anywhere other than the principal diagnosis is uncommon: ORLS data indicate that this occurs in about 3 per cent of cases.

Indicators relating to death need precise definitions. In the calculation of case fatality rates, indicator 4, one issue is whether it is only possible reliably to identify deaths in the hospital admission for the fracture; or whether deaths following transfer or discharge can also be identified. A further consideration is the time interval from fracture to death.

When deaths can only be identified when they occur in the admission episode for the fracture, they are typically called 'in-hospital' deaths; and they are conventionally calculated as deaths that occur within 30 days of admission. When deaths outside hospital can be identified reliably, there is merit in calculating case fatality rates at longer time intervals. ORLS data show that, in the first 30 days following fractured neck of femur, death rates are about ten times higher than deaths rates in a 30-day period in the general population of the same age. They remain significantly elevated, above the general population level, for at least 120 days after fracture.

ORLS data also show that comparisons of death rates between hospitals, following fractured proximal femur, can be seriously misleading unless deaths following transfer and discharge are included in the calculations. This is because, in particular, transfer and discharge practices vary between hospitals.

Considering all patients with fractured proximal femur aged 65 years and over, ORLS data show that 12 per cent are dead within 30 days, and 24 per cent are dead within 120 days, of admission.

When data from death certificates are available and linked to records of people with fracture, a question arises of whether case fatality rates should be calculated for all causes of death or for just those deaths where the certifying doctor has attributed the death to the fracture. There is a considerable literature that shows that doctors are reluctant to certify fractured proximal femur as a cause of death even in patients who die within (say) 30 days of fracture. For example, data from ORLS have been used to show that only 17 per cent of 992 people who died within 30 days of fractured proximal femur had the diagnosis recorded as the underlying cause of death; and that only a further 8 per cent had the diagnosis recorded anywhere else on the death certificate (Goldacre 1993). In our view, 'all-causes' mortality is the right measure.

The under-recording of the diagnosis on death certificates also means that population-based mortality based on data on death certificates alone has very limited value. The best measure of population-based mortality, as defined for indicator 3, is to construct a numerator from 'all people who have fractured proximal femur and who die within 30 days of the fracture' and relate that to the denominator of the whole population from which the fracture patients derive.

Calculation of re-admission rates, based on an initial group of people admitted with fractured proximal femur, should exclude those who die in hospital. Apart from this adjustment to the denominator, similar considerations to those discussed above apply to the identification and calculation of re-admission rates.

The investigator needs to decide whether to count re-admissions as consultant episodes or in-patient spells (the latter is almost invariably preferable); and, if someone is re-admitted more than once, whether to count each re-admission or count the person once only as a 'person re-admitted'.

Decisions are also needed about the time interval between the initial hospital episode and the date of re-admission; and about whether the counting of the time interval should start from the date of admission with the fracture or the date of discharge from the initial admission.

Further decisions are required about whether to count all sources of re-admission or emergency re-admissions only; and about whether to count all re-admissions or only those for particular conditions (e.g. thromboembolism; specific complications of fracture). As an example, ORLS data show re-admission rates, for all causes of emergency re-admission following fractured proximal femur, of 4.3 per cent within 30 days and 8.3 per cent within 120 days of discharge.

CANDIDATE INDICATORS TO BE DERIVED FROM SURVEYS

Five of the candidate indicators can be derived from surveys, involving patients, carried out about 120 days after surgery.

Post-surgery pain (indicator 10) was recommended by the working group to be measured by the Charnley Hip Score (Charnley 1972). It is widely used following hip surgery, and has a straightforward scoring system that correlates well with the degree of mobility and ability to walk (Sutton et al. 1996). There are other more sophisticated measures available, but they are longer and more time-consuming for elderly patients.

Two of the measures are longitudinal (indicators 11 and 13), and these have particular derivation problems as they require a baseline as well as a 120-day assessment. As there is difficulty in achieving completeness, the number lost to follow-up should be presented with the results. The baseline measures have to be made on retrospective data about the pre-fracture situation collected during the hospital admission.

In order to measure social integration (indicator 11) the working group recommended using the adapted, unweighted Social Isolation Scale from the Nottingham Health Profile (Sutton et al. 1996).

The two-item social function scale of the SF-36 could also be used (Ware and Sherbourne 1992).

The working group recommended that return to pre-fracture mobility (indicator 13) should be measured by the use of two ordinal scales assessing walking ability and walking aids requirements (Parker et al. 1998). Mobility can also be measured by the Oxford Hip Score (OHS) (Dawson et al. 1996); this was developed particularly for total hip replacement and provides a short, reliable and valid measure sensitive to clinically important changes. The inclusion of OHS would make up for the information lost by not using indicator 12 relating to the activities of daily living measured by the Barthel score.

The attainment of patient-specified outcome goals (indicator 14) was identified as an important outcome measure. The working group were unable to recommend a single measure, although they favoured the Binary Individualised Outcome Measure (Spreadbury and Cook 1995) and the Canadian Occupational Performance Measure (Law et al. 1994).

It should be possible to identify whether patients have returned post-discharge to their pre-fracture category of accommodation (indicator 15) from hospital patient administration systems, but their status at 120 days will need to be obtained by survey. Currently, accommodation categories are not part of an ordinal scale, so the indicator only identifies those who return to their pre-fracture category and not those who have been able to obtain a more independent accommodation setting. A three-point accommodation ladder has been used to summarize discharge destinations for elderly people (Parker et al. 1994), and this could be used for patients with fractured proximal femur.

CONCLUSIONS

In any given situation, the purposes for which indicators are used need to be clearly thought through. The indicators which are most relevant to each purpose need to be selected. Ideally, they should conform to agreed definitions so that data and results can be shared and compared. Linkage of hospital statistics, including linkage to death certificate data, will be an important step forward in the development of routine information and audit systems. Developments of sample surveys are warranted to measure patient-assessed outcomes on a more routine basis than is currently generally the case.

ACKNOWLEDGEMENTS

Alastair Mason, Andrew Garratt and Edel Daly are funded by the Department of Health as part of its funding of the National Centre for Health Outcomes Development. The views expressed in this chapter are those of the authors and not necessarily those of the Department of Health.

REFERENCES

Audit Commission (1995): *United They Stand: Co-ordinating care for elderly patients with hip fracture.* HMSO, London.

Charnley, J. (1972): The long term results of low friction arthroplasty of the hip performed as a primary intervention. *J Bone Joint Surg* **54-B**, 61–76.

Dawson, J., Fitzpatrick, R., Carr, A., and Murray, D. (1996): Questionnaire on the perceptions of patients about total hip replacement. *J Bone Joint Surg* **78**, 185–90.

Department of Health (1993): *Population Health Outcome Indicators for the NHS: Consultation document.* University of Surrey, Institute of Public Health.

Department of Health (2000): *Quality and Performance in the NHS: NHS performance indicators.* Department of Health, Leeds.

Department of Health (2001): *NHS Performance Indicators: A consultation.* Department of Health, London.

Fairbank, J., Goldacre, M., Mason, A., Wilkinson, E., Fletcher, J., Amess, M., Eastwood, A., and Cleary, R. (1999): *Health Outcome Indicators: Fractured proximal femur. Report of a working group to the Department of Health.* National Centre for Health Outcomes Development, Oxford.

Goldacre, M. J. (1993): Cause-specific mortality: understanding uncertain tips of the iceberg. *J Epidemiol Community Health* **47**, 491–6.

Hamilton, B. H., and Bramley-Harker, R. E. (1999): The impact of the NHS reforms on queues and surgical outcomes in England: evidence from hip fracture patients. *Economic J* **109**, 437–62.

Handoll, H. H. G., McBirnie, J. F. M., Tytherleigh-Strong, G., Awal, K. A., Milne, A. A., and Gillespie, W. J. (2000): *Heparin, Low Molecular Weight Heparin and Physical Methods for Preventing Deep Vein Thrombosis and Pulmonary Embolism Following Surgery for Hip Fractures* (Cochrane Review). The Cochrane Library Issue 4, Update Software, Oxford.

Law, M., Baptiste, S., Carswell, A., McColl, M. A., Polatajko, H., and Pollock, N. (1994): *Canadian Occupational Performance Measure.* Canadian Association of Occupational Therapists, Canada.

Mahoney, F. I., and Barthel, D. W. (1965): Functional evaluation: the Barthel Index. *Maryland State Med J* **14**, 61–5.

Mant, J. (2000): Public health perspective. In: Rudd, A., and Pearson, M. (eds), *Measuring Clinical Outcomes in Stroke, Acute Care.* Royal College of Physicians Clinical Effectiveness and Evaluation Unit, London.

Mason, A. (2000): Using existing information databases to measure outcomes in fractured proximal femur. In: Potter, J., Georgiou, A., and Pearson, M. (eds), *Measuring the Quality of Care for Older People.* Royal College of Physicians Clinical Effectiveness and Evaluation Unit, London.

McColl, A. J., and Gulliford, M. C. (1993): *Population Health Outcome Indicators for the NHS: A feasibility study.* Faculty of Public Health Medicine, London.

NHS Executive (1999a): *Quality and Performance in the NHS: Clinical indicators.* Department of Health, London.

NHS Executive (1999b): *Quality and Performance in the NHS: High level performance indicators.* Department of Health, London.

Parker, M. J., Currie, C. T., Mountain, J. A., and Thorngren, K. G. (1998): Standardisation audit of hip fracture in Europe (SAHFE). *Hip Int* **8**, 10–15.

Parker, S. G., Du, X., Bardsley, M. J., Goodfellow, J., Cooper, R. G., Cleary, R., Broughton, S. G., Streit, C., and James, O. F. W. (1994): Measuring outcomes in care of the elderly. *J R Coll Physicians Lond* **28**, 428–33.

Public Health Development Unit NHS Executive (1998): *Clinical Effectiveness Indicators: A consultation document*. Department of Health, London.

Pulmonary Embolism Prevention Trial Collaborative Group (2000): Prevention of pulmonary embolism and deep vein thrombosis with low dose aspirin: pulmonary embolism prevention trial. *Lancet* **355**, 1295–302.

Rudd, A., Irwin, P., Rutledge, Z., Lowe, D., Wade, D., Morris, R., and Pearson, M. (1999): The national sentinel audit for stroke: a tool for raising standards of care. *J R Coll Physicians Lond* **33**, 460–4.

Secretary of State for Health (1998): *Our Healthier Nation: A contract for health*. HMSO, London.

Spreadbury, P., and Cook, S. (1995): *Measuring the Outcomes of Individualised Care: The Binary Individualised Outcome Measure*. City Hospital NHS Trust, Nottingham.

Sutton, G., Foan, J., Hyndman, S., Todd, C., Rushton, N., and Palmer, R. (1996): *Developing Measurable Indicators for the Quality of Care of Hip Fracture Patients*. Institute of Public Health, Cambridge.

Ware, J. E., and Sherbourne, C. D. (1992): The MOS 36-item short-form health survey (SF-36): conceptual framework and item selection. *Med Care* **30**, 473–83.

3

Economic evaluation
Nikos Maniadakis and Alastair Gray

INTRODUCTION

Due to recent technological advances, epidemiological and demographic trends and rising public expectations, the demand for and consequently the expenditure on healthcare services has rapidly increased over the past three decades. Because resources are scarce and cannot meet all demands, it is important to ensure that the available resources are allocated in ways that maximize overall societal benefit. Thus, the decision on which healthcare interventions to use should be based upon an assessment of their benefit in relation to their cost, and this defines the realm of economic evaluation. In particular, economic evaluation is concerned with the systematic comparison of the resource costs and health effects of alternative healthcare interventions, including: drugs, devices, equipment, procedures and organizational and managerial systems.

In a number of countries, for example Australia, Canada, Netherlands, Sweden, Portugal, Finland, Denmark and France, economic evaluation plays a part in the decision-making criteria employed by governments to decide upon the price or the reimbursement level of pharmaceuticals and other interventions. The establishment of the National Institute of Clinical Excellence (NICE) in 2000 has taken the UK in this direction also; NICE is commissioned to assess the clinical effectiveness and cost-effectiveness of healthcare interventions and advise the National Health Service on their use. In other countries, such as the US and Germany, managed care organizations, sickness funds and other healthcare providers are increasingly taking economic criteria into account when deciding which interventions to include in

their formularies. Finally, new treatment guidelines and disease management programmes are increasingly taking into account economic evidence.

For these reasons, the economic evaluation of healthcare interventions is becoming increasingly common. The number of studies undertaken and published each year is rising exponentially, and the body of literature in the area of health economics dealing with economic evaluation and its methods is growing rapidly. Accompanying this growth, there has been increased interest in developing and standardizing the methodologies used. The university teaching of economics, epidemiology, medicine, pharmacy, health sciences and public health increasingly includes components dealing with economic evaluation, and there are now several postgraduate courses, professional associations and journals dedicated to this field. The present chapter takes the reader though the basic principles of economic evaluation, where possible illustrating these with examples drawn from the orthopaedics literature.

THE FRAMEWORK

Economic evaluation compares the costs and health outcomes associated with different health interventions, in order to help select from a range of options those that maximize the health benefit attained from given resources. Assume for instance that the aim is to find whether a new treatment for back pain is preferable to one that currently constitutes the commonly used practice or standard of care – the comparator. If we measure and compare the cost and effect associated with each treatment,

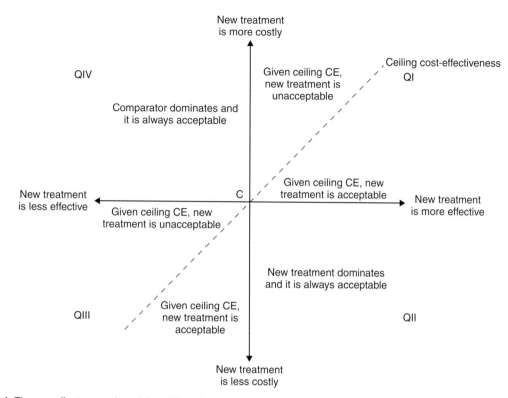

Figure 3.1 The cost-effectiveness plane. Adapted from Anderson *et al.* (1986); Black (1990) and Maniadakis and Gray (2000).

we may face one of four situations, each represented graphically by the quadrants of the cost-effectiveness plane in Fig. 3.1 (Anderson *et al.* 1986; Black 1990; Maniadakis and Gray 2000). In this diagram, the horizontal axis represents the difference in the effect between the new intervention and the comparator, and the vertical axis represents the difference in costs. The second quadrant of the plane represents a situation where the new treatment 'dominates' its comparator because it is less costly and more effective. The opposite happens in the fourth quadrant, where the comparator – existing therapy – dominates the new treatment. It is apparent in such cases that the dominant therapy should be always preferred.

By contrast, the decision is not so straightforward in the other two quadrants. As is often the case in reality, the first quadrant depicts a situation where the new treatment is more effective but also more costly, whilst the third quadrant depicts a situation where it is less effective and less costly. In these circumstances, there is a trade-off between costs

and effects, and the decision on which treatment to accept depends upon the maximum amount that the decision-maker is willing to pay for a gain in effectiveness. This is depicted graphically in Fig. 3.1 by the dotted line that goes through the origin. In essence, much of economic evaluation is concerned to locate interventions on this cost-effectiveness plane and help decision-makers decide whether or not to allocate funds to particular therapies. The remainder of the chapter discusses some of the main steps required to do this.

HEALTH OUTCOME MEASUREMENT AND VALUATION

The choice of the outcome measure used to quantify treatment effectiveness dictates the form of the economic analysis to be performed, namely cost-effectiveness, cost-utility or cost-benefit analysis. In cost-effectiveness analysis a single outcome of therapy is typically measured in terms of physical or natural units, such as: number of complications avoided (Borghi and Lazzaro 1996), score in the Locomotion scale (Jonsson and Larsson 1991), and lives or life-years saved (O'Brien *et al.* 1994). If the effectiveness of the treatments under consideration is shown to be equivalent (or almost equivalent), then the objective becomes to find the alternative that minimizes costs. This is sometimes referred to as cost-minimization analysis (Grimer *et al.* 1997). Sometimes, studies report costs and multiple outcomes separately, leaving their aggregation to the reader; these are referred to as cost-consequence analyses (Powell *et al.* 1994; Javid 1995).

In cost-utility analysis the multiple effects of an intervention are quantified in terms of a single composite outcome measure, often termed by economists a 'utility index'. This composite measure reflects the valuations that individuals place on particular states of health and consequently the well-being they derived from them. Utility is typically scaled from 0 to 1 (or 0 to 100), where 0 relates to worst and 1 (or 100) to the best imaginable state of health. The product of the time in a particular health state, times the utility associated with that health state is often referred to as a Quality Adjusted Life Year or QALY. If, for instance, having a vertebral deformity is associated with a utility value of 0.75, then a year of life with that fracture is equivalent to 0.75 quality adjusted life-years.

Various methodologies and instruments exist for valuing health states. Disease-specific measures focus on specific diseases, for example osteoporosis (Lips *et al.* 1997; Oleksisk *et al.* 2000), as opposed to generic measures that can be applied in a range of different disease or treatment settings to try to capture overall health status. Techniques for eliciting valuations include the rating scale, magnitude estimation, standard gamble, time trade-off and person trade-off approaches. The subjects questioned can include patients, professional groups such as nurses and doctors, or the general public. Evaluations can measure health state utility directly or indirectly though use of multi-attribute utility systems for which empirical utility functions and tariffs have been estimated through research. Such systems for instance include the EuroQol EQ-5D, the Health

Utility Index (HUI) and the Quality of Well-Being Scale (QWB). These methodologies and instruments are discussed in detail elsewhere (Sloan 1995; Gold *et al.* 1996; Johannesson 1996; Bowling 1997; Drummond *et al.* 1997). Because quality of life is important, but also because this type of analysis facilitates broad comparisons between health care interventions, cost-utility analyses are increasingly common and many agencies such as NICE encourage its use. Studies of this type are increasingly common in orthopaedics (Parker *et al.* 1992; James *et al.* 1996).

Finally, cost-benefit analysis attempts to report all costs and effects associated with an intervention in monetary terms, for example by estimating the value of life, thereby estimating the value of any gains from an intervention, and comparing this with the costs of the intervention. Various approaches can be used to convert health effects into monetary terms. In early research, according to the human capital approach, average earnings were attached to healthy working time gained as a result of an intervention and the total value was then computed as the present value of future earnings. There are few examples of this approach in this area of orthopaedics (Tunturi *et al.* 1979; Tredwell 1990; Brown *et al.* 1992; Versloot *et al.* 1992). A variant of this approach assumes that, after a certain period called the 'friction period' (hence the name of the approach), any individual will be replaced at work and hence society will occur no further loss from her or his absence (Koopmanschap *et al.* 1995). The human capital approach is not without shortcomings, as it assumes that earnings reflect productivity, and places low valuations on those unemployed or on low incomes.

An alternative approach is to measure patient willingness to pay for a certain health state or for an intervention. This approach is underpinned by the idea that in the absence of a perfect market – where prices reflect the value of different commodities – one can create hypothetical market situations and ask subjects to express preferences and attach values to health states in terms of their willingness to pay to attain them, or their willingness to accept payment to forego them. These methods of eliciting valuations are referred to as contingent valuation. This approach has well-established links with the broader theoretical base of welfare economics, but because of methodological and measurement drawbacks is not commonly used. However, in recent years there has been renewed interest in this field (Bala *et al.* 1999).

It is important to choose the outcome and type of economic evaluation that will best illuminate the subject matter of the study. In general, cost-effectiveness analysis is more appropriate when the health effect of the treatments considered can be captured by a single measure. It is simpler to perform and easier to understand, but cannot be used when interventions have multiple health effects, and does not permit comparisons between treatments that affect different health dimensions. If quality of life *and* survival are important outcomes, cost-utility analysis is preferable. This is a more complex form of analysis, but it can be used to capture multiple health effects and can be also used to compare different treatments when a standard outcome measure such as QALY is used. Because it captures multiple effects and patient health state-related utility, cost-utility analysis is broader than cost-effectiveness analysis. For comparative purposes it is recommended that analyses should aim to produce results in terms of the cost per QALY (Canadian Co-ordinating Office for Health Technology Assessment (CCOHTA) 1997).

THE PERSPECTIVE

A health intervention may affect a large number of parties including patients and their families, the healthcare sector, other sectors and society as a whole (Brown *et al.* 1992; Versloot *et al.* 1992; Goossens *et al.* 1998). In theory, economic evaluation should consider all effects and resource consequences of the treatments assessed. In practice, however, the effects and resource consequences considered often depend on the purpose and ultimate use of the evaluation. Nonetheless, the effects and costs of an intervention may be experienced quite differently by different users, and so the perspective adopted should be clearly defined and justified.

Table 3.1: Cost (US$ 1989) of surgery versus conservative treatment for the management of herniated lumbar intervertebral disc

Treatment	Cost of treatment	Compensation cost	Total cost
Surgery	26 643	29 411	56 054
Conservative	16 572	37 066	53 638

Source: Adapted from Shvartzman *et al.* (1992).

Consider, for example, a study comparing surgery with conservative treatment for the management of herniated lumbar intervertebral disc (Shvartzman *et al.* 1992). From a societal perspective, the study found no significant cost or effect differences and thus none of the treatments was preferable over the other. However, as shown in Table 3.1, the total cost consisted of the cost of the treatment and the compensation cost related to absenteeism. Therefore, as the outcome was the same, from a hospital point of view the conservative treatment is more cost-effective, whereas from the point of view of an insurance scheme paying compensation costs, surgery is more cost-effective.

Most published economic evaluations in the UK adopt the perspective of the healthcare provider and do not adopt a broader perspective. However, in many cases health interventions will have broad implications and narrow perspectives will not give the full picture. Thus, for comparative and policy-making purposes, the societal approach will generally be the preferred option; consequences can then be rearranged into multiple viewpoints depending on the use of the study (Canadian Co-ordinating Office for Health Technology Assessment (CCOHTA) 1997).

HEALTH OUTCOME DATA SOURCES

Economic evaluations rely on good evidence of treatment effectiveness and outcome. The most reliable study design for obtaining such information is the randomized double-blind controlled trial, with other study designs ranked thereafter (Sheldon *et al.* 1993). Despite their advantages, the orthopaedics literature contains very few economic evaluations alongside randomized trials (Bourne *et al.* 1994; Borghi and Lazzaro 1996; Faulkner *et al.* 1998; Fitzpatrick *et al.* 1998; Goossens *et al.* 1998). This may be due to the fact that these can sometimes be unnecessary, inappropriate, impossible, inadequate or very costly to pursue (Black 1996). In addition, trials are often concerned with efficacy as opposed to effectiveness, that is, efficacy in real-life terms. Trials may give robust answers and thus have high internal validity, but may not fully represent reality for a wide range of reasons: they are often carried out in centres of excellence, frequently not representing the average practice; they may not recruit the average patient population because of strict entry criteria; and they may (as in many phase III trials of pharmaceuticals) compare new active treatments with placebos, the latter not being an option in reality. Thus, it is often argued that randomized trials may be the best venue for proving efficacy, safety and treatment quality, but not the best venue for providing evidence on treatment use and cost-effectiveness. Phase IV randomized and non-randomized naturalistic or observational trials may have higher external validity, may reflect reality to a great degree, and they may also capture the effect of learning curves. In cases where trials are not available or feasible, the next best source of evidence may be cohort or case-control studies, followed by case reports and expert panels. However, such studies are very vulnerable to bias and errors in inference, and this increases uncertainty around their results, especially when small samples are involved.

Finally, evidence on effectiveness may come from a literature review or from a meta-analysis: that is, a study which synthesizes data from a variety of primary clinical studies (Cutler *et al.* 1994; O'Brien *et al.* 1994; Borris and Lassen 1996; Grimer *et al.* 1997). By pooling a number of primary studies, meta-analyses achieve large sample sizes and thus make it possible to detect small differences in effects. It is crucial, however, to ensure that treatments are comparable, that the original studies have been conducted properly, that the biases to which they are subject have been minimized, and that differences in setting are acknowledged. It is also important to test for homogeneity before pooling results (Gillespie *et al.* 1995; Sheldon 1996).

COSTING

Costs associated with an intervention can be classified into various categories. Direct medical costs are associated with the patient's medical care, and may include items such as hospitalizations, medications and visits to professionals. Direct non-medical costs include costs not directly associated with patient treatment, such as costs occurring in other sectors (nursing, residential, social care) or carried by patients and their families, such as out-of-pocket expenses for various items associated with care. Next, productivity losses are opportunity costs reflecting the loss to the society caused by patients' inability to work during treatment, as a result of their illness or side effects, or because of premature mortality, or because relatives need to take time off work to provide informal care.

Costing involves measuring the quantities of resources consumed, and assigning unit costs (prices) to these quantities to obtain a cost per patient. Often economic evaluations make use of average costs published at a national level. However, micro-costing based on accurate resource utilization data specific to the interventions under consideration, although time-consuming and laborious to collect, is likely be more accurate and reliable. Resource utilization data such as hospital length of stay, numbers of consultations or time in operating theatre, and medications given can be collected within the context of a randomized controlled trial, a naturalistic or observational trial, from hospital information systems and primary care databases, from databases of managed care organizations and sickness funds, or from patient chart reviews and other records.

The theoretically correct price for a resource is its opportunity cost – that is, the value of the opportunities foregone by not using the resources in the best alternative way – but in practice market prices

Table 3.2: Average yearly total cost (US$ 1989) of treatment for the management of herniated lumbar intervertebral disc

Treatment	Year 1	Year 2	Year 3	Year 4	Year 5	Total
Surgical	36 761	8350	5560	3650	1733	56 054
Conservative	25 510	14 546	5412	4170	4000	53 638

Source: Adapted from Shvartzman et al. (1992).

are often used instead. In most cases these are easily obtainable, but some difficulty surrounds the valuation of resources such as volunteer, family, or leisure time, where one may argue that the opportunity cost is anything between zero, average earnings or average overtime earnings (Posnett and Jan 1996). It is also difficult in many instances to estimate the costs of capital outlays such as building and equipment, and the overhead costs of resources such as administration which are not directly related to the treatment. Alternative ways of treating such costs are discussed by several authors (Sloan 1995; Gold et al. 1996; Johannesson 1996; Posnett and Jan 1996; Drummond et al. 1997).

The costs measured in an evaluation depend on the perspective adopted. Most evaluations in orthopaedics are confined to direct medical costs, and few studies have attempted to value costs incurred outside the hospital sector. However, as noted before, it is possible that a treatment may transfer costs from the hospital sector to the patients and their families or to other sectors, and so these costs should also be considered. This again underlines the desirability of adopting a broad societal approach in an economic evaluation.

ANALYTIC HORIZON AND DISCOUNTING

The time horizon of the study needs to be long enough to capture all the major resource implications and health effects associated with the treatments assessed and the cut-off points should be clearly defined. The results of a study on the management of herniated lumbar intervertebral disc

where, during a five-year period, the costs of surgery are initially higher than the comparator, but are subsequently much lower, are shown in Table 3.2 (Shvartzman et al. 1992). Hence a study with a shorter follow-up period might well have reached a different (misleading) conclusion. Unfortunately, it is not always easy to determine in advance the appropriate cut-off point, and this is manifested in disagreements between studies on the appropriate time horizon for an evaluation, even when they are focused on similar conditions (Javid 1995; James et al. 1996; Goossens et al. 1998).

Because it is often difficult or uneconomical to undertake a study with appropriate long-term measured endpoints, intermediate or surrogate points may be used instead. Typical examples of intermediate endpoints include blood pressure, serum cholesterol or haemoglobin – changes in which may be good predictors of longer-term costs and health effects that occur over the course of decades. Because evidence on treatment effectiveness is frequently based on such intermediate endpoints, and because the time horizon of an economic evaluation needs to extend a long way beyond these endpoints and ideally needs to cover the patients' lifetimes, it is frequently necessary to extrapolate from intermediate to final endpoints using a range of mathematical models (O'Brien et al. 1994; Gillespie et al. 1995; James et al. 1996; Faulkner et al. 1998; Fitzpatrick et al. 1998). Extrapolation beyond the period observed in a clinical study is not always straightforward, and the assumptions used should be justified and thoroughly tested.

Moreover, as comparisons are made in the present, measurements have to be adjusted for timing. This is because individuals have a positive rate of time

Table 3.3: Cost-effectiveness in the treatment of undisplaced subcapital fractures

Treatment	Life expectancy	Survival rate	Utility score	QALYs	Cost (£1988/9)	Average cost-effectiveness	Incremental cost-effectiveness
A. Do-nothing	8.6	0.6	0.95	4.902	0	0	–
B. Conservative	8.6	0.7	0.97	5.839	2500	428	–
C. Operative	8.6	0.7	0.98	5.899	2800	475	–
B versus A	–	–	–	–	–	–	2667
C versus A	–	–	–	–	–	–	2807
C versus B	–	–	–	–	–	–	4983

Source: Adapted from Parker *et al.* (1992).

preference: in other words, people in general prefer desirable consequences (such as health improvements) to occur earlier and undesirable consequences (such as costs) to occur later. Therefore, future effects and costs have to be discounted to the present. Discounting rates vary from one country over to the next. In the UK, for many years the consensus among economists was that both costs and outcomes should be discounted at the Treasury recommended rate of 6 per cent per annum. Recently, however, NICE has issued guidance indicating that costs should be discounted at 6 per cent per annum and health outcomes at 1.5 per cent per annum. In contrast, in the USA the rate recommended is 3 per cent for costs and outcomes, while in many European countries the discount rate is 4–5 per cent. Thus, for comparative purposes analyses should be performed and reported using a range of rates (including 0 per cent).

THE COMPARATOR AND INCREMENTAL ANALYSIS

Economic evaluation is based on comparisons between alternative courses of action. Thus, the cost-effectiveness of a treatment should always be established relative to an appropriate comparator, which may be current practice, the least costly or most effective existing alternative, or – where it is meaningful – a do-nothing option. The choice of the comparator needs to be justified, and the evaluation should always report incremental results, that is the additional costs which a treatment imposes relative to a comparator over the additional benefits it delivers (Karlsson and Johannesson 1996; Briggs and Fenn 1997; Weinstein and Stason 1977). The literature provides many examples of average cost-effectiveness ratios which can be misleading. Consider for instance Table 3.3, which displays the costs and effects associated with treatments for hip replacement in the case of undisplaced subcapital fracture (Parker *et al.* 1992). The incremental analysis indicates that quality adjusted life gains come at much higher cost than indicated by the average analysis, the reason being that the do-nothing option still yields some quality adjusted life years, so attributing all the health outcome to the intervention is to overstate its effect.

MATHEMATICAL MODELLING

It was noted earlier that, where the costs and effects of an intervention take many years to occur, modelling can be used to extrapolate in time. Modelling is also useful where diseases are characterized by multiple stages, when data and results need to be extrapolated from one setting to another, or where research needs to compare two treatments that previously have been individually assessed against a common option such as a placebo. Modelling can be used early in a study to investigate whether it is worth proceeding with the evaluation, to identify the key variables that should attract attention, and to estimate the sample sizes needed to detect significant cost-effectiveness differences.

For these reasons, some commentators argue that models are an unavoidable fact of life in economic evaluation (Buxton *et al.* 1997) and orthopaedics is an area in which this is very true, as indicated by many published studies that have used this approach (O'Brien *et al.* 1994; Chang *et al.* 1996; Pynsent *et al.* 1996; Faulkner *et al.* 1998; Fitzpatrick *et al.* 1998). Different types of model exist, of which decision trees represent the simplest form, while more complex forms of modelling involve Markov models, which are able to represent different stages of a disease and the impact of interventions on costs and outcomes more accurately. Decision trees represent the progression of a patient into different stages of a disease by means of branches of a tree, each branch being associated with different probabilities, costs and health outcomes. Interventions affect the management of patients and their progression to different disease states, costs and outcomes. The expected cost, effectiveness and cost-effectiveness of different therapy options can then be derived mathematically or with the assistance of software. In more sophisticated forms of analysis, repeated simulations are used to represent the passage of individual patients or patient cohorts through different states of the model, and results are computed each time to derive estimates of the uncertainty around the resulting costs, effects and cost-effectiveness of different interventions. It should be kept in mind that, despite their advantages, models also have shortcomings; particular attention should be paid to sources of information, underlying assumptions, and the overall validity of models (O'Brien 1996; Sheldon 1996).

DATA ANALYSIS METHODS

Early economic evaluations were simply confined to computing an incremental cost-effectiveness ratio without much consideration of the limitations, complexity, distributional form or other peculiarities of

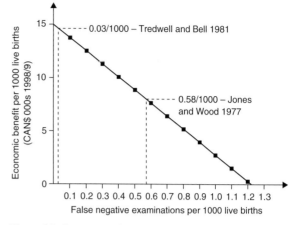

Figure 3.2 Sensitivity analysis in neonatal screening for hip dislocation. Reprinted from Tredwell (1990).

the cost and effect data and of the cost-effectiveness ratio. In practice, however, economic evaluations are often based on cost and effect data from various sources, and these data may be imprecise, subject to variation, or involve guesses and assumptions. The samples used may also be very small, increasing the uncertainty around any results obtained. A simple way of testing the robustness of the results is a one-way sensitivity analysis, where each component of an analysis is varied over a certain range to assess the impact on the results. An example of this approach is shown in Fig. 3.2, which relates to a study of neonatal screening for dislocation of the hip (Tredwell 1990). The authors calculated the net benefit (per 1000 babies screened) for a range of false-negative rates used in different studies, to demonstrate the conditions under which a screening programme would be cost-effective (Jones and Wood 1977; Tredwell and Bell 1981). This is the approach used predominately not only in orthopaedic evaluations (O'Brien *et al.* 1994; Gillespie *et al.* 1995) but also in evaluations in other therapy areas (Briggs and Sculpher 1995).

More sophisticated methods of dealing with uncertainty include changing two or more variables simultaneously, or employing statistical methods to calculate confidence intervals around costs, effects and the estimated incremental cost-effectiveness ratio. This is illustrated in Fig. 3.3, where the horizontal and vertical 'I' bars show the 95 per cent confidence

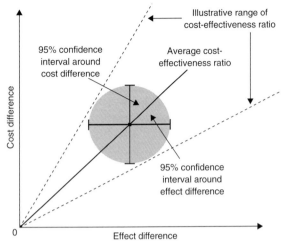

Figure 3.3 Confidence region for the cost-effectiveness ratio. Adapted from O'Brien *et al.* (1994); Van Hout *et al.* (1994); Chaudhary and Stearns (1996) and Briggs *et al.* (1997).

intervals around the effect difference and cost difference, respectively. The ray that connects the intersection of the two 'I' bars with the origin of the plane has a slope equal to the estimated cost-effectiveness ratio, and the spherical area gives an approximate idea of the variance around this ratio. Methods exist to measure the confidence interval around the cost-effectiveness ratio precisely (O'Brien *et al.* 1994; Van Hout *et al.* 1994; Chaudhary and Stearns 1996; Briggs *et al.* 1997).

In recent years the field has experienced many other methodological advances, concerned with the handling of missing and censored data, the possible interactions between health outcomes and treatment resources, the estimation of sample sizes on the basis of incremental cost-effectiveness ratios, the analysis of complex data sets collected alongside large multinational trials, and the application of Bayesian methods to economic evaluation (Wilke *et al.* 1998; Claxton 1999; Willan and O'Brien 1999).

CONCLUSIONS

Economic evaluations of healthcare interventions are becoming more unavoidable and more common. Despite its relative size and importance, orthopaedics as a field has seen only a limited number of economic evaluations so far, but in the future this will change. For comparative, quality and transparency reasons it is important that these studies should be standardized and should comply with certain underlying principles. Thus, several guidelines and articles have recently been published on how to perform, report and referee economic evaluations, and several parties are working towards a greater harmonization of the methodologies used in economic evaluation. A checklist of important elements of an economic evaluation and a general glossary of terms follow.

CHECKLIST FOR ECONOMIC EVALUATION

A: The Framework

☐ The background of the problem being addressed and the general design of the programme under investigation, including the target population, should be stated.

☐ The type of analysis being performed should be clearly stated and justified.

☐ The comparator programme should be justified and properly described.

☐ The perspective and the time horizon of the study should be justified and stated.

B: Data and methods

☐ All resources of interest in the analysis should be clearly identified, measured and valued.

☐ All outcomes of interest in the analysis should be clearly identified, measured and valued.

☐ Methods of obtaining estimates of effectiveness, costs and quality of life valuations and the sources of information should be given.

C: Results

☐ The base case results in terms of costs, effectiveness and incremental cost-effectiveness ratios should be clearly set out.

☐ The sensitivity of the results and the assumptions and uncertainties should be reported.

D: Discussion

☐ The results should be placed in the context of other relevant economic evaluations.

☐ The relevance of the study and policy questions and any ethical or distributive implications should be discussed.

A GENERAL GLOSSARY OF TERMS

Analytic (time) horizon   Period over which outcomes and costs are measured

Average cost   Total cost of a treatment or a programme divided by the total quantity of treatment units provided

Comparator   Treatment selected for comparison in cost-effectiveness analysis; usually the most commonly used, the do-nothing, the most cost-effective, the most effective or the least costly

Cost-benefit analysis   Type of analysis that measures costs and benefits in pecuniary units and computes a net monetary gain or loss

Cost-consequence analysis   Type of analysis that lists the costs and outcomes of treatments in a disaggregated form

Cost-effectiveness analysis   Type of analysis in which costs are contrasted to a single outcome typically measured in terms of physical or natural units such as years of life gained

Cost-effectiveness plane   A two-dimensional plane depicting the possible cost-effectiveness differences between alternative treatments

Cost-minimization analysis   Type of analysis which compares only the costs of treatments in the case of equal effectiveness

Cost-utility analysis   Type of analysis in which costs are contrasted to a single health index measure – called utility – which reflects quantity as well as quality of life

Direct cost   Costs related directly to the treatment under consideration, e.g. drug costs, doctor salaries

Discounting rate   Rate used to convert future costs or outcomes into equivalent present values

Economic evaluation   The systematic comparison of the costs and health outcomes of healthcare interventions and programmes

Effectiveness   The degree to which a therapeutic outcome is achieved in real-world patient populations under actual or average conditions of treatment provision

Efficacy   The degree to which a therapeutic outcome is achieved in a patient population under rigorously controlled and monitored circumstances, such as controlled clinical trials

Human capital approach   Method of quantifying the indirect cost of an illness in terms of production loss measured by remaining lifetime market earnings lost

Incremental cost effectiveness   The ratio of the incremental cost over the incremental effectiveness of a treatment relative to a comparator

Indirect cost   Costs not directly related to provision of a treatment, such as production losses due to morbidity, mortality or care giving

Intangible costs   Costs associated with the suffering, pain and loss of health due to a disease or a healthcare intervention

Marginal cost   Additional cost of producing one additional unit

Modelling   An analytic technique used to simulate real-world processes and events and account for the uncertainties in the probabilities, costs and outcomes related to specific treatments

Opportunity cost   The value of forgone benefits because a certain healthcare resource is not deployed to its best alternative use

Overhead cost   Costs incurred when providing services but not directly related to specific treatment, such as building maintenance

Perspective   View point chosen for the analysis when reporting the costs and healthcare outcomes of an intervention; typical examples include healthcare system, government, society or insurer

Productivity cost   The cost associated with lost or impaired ability to work or engage in leisure activities due to morbidity and mortality

Quality Adjusted Life Year (QALY)   A life-year adjusted for the utility (quality) associated with the state of health during that year

Scenario analysis   Method of examining changes in results of an economic analysis when key variables are varied simultaneously

Sensitivity analysis   Method of establishing the robustness of economic analysis, which examines the changes in the results of the analysis when key variables are varied over a specified range

Threshold analysis   Process which identifies the values of key variables which alter the results of an economic analysis

Time preference   Degree to which individuals or society are willing to trade present for future consumption of a commodity of interest

Utility   Composite measure which refers to the valuation placed by individuals to a particular state of health; it usually takes a value between 0 (death) and 1 (perfect health)

(Adapted from: ISPOR LEXICON, Pashos C.L., Klein E.G., and L.A. Wanke, International Society for Pharmacoeconomics and Outcomes Research, Princeton, USA, 1998.)

REFERENCES

Anderson, J. P., Bush, J. W., Chen, M., and Dolenc, D. (1986): Policy space areas and properties of benefit-cost/utility analysis. *JAMA* **255**, 794–5.

Bala, M. V., Mauskopf, J. A., and Wood, L. L. (1999): Willingness to pay as a measure of health benefits. *Pharmacoeconomics* **15**, 9–18.

Black, N. (1996): Why we need observational studies to evaluate the effectiveness of health care. *Br Med J* **1**, 76–9.

Black, W. C. (1990): The cost-effectiveness plane: a graphic representation of cost-effectiveness. *Med Dec Mak* **10**, 212–15.

Borghi, B., and Lazzaro, C. (1996): Indobufen in the prevention of complications in orthopaedic surgery: a pharmacoeconomic assessment. *Br J Med Econ* **10**, 129–44.

Borris, L. C., and Lassen, M. R. (1996): Thrombo-prophylaxis with low molecular weight heparin after major orthopaedic surgery is cost effective. *Drugs* **52**, 42–6.

Bourne, R. B., Rorabeck, C. H., Laupacis, A., *et al.* (1994): A randomised clinical trial comparing cemented to cementless total hip replacement in 250 osteoarthritic patients: the impact on health related quality of life and cost effectiveness. *Iowa Orthop J* **14**, 108–14.

Bowling, A. (1997): *Measuring Health: A review of quality of life measurement scales*. Open University Press, Buckingham.

Briggs, A. H., and Fenn, P. (1997): Trying to do better than average: a commentary on 'statistical inference for cost-effectiveness ratios'. *Health Economics* **6**, 491–5.

Briggs, A. H., and Sculpher, M. J. (1995): Sensitivity analysis in economic evaluation: a review of published studies. *Health Economics* **4**, 355–71.

Briggs, A. H., Wonderling, D. E., and Mooney, C. Z. (1997): Pulling cost-effectiveness analysis up by its bootstraps: a non-parametric approach to confidence interval estimation. *Health Economics* **6**, 327–40.

Brown, K. C., Sirles, A. T., Hilyer, J. C., and Thomas, M. J. (1992): Cost-effectiveness of a back school intervention for municipal employees. *Spine* **17**, 1224–8.

Buxton, M. J., Drummond, M. F., van Hout, B. A., *et al.* (1997): Modelling in economic evaluation: an unavoidable fact of life. *Health Economics* **6**, 217–27.

Canadian Co-ordinating Office for Health Technology Assessment (CCOHTA) (1997): *Guidelines for the Economic Evaluation of Pharmaceuticals*. CCOHTA. Ottawa.

Chang, R. W., Pellissier, J. M., and Hazen, G. B. (1996): A cost-effectiveness analysis of total hip arthroplasty for osteoarthritis of the hip. *JAMA* **275**, 858–65.

Chaudhary, M. A., and Stearns, S. C. (1996): Estimating confidence intervals for cost-effectiveness ratios: an example from a randomised trial. *Stat Med* **15**, 1447–58.

Claxton, C. (1999): The irrelevance of inference: a decision-making approach to the stochastic evaluation of health care technologies. *Health Economics* **8**, 341–64.

Cutler, R. B., Fishbain, D. A., Rosomoff, H. L., Abdel-Moty, E., Khalil, T. M., and Rosomoff, R. S. (1994): Does nonsurgical pain center treatment of chronic pain return patients to work?

A review and meta-analysis of the literature. *Spine* **19**, 643–52.

Drummond, M. F., O'Brien, B., Stoddart, G. L., and Torrance, G. W. (1997): *Methods for the Economic Evaluation of Health Care Programmes*. Oxford Medical Publications, Oxford University Press, New York.

Faulkner, A., Kennedy, L. G., Baxter, K., *et al.* (1998): Effectiveness in primary hip replacement: a critical review of evidence and an economic model. *Health Technology Assessment* **2**(6), 1–134.

Fitzpatrick, R., Shortall, E., Sculpher, M., *et al.* (1998): Primary total hip replacement surgery: a systematic review of outcomes and modelling of cost-effectiveness associated with different prostheses. *Health Technology Assessment* **2**(20), 1–64.

Gillespie, W. J., Pekarsky, B., and O'Connell, D. L. (1995): Evaluation of new technologies for total hip replacement. Economic modelling and clinical trials. *J Bone Joint Surg Br* **77-B**, 528–33.

Gold, M. R., Siegel, J. E., Russell, L. B., and Weinstein, M. C. (1996): *Cost-effectiveness in Health and Medicine*. Oxford University Press, New York.

Goossens, M., Rutten-Van Molken, M., Kole-Snijders, A., Vlaeyen, J., Van Breukelen, J., and Leidl, R. (1998): Health economic assessment of behavioural rehabilitation in chronic low back pain: a randomised clinical trial. *Health Economics* **7**, 39–51.

Grimer, R. J., Carter, S. R., and Pynsent, P. B. (1997): The cost-effectiveness of limb salvage for bone tumours. *J Bone Joint Surg Br* **79-B**, 558–61.

James, M., St-Leger, L. S., and Rowsell, K. V. (1996): Prioritising elective care: a cost utility analysis of orthopaedics in the north west of England. *J Epidemiol Community Health* **50**, 2–9.

Javid, M. J. (1995): Chemonucleolysis versus laminectomy: a cohort comparison of effectiveness and charges. *Spine* **20**, 2016–222.

Johannesson, M. (1996): *Theory and Methods of Economic Evaluation in Health Care*. Kluwer, Dordrecht.

Jones, D., and Wood, B. (1977): An assessment of the value of examination of the hip in the newborn. *J Bone Joint Surg Br* **59-B**, 318–22.

Jonsson, B., and Larsson, S. E. (1991): Functional improvement and costs of hip and knee arthroplasty in destructive rheumatoid arthritis. *Scand J Rheumatol* **20**, 351–7.

Karlsson, G., and Johannesson, J. (1996): The decision rules of cost-effectiveness analysis. *Pharmacoeconomics* **9**, 113–20.

Koopmanschap, M. A., Rutten, F. F. H., van Ineveld, B. M., and van Roijen, L. (1995): The friction cost method for measuring indirect costs of disease. *J Health Econ* **14**, 171–89.

Lips, P., Cooper, C., Agnusdei, D., Caulin, F., Egger, P., Johnell, O., Kanis, J. A., Liberman, U., Minne, H., Reeve, J., Reginster, J. Y., de Vernejoul, M. C., and Wiklund, I. (1997): Quality of life as outcome in the treatment of osteoporosis: the development of a questionnaire for quality of life by the European Foundation for Osteoporosis. *Osteoporos Int* **7**, 36–8.

Maniadakis, N., and Gray, A. (2000): Health economics and orthopaedics. *J Bone Joint Surg* **82-B**, 2–8.

O'Brien, B. J. (1996): Economic evaluation of pharmaceuticals. Frankenstein's monster or Vampire of Trials? *Medical Care* **34**, DS99–108.

O'Brien, B. J., Anderson, D. R., and Goeree, R. (1994): Cost-effectiveness of enoxaparin versus warfarin prophylaxis against deep-vein thrombosis after total hip replacement. *Can Med Assoc J* **150**, 1083–90.

Oleksisk, A. M., Lips, P., and Dawson, A. (2000): Health-related quality of life (HRQOL) in postmenopausal women with low BMD with or without prevalent vertebral fractures. *J Bone Miner Res* **15**, 1384–92.

Parker, M. J., Myles, J. W., Anand, J. K., and Drewett, R. (1992): Cost-benefit analysis of hip fracture treatment. *J Bone Joint Surg Br* **74-B**, 261–4.

Posnett, J., and Jan, S. (1996): Indirect cost in economic evaluation: the opportunity cost of unpaid inputs. *Health Economics* **5**, 13–23.

Powell, E. T., Krengel, W. F., King, H. A., and Lagrone, M. O. (1994): Comparison of same-day sequential anterior and posterior spinal fusion with delayed two-stage anterior and posterior spinal fusion. *Spine* **19**, 1256–9.

Pynsent, P. B., Carter, S. R., and Bulstrode, C. J. K. (1996): The total cost of hip joint replacement: a model for purchasers. *J Public Health* **18**, 157–68.

Sheldon, T. A. (1996): Problems of using modelling in the economic evaluation of health care. *Health Economics* **5**, 1–11.

Sheldon, T. A., Song, F., and Smith, G. D. (1993): Critical appraisal in health and medicine: how to assess whether health-care interventions do more good than harm. In: Drummond, M., and Maynard, A. (eds), *Purchasing and Providing Cost-effective Health Care*. Churchill Livingstone, London.

Shvartzman, L., Weingarten, E., Sherry, H., Levin, S., and Persaud, A. (1992): Cost-effectiveness analysis of extended conservative therapy versus surgical intervention in the management of herniated lumbar intervertebral disc. *Spine* **17**, 2–82.

Sloan, F. (1995): *Valuing Health Care*. Cambridge University Press.

Tredwell, S. J. (1990): Economic evaluation of neonatal screening for congenital dislocation of the hip. *J Pediatr Orthop* **10**, 327–30.

Tredwell, S. J., and Bell, H. M. (1981): Efficacy of neonatal hip examination. *J Pediatr Orthop* **1**, 61–5.

Tunturi, T., Niemela, P., Laurinkari, J., Patiala, H., and Rokkanen, P. (1979): Cost-benefit analysis of posterior fusion of the lumbosacral spine. *Acta Orthop Scand* **50**, 427–32.

Van Hout, B. A., Gordon, G. S., and Rutten, F. F. (1994): Costs, effects and C/E ratios along side a clinical trial. *Health Economics* **3**, 309–19.

Versloot, J. M., Rozeman, A., van Son, A. M., and van Akkerveeken, P. F. (1992): The cost-effectiveness of a back school programme for the industry: a longitudinal controlled field study. *Spine* **17**, 22–7.

Weinstein, M. C., and Stason, W. B. (1977): Foundations of cost-effectiveness analysis for health and medical practices. *N Engl J Med* **296**, 716–21.

Wilke, R. J., Glick, H. A., Polsky, D., and Schulman, K. (1998): Estimating country-specific cost-effectiveness from multinational clinical trials. *Health Economics* **7**, 481–93.

Willan, A., and O'Brien, B. (1999): Sample size and power issues in estimating incremental cost-effectiveness ratios from clinical trials data. *Health Economics* **8**, 203–11.

4

Randomized controlled trials
Jeremy C. T. Fairbank

INTRODUCTION

Orthopaedic clinical practice is largely based on empirical knowledge. We have relied on observational studies and personal experience. Our teachers learned this way, and we have modified or occasionally revolutionized their ideas. We apply these ideas to individual patients in an often arbitrary or idiosyncratic fashion. Usually, a 'reasonable body' of opinion can be rallied round to support our clinical judgement when things go wrong. In contrast, the rest of medicine (but less obviously surgery) is advancing down an 'evidence-based' route, which is empowered by the Randomized Controlled Trial (RCT), which is generally agreed to be the most powerful method of establishing the optimal management. Other generic trial designs are shown in Table 4.1.

In this Chapter I review the practicalities of performing RCTs in surgical practice, and their relationship with observational studies (Baum 1999; Fairbank 1999). The precision of outcome measures has a major effect on the power of studies and what clinical value may be placed on them.

EPIDEMIOLOGY

The following points should be made:

- Orthopaedic surgeons, perhaps more than any other doctor, have to live for years with the consequences of their decisions about each patient. Few of our patients die because of what we do to them. Many have their quality of life profoundly affected for better or worse. We, as others do, learn from our mistakes.

Table 4.1: A classification of biomedical research reports (Modified from Bailar and Mosteller 1986; Campbell and Machin 1993)

1. **Longitudinal studies**
   A. Prospective
      1. Deliberate intervention
         a Randomized (RCT)
         b Non-randomized
2. **Observational studies**
   A. Retrospective
      1. Deliberate intervention
      2. Observational studies
   B. Prospective
      1. Deliberate intervention
      2. Observational studies
3. **Cross-sectional**
   A. Disease description
   B. Diagnosis and staging
      1. Abnormal ranges
      2. Disease severity
   C. Disease process

RCT, Randomized clinical trial.

Perhaps too strongly are we influenced by the outcome of a difficult or memorable case.

- Orthopaedic surgeons and epidemiologists both argue from the particular to the general, the process of induction. We often argue from one particular to another, an anathema to the epidemiologist.

- RCTs have influenced epidemiologists more than orthopaedic surgeons.

- In spite of this, RCTs are not often used in the surgical practice. There are a number of reasons why this might be, and these are discussed below.

OBSERVATIONAL VERSUS RANDOMIZED TRIALS

Trialists have strongly held the view that the treatment effect seen in observational studies is much larger than that seen in RCTs. It is usually easier to perform an observational study, although few have been carried out to the technical standard of RCTs. This view has been challenged by Britton *et al.* (1998) in a study for NHS Health Technology assessment. This view has been supported by a series of studies published in the *New England Journal of Medicine* in 2000 (Benson and Hartz 2000; Concato *et al.* 2000; Pocock and Elbourne 2000). No formal study has been set up to test this hypothesis.

An article which was strongly against observational studies (MacMahon and Collins 2001) provoked a storm of correspondence. Jahn and Razum (2001) pointed out that observational studies tested real life when treatment depends on the individual performance of a health worker (AKA a surgeon!). Coomber and Perry (2001) suggested that an experiment (a trial) is fundamentally different from an observation, in that an experiment is designed to test a hypothesis. Observation is to view the 'real world', and the latter should follow the former to test the experiment's applicability – the two processes are complementary. These authors also emphasize that most observational studies are poorly supported (Coomber and Perry 2001).

RANDOMIZED TRIALS IN SURGERY

In 1992, Stirrat and colleagues spelled out some of the problems that arise with RCTs in surgery (Stirrat *et al.* 1992):

- Placebo operations are unethical. There are at least two examples where placebo operations

have been used in RCTs: Ligation of the internal mammary artery for angina (Cobb 1959) and arthroscopic surgery for osteoarthritis of the knee (Moseley and O'Malley 2002). This has to be accepted as a limitation of all surgical RCTs, as special difficulties arise when comparing surgical and non-surgical treatments.

- Blinding of the patient is usually impossible, although sometimes it is possible to mislead observers with dummy dressings or to keep patients clothed. It is important to develop outcomes which are unlikely to be biased by the unblinded observer, such as questionnaires which are scored by someone else.

- There are a number of problems surrounding surgical skills. If two operations are being compared, a surgeon may be much better at one operation than another. An example is the recent fastidious trial in Finland comparing three techniques of managing cervical disc disease. This involved the surgeons in using an autograft-based interbody fusion, a technique that they had abandoned years before in preference for allografts. They had to relearn the old technique to complete the trial. There was little to choose between the three groups, except that 80 per cent of their patients had donor site pain (which seems very high, and might be blamed on surgical incompetence) (Savolainen *et al.* 1998). However we can look back to an observational study followed by a trial in Bristol which suggests that this finding is unexceptional (Rawlinson 1994). The real problem here is that the Finnish trial had only about 30 patients in each group, which may well be insufficient to reveal significant complications or to demonstrate important differences between the treatment groups. Surgeons undoubtedly vary in their skills, and this leads to problems of applicability. In other words, just because one surgeon can get good results, it does not mean that others can. In my view, this is one of the great arguments for the multicentre trial.

- New operations take time to develop and to overcome the 'learning curve'. It is impractical to randomize all new interventions from 'the first patient', as has been quoted by Chalmers (Collins *et al.* 1996).

- Because operations have to take place in operating theatres constrained by schedules, availability and money, an RCT in surgery can be very difficult to organize. For example, the MRC Spine Stabilization Trial had difficulties because the surgical budget and the physiotherapy budget were rigid and distinct (Frost *et al.* 1997).

- Patients and surgeons are prejudiced over the choice of procedure, which seriously interfere with recruitment.

- Outcome measures are not straightforward. Death is fortunately not a normal feature of orthopaedic practice, and in surgical specialities where it is, death may not necessarily be attributable to the intervention. Condition-specific and general health questionnaires are widely available, but their sensitivity to change and validity is often open to question.

- Follow-up is prolonged. When do you stop? How many grant-givers will fund this? Will your successors be prepared to continue the study after you retire?

- It is part of the surgeons' ethos to believe in themselves and their surgical skills. This was written over a decade ago, and things are changing. In the UK, confidence in doctors has been shaken by a number of events. It is difficult for surgeons to say to their patients that they 'don't know' the best treatment.

- Because trials are difficult to mount, and surgeons are too busy they do not get done – sadly all too true.

- Patients are perceived as being reluctant to become 'guinea pigs', and this is a view that should be rejected. In my view, the altruistic motive for patients to join trials should not be promoted. Trials can be about defining the best treatment for that individual patient, although general conclusions can only be drawn once the study is complete.

- Surgeons lose money and kudos by submitting a new procedure to a trial. This also may be true.

- Protocols are difficult to agree. Entry criteria are too tight.

Although surgeons prefer randomization by centre, this develops many biases and is unacceptable. It is important that a multicentre trial uses stratification to ensure that there is an even distribution of patients between treatment groups in each centre.

BIAS

Bias is defined as something other than the experimental therapy interfering with the outcome between groups in a RCT. There are three broad categories of explanation for observed results: treatment effect; the play of chance; and bias. The most delicate of these is the treatment effect, and considerable lengths must be taken to protect it from masking by the other two effects. Causes of bias are wide and various, but many boil down to failures in the randomization process. Randomization by hospital record number, date of birth or any system which allows prediction by even the most honest investigator is asking for bias to be introduced at the most fundamental part of the process of an RCT. If randomization allows the patient or surgeon to select treatment before the trial treatment has started, this will introduce bias.

Randomization bias

This is bias developed in the process of randomization. Randomization should allow the even distribution of confounding factors in each group. Confounders are those factors which have a strong effect on the outcome, such as age or smoking in a trial of spinal fusion. However, as all gamblers know, the play of chance can work strongly in one direction over a long time, particularly when numbers are small. Even large trials are not immune to this. An extreme example is the ISIS2 trial (The role of aspirin in the management of myocardial infarction). This showed that even when they had recruited 18 000 patients that the play of chance suggested that this treatment was ineffective in those patients whose birth sign was either Libra or Gemini (Collins *et al.* 1996). Others would argue that this is an extreme example of 'data-dredging', rather than randomization bias. This example also demonstrates the danger of subgroup analysis that should be avoided at all costs, because it can easily lead to erroneous conclusions. Subgroups may only be analysed if they are designed into the trial from its outset.

Intention to treat analysis

Clinical trials are subject to bias through both expected and unexpected confounding factors. The most potent weapon against this is a proper randomization system. The object of an intention to treat analysis is that patients are analysed on the basis of the treatment group to which they were initially randomized, regardless of what happened afterwards. This may be seen as a comparison of treatment strategies. Randomization should take place as close to treatment as possible, to reduce the temptation by clinician or patient to alter the allocation. In practice, treatment plans may be altered by circumstances not apparent when the original treatment plan was conceived. An 'intention to treat' analysis prevents post-randomization reallocation bias, which is the picking out of patients who have been moved from one group to another for various reasons and using these to illustrate the discussion.

PROBLEMS OF RCTS IN SURGERY

At this point, it is opportune to examine some large surgical trials to see what lessons they carry for orthopaedic surgery. The first example is concerned with carotid endarterectomy for transient ischaemic attacks (TIA) (Group ECSTC 1998). This condition has the advantage that disease severity can be assessed by a carotid angiogram, and an estimation of percentage stenosis obtained (even here there is a problem, as North America uses a different method of calculating stenosis from Europe!). This means that any patient who satisfies the clinical criteria for TIA can have a radiological stenosis from 0 to 100 per cent. Surgeons admitted to a degree of uncertainty as to the percentage occlusion that justified the risks attached to surgery, and few agreed where that point lay. Surgeons admitted patients to the trial when they were 'uncertain' of the outcome. This allowed the trialists to build up a picture of outcome versus percentage occlusion. The trial randomized patients into immediate surgery versus 'watchful waiting'. Where the treating surgeon was 'certain' of the outcome either for or against surgery, then the patient would be treated in that way. It rapidly became apparent that the spectrum of uncertainty varied very considerably from one surgeon to another. By the time 3000 patients had been randomized it was clear that there was little benefit to surgery for patients with mild stenosis (0 to 29% occlusion), whereas for those with severe stenosis (70–99%), there was substantial benefit to surgery (Group ECSTC 1991). The final result of the trial, which involved the randomization of a total of 4000 patients, has shown no advantage for surgery over medical treatment in this zone of uncertainty (30–70% occlusion) (the break point was around 65%). This trial took 13 years to recruit 4000 patients from over 90 hospitals (Group ECSTC 1998), with most of the patients recruited in Europe. A single patient was recruited in Australia, which in no way repays the efforts that must have been taken to set the trial up in that country. The principal outcome measures were death or stroke.

The next example trial also comes from vascular surgery (Participants TUSAT 1998a), and concerns small abdominal aneurysms. Should you operate straightaway or watch and wait to see if the aneurysm gets bigger? Here again there is something (aortic diameter) which can be measured fairly easily with either ultrasound or computed tomography (CT). There was a clear answer from 1090 patients. This trial took seven years to complete, and there was little to choose between the two strategies, the conclusion being that watchful waiting is better and safer. A second report shows that this strategy is also cheaper (Participants TUSAT 1998b). This illustrates another point – that these trials now have an economic analysis as an important component.

It is of considerable importance that a number of apparently well-established surgical methods of treatment have been found wanting through RCTs. Examples of these, mainly from general surgery, are gastric freezing for bleeding peptic ulcers, carotid body denervation for asthma, prophylactic portalcaval shunting for oesophageal bleeding, nephroplexy for visceroptosis, appendicectomy for chronic inflamed appendix and peri-arterial sympathectomy (Salzman 1985).

Now it is obvious that these trials are tedious and expensive to complete. If they address important questions, they are likely to have a significant impact on practice. To my knowledge, in the UK there are two large trials involving orthopaedic surgeons either in progress or about to start – the Spine Stabilisation Trial and the Knee Replacement Trial (KAT).

Many large trials are about treatment strategies. Others such as KAT, compare one implant or technique with another. Treatment strategies might be early surgery against delayed surgery, or perhaps surgery against rehabilitation. They recognize that there is a diversity of skills between individuals and institutions. They are testing 'real life' in the sense that if you had the misfortune to have any of these conditions, you may not encounter the best surgeon ever. You would hope to encounter one who was aware of the significance of these studies, and was perhaps auditing results against the reported results of these trials. It is common to find that large trials do not report the spectacular results seen in observational studies. It is likely that the results reflect reality. In orthopaedics and trauma there are number of issues that might be amenable to this approach, and a few small trials are in progress. Unfortunately, when the answer is not obvious, it is likely that large numbers are needed to obtain a robust result, as the differences may be small.

THE DESIGN OF A SURGICAL RCT

The design and execution of RCTs is not easy, particularly if surgical treatment is involved (Stirrat *et al.* 1992). The concepts involved are complex, and even if the trial is well designed, recruitment may be difficult. Doctors and patients are unhappy with the loss of autonomy implied by randomization of treatment. However, it can be strongly argued that in a field where both the 'correct' treatment and its outcome is open to substantial uncertainty, it is unethical *not* to use a RCT format when offering treatment. It follows that it is in the patient's best interest to have treatment dictated within a methodological framework which maximizes their chances of receiving the best treatment. A well-designed RCT does just this. Treatment may cause harm as well as benefit, and this harm may occur on either arm of the treatment protocol. The placebo arm may cause harm through denying an effective treatment, as well as benefit through avoidance of a treatment which might make them worse. This argument has to be balanced by the ethical demand that the patient is not forced into a trial by denying them treatment if they refuse to join the trial. It has to be stressed that 'normal' treatment can continue if the patient does not enter the trial, and this leads to the uncertainty principle (see below).

The CONSORT statement (Begg *et al.* 1996) is a valuable starting point for trial designers, although it is aimed specifically at harmonizing the presentation of results. It does highlight many of the hurdles over which trial designers have to jump before publishing their results, and it is most important that the design takes into account those questions from its earliest stages of development. The elements of a trial design are summarized in Fig. 4.1. There is a great temptation when setting up a trial to over-collect data; this means that every morsel of the patient's condition is collected together and analysed. Unfortunately, even with very large numbers, this leads to subgroup analysis that often produces inappropriate conclusions.

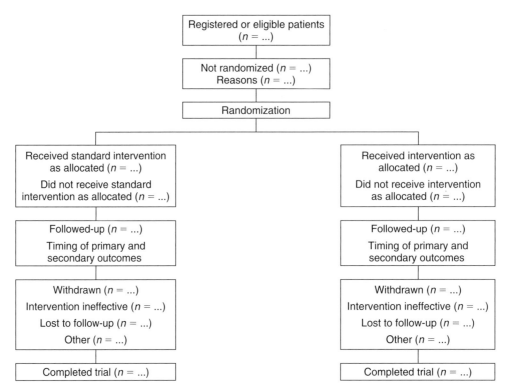

Figure 4.1 The CONSORT statement (From: Begg, C., *et al.* (1996): *JAMA* **276**, 637–9; and Moher, D., *et al.* (2001): *JAMA* **285**, 1987–91).

Trial design

Trial design is not easy, and a legion of difficulties confront the trialist. This chapter can only allude to some of these, but some notes follow on important aspects of running a multicentre trial:

- It is essential to clarify and refine the clinical question into one that can reasonably be answered, and the trial design stems from this process.

- Two-arm trials are superior to all others. Multi-arm trials often require more patients than the total of a series of two-arm studies.

- Subgroup analysis at the end of the trial is tempting, but often misleading. The subgroups that are to be analysed should be defined at the design stage, so that sufficient numbers of patients will be in those groups for useful analysis.

- The data collected at the time of randomization should form the basis for this analysis.

- As much advice as possible should be sought from as many experienced trialists as possible before starting.

- Advisors should include: trial coordinators; outcomes experts; statisticians; trialists in the field and outside it; trials experts in the grant-giving organizations.

- Public funders usually require a health economic analysis as part of the trial. Health economists should be part of the design team, as their agenda may be different from the clinical investigators. However, care should be taken that this does not create additional work for trial collaborators.

- The protocol needs multiple revisions and refinements. It should be shown around, and its publication considered in advance of the trial.

- The fine detail and organization behind a trial will make or break it.

- All collaborators involved in a trial should be aware of the commitment of time and effort involved in the trial. If they do not, the trial will fail.

- Good communications are essential, particularly in large multicentre trials.

- All treatment costs should be accounted for in the initial budget, and this depends on the local healthcare system. The majority of systems are not 'trial friendly'!

- The same applies to contracting systems for purchasing healthcare.

Recruitment

The following points should be considered:

- A successful trial depends on recruitment. Patients need to be convinced that joining a trial is in their best interest. This depends on clinicians and others counselling patients, and the use of well-designed hand-outs, videos and other media. Press and other publicity may be useful.

- Recruitment depends on hard-worked clinicians, who will obtain only limited kudos from the enterprise, however much they may be convinced of the validity of the question. Publication may be best achieved under a collective banner with a long list of credits.

- It is essential to minimize the work done by the recruiting physician. The data set they are asked to collect should be minimized.

- Well-designed paperwork and skilled local trial staff who are dedicated to making the trial work are essential.

- Clinicians exaggerate the number of eligible patients. All estimates of eligible patients should be halved. The trial will be doing well if it can recruit half of these into the trial. Efforts should be made to confirm the numbers from hospital data sets.

There are always problems in recruiting patients to clinical trials, even if the details are well explained.

It may well be in the patients best interests to have their treatment within the format of a clinical trial. However, the loss of autonomy involved may be more than can be tolerated. In theory, if there is a well-designed trial with two treatment arms about which there is significant uncertainty that has been reviewed in detail by a wide body of clinicians and also by ethical committees, then the patient is maximizing his/her chance that the treatment is optimal by joining the trial.

This is a crucial point. A treatment may improve or occasionally cure symptoms. It may also make no difference or even make things worse or kill the patient. The stakes are high: whether the alternative is a well-established treatment or a placebo, the outcome of either arm of the protocol may be beneficial or do harm. If we, the doctors, genuinely do not know which is the best treatment, then how can our patients decide? I believe that a strong case can be made that since no-one knows the answer, the patient's uncertainty is best resolved in terms of a well-designed RCT, and it is in their best interest to join the trial. An RCT does not have to be 'sold' on the basis of altruism to others with the same condition. How do we persuade our patients (and our colleagues) that using a RCT is a reasonable approach? First, we must have a good clinical case where there is genuine uncertainty (disagreement amongst experts) about the best strategy. If this is comparing the strategy of early surgery against watchful waiting, it is important to stress to patients that they will get the operation if it is needed. The abdominal aneurysm trial is a good example of a study which shows a disadvantage of early surgery, though many of the patients who were in the watchful waiting group eventually came to surgery, this did not appear to disadvantage them, with a significant proportion avoiding surgery altogether. We have to explain that it means that neither the treating surgeon or the patient can choose which treatment strategy they get. It is important to stress that this approach is good practice, and reflects the careful thought of many surgeons, grant-givers and ethics committees. The public needs to be educated about clinical trials. Ultimately, it should be in the self-interest of both the patient and the surgeon to be involved in the trial. Perhaps we should find a new word for trial, and we should be on the lookout for trial designs that make it easier for patients to become involved. There is some evidence from cancer trials that outcome is better in patients involved than in those not involved in trials. We are unlikely to gather this sort of evidence in orthopaedics, but we do need to enhance the kudos attached to participating in a trial, since there is no way that the individual is going to be featured at the top of the paper. Perhaps merit awards or their successors should be awarded to participants.

Stratification

Unfortunately, the play of chance is such that a strong confounding factor, is that it may cause an eccentrically distribution of pre-defined subgroups. If there are well-recognized confounding factors, the randomization process can be stratified, so that a guaranteed equivalent number of individuals arrives in each group.

The uncertainty principle

It is ethical to enter a trial where both the patient and clinician are 'uncertain' as to the outcome of treatment in either arm. It is unethical to enter a trial where either the patient or clinician is 'certain' of either a successful or unsuccessful outcome of one or other treatment arm. 'Uncertainty' does not come easily to surgeons, although, in honesty, few of us can be totally confident of an outcome in any case. Similarly, patients must have confidence in their surgeon. Expressions of uncertainty have to be explained with care, and this requires that a patient is able to grasp the concepts involved.

Outcome measures

Having identified the question, condition-specific outcome measures are needed. This is not easy, and is the main focus of this book. What are these measures really measuring? How sensitive are they to change? What change carries clinical significance? We also need generic outcome measures. Our patients often demonstrate high scores on these questionnaires compared with the 'normal' population, and this is one of the fighting grounds of health resource distribution. Orthopaedics and orthopaedic patients will lose out if we do not gather evidence of the efficacy of our treatments (Elliott *et al.* 1999; Sprangers *et al.* 2000).

Power

The issues surrounding the application of trial finding to clinical practice reflect a difference in perception between clinicians and epidemiologists. Trials are built on classical statistics where the trial result is compared with a null hypothesis that there is no difference between the outcome of two or more treatment groups. The conventional criteria of $P \leq 0.05$ represents a better than 1 in 20 chance that the difference is not one caused by chance. A classic power calculation is shown in Table 4.2. Sterne and Smith (2001) have argued that in a world where thousands of trials are performed this is insufficient to be convincing. They suggest much higher levels of probability (say $P > 0.001$) should become the normal threshold. The probability should be presented as a precise value and seen in the context of the study and other work, and not just in isolation. These authors advocated fewer, bigger and more powerful studies – echoing a longstanding theme from Richard Peto and his colleagues in Oxford (Collins *et al.* 1996).

Trial size

How large is large? The size of the trial depends on the expected differences and outcome between two groups which are of clinical significance. Both increased variability and small differences to detect independently mean that more numbers are needed. Often, reliable data are difficult to come by in this

Table 4.2: Power calculations for Oswestry Disability Index as an outcome measure for the Spine Stabilisation Trial (Change of 50% to 30%; cf. 50% to 34%). Number of patients per group

Number of subjects required per treatment group	Standard deviation = 10	Standard deviation = 15
$P = 0.01$		
90% Power	188 patients	420 patients
80% Power	148 patients	330 patients
$P = 0.05$		
90% Power	133 patients	296 patients
80% Power	100 patients	222 patients

area, and indeed this is one of the reasons the trial has been carried out in the first place. Pilot studies are sometimes useful not only in defining the differences in outcome but also in ironing out methodological difficulties in the principal trial design. It has been the universal experience of the large trialists that 'larger is better', and some of these trials have recruited more than 60 000 patients. Studies should be designed to differentiate between clinically worthwhile differences of outcome and clinically immaterial differences of outcome. The major theme of this book is to identify appropriate outcome measures. The clinical relevance of the outcome measure is of crucial importance. Lack of change of an outcome measure in an individual patient may conceal an important clinical benefit.

Trial coordination

The trial administrator is a key person. He/she should have had experience in other clinical trials before running a trial. The trial office will require expertise in data management, data entry, computing and, above all, good communications with other trial centres. A computer programmer is essential. There are many commercial databases available, but all require careful management. The collected data is a most precious resource. Double entry with programmed cross-checks is essential. The data management committee needs access to the data, which cannot be shown to the trialists until the trial is completed. This means that there has to be someone expert in accessing the database who is not a trialist. Regular data backups with copies held in different locations are essential.

Ethics committees

If the clinical question is valid, an ethical trial should be constructable. Arrangements differ from country to country. Where local ethics committees or Review Boards exist, a new submission will have to be made to each committee, which may be a lot of work for either the local clinicians, trialists or trial coordinator.

Funding

Multicentre trials are very expensive. Talk to potential donors from the start, and take their advice. Beware of conflict of interest with commercial sponsors, and obtain guarantees of funding through the trial. The trialists need to be in control of the final publications.

REFERENCES

Bailar, J., and Mosteller, F. (1986): *Medical Uses of Statistics.* NEJM Books, Boston, Massachusetts.

Baum, M. (1999): Reflections on randomised controlled trials in surgery. *Lancet* **353** (Suppl. 1), 6–8.

Begg, C., Cho, M., Eastwood, S., *et al.* (1996): Improving the quality of reporting of randomised controlled trials: the CONSORT statement. *JAMA* **276**, 637–9.

Benson, K., and Hartz, A. (2000): A comparison of observational studies and randomized, controlled trials. *New Engl J Med* **342**, 1878–86.

Britton, A., McKee, M., Black, N., McPherson, K., Sanderson, C., and Bain, C. (1998): Choosing between randomised and non-randomised studies: a systematic review. *Health Technology Assessment* **2**, 13.

Campbell, M., and Machin, D. (1993): *Medical Statistics: A common sense approach*. John Wiley & Sons, Chichester.

Cobb, J. (1959): Prophylactic sclerotherapy injection of bleeding oesophageal varices. *N Engl J Med* **260**, 1115–18.

Collins, R., Peto, R., Gray, R., and Parish, S. (1996): Clinical trials. In: Weatherall, D., Ledingham, J.G.G., and Warell, D.A. (eds), *Oxford Textbook of Medicine*. Oxford University Press, Oxford, pp. 21–32.

Concato, J., Shah, N., and Horwitz, R. (2000): Randomized, controlled trials, observational studies, and the hierarchy of research design. *N Engl J Med* **342**, 1887–92.

Coomber, H., and Perry, I. (2001): Observational studies for health assessment (Letter). *Lancet* **357**, 2140–1.

Elliott, A., Smith, B., Penny, K., Smith, W., and Chambers, W. (1999): The epidemiology of chronic pain in the community. *Lancet* **354**, 1248–52.

Fairbank, J. (1999): Randomised controlled trials in surgery. *Lancet* **354**, 257.

Frost, H., Fairbank, J., and MacDonald, J. (1997): Spine stabilisation trial. Implementation of a multicentre randomised controlled trial. *Physiotherapy* **83**, 645.

Group ECSTC (1991): MRC European Carotid Surgery Trial, interim results for symptomatic patients with severe (70–99%) or with mild (0–29%) carotid stenosis. *Lancet* **337**, 1235–43.

Group ECSTC (1998): Randomised trial of endarterectomy for recently symptomatic carotid stenosis; final results of the MRC European Carotid Surgery Trial (ECST). *Lancet* **351**, 1379–87.

Jahn, A., and Razum, O. (2001): Observational studies for intervention assessment (Letter). *Lancet* **357**, 2141.

MacMahon, S., and Collins, R. (2001): Reliable assessment of the effects of treatment on mortality and major morbidity II: observational studies. *Lancet* **357**, 455–62.

Moher, D., Schulz, K. F., Altman, D., *et al*. (2001): The CONSORT Statement: revised recommendations for improving the quality of reports of parallel-group randomized trials. *JAMA* **285**, 1987–91.

Moseley, J. K., and O'Malley, K. (2002): A controlled trial of arthroscopic surgery for osteoarthritis of the knee. *N Engl J Med* **347**, 81–8.

Participants TUSAT (1998a): Mortality results for randomised controlled trial of early elective surgery or ultrasonographic surveillance for small abdominal aortic aneurysms. *Lancet* **352**, 1649–55.

Participants TUSAT (1998b): Health service costs and quality of life for early elective surgery or ultrasonographic surveillance for small abdominal aortic aneurysms. *Lancet* **352**, 1656–60.

Pocock, S., and Elbourne, D. (2000): Randomized trials or observational tribulations? *N Engl J Med* **342**, 1907–9.

Rawlinson, J. (1994): Morbidity after anterior cervical decompression and fusion. The influence of the donor site on recovery, and the results of a trial of Surgibone compared to autologous bone. *Acta Neurochir (Wein)* **13**, 106–18.

Salzman, E. (1985): Is surgery worthwhile? *Arch Surg* **120**, 771–6.

Savolainen, S., Rinne, J., and Hernesniemi, J. (1998): A prospective randomized study of anterior single-level cervical disc operations with long-term follow-up: surgical fusion is unnecessary. *Neurosurgery* **43**, 51–5.

Sprangers, M., de Regt, E., Andreis, F., *et al*. (2000): Which chronic conditions are associated with better or poorer quality of life? *J Clin Epidemiol* **53**, 895–907.

Sterne, J., and Smith, G. (2001): Sifting the evidence – what's wrong with significance tests? *Br Med J* **322**, 226–31.

Stirrat, G., Farndon, J., Farrow, S., and Dwyer, N. (1992): The challenge of evaluating surgical procedures. *Ann Roy Coll Surg* **74**, 80–4.

5

Register studies

Leif I. Havelin, Birgitte Espehaug, Ove Furnes, Lars B. Engesæter, Stein A. Lie and Stein E. Vollset

INTRODUCTION

In orthopaedics, register studies have most commonly been used in joint replacement surgery for the surveillance of the quality of the large numbers of different prostheses and techniques in use, many of which are otherwise undocumented. Registers usually record patients with certain diagnoses or treatments in a defined population, and their outcome is assessed. Registers can be valuable tools both in research and in quality control, and they could most likely also be beneficial in most orthopaedic fields.

Too few randomized controlled trials (RCTs) are performed in orthopaedics. Since results from clinical trials with satisfactory follow-up do not exist for the majority of orthopaedic devices and treatments, one alternative is to use register studies. The workload for the reporting surgeons in register studies is usually less than in randomized trials. Register studies can therefore more easily cover long time periods with large numbers of patients and participating surgeons. However, as register studies are observational and not experimental – as factors are RCTs – analytic approaches to handle confounding factors are important.

The present chapter is based on the authors' experiences from running the Norwegian Arthroplasty Register (Havelin *et al.* 2000), and examples from this register will be presented. Norway has 4.4 million inhabitants, and annually about 7500 joint replacement operations are reported. In the year

2001, the registry contained information on approximately 90 000 joint arthroplasty operations.

DEFINITION

Medical registers usually cover patients of one or a few diagnostic groups, or patients who receive certain treatments (e.g. operations). Registers may cover patients from a whole country, a region, a group of hospitals, or from a group of surgeons. The patients are followed until death or during a limited time period. The results of the different treatment modalities are assessed and compared on the basis of the collected data.

Comment

Some orthopaedic registers record only failures (e.g. revisions) and not the primary surgery. In such outcome registers, with few or no data from the population from which the cases were recruited, there will be insufficient data from the patients at risk, and the possibility to adequately identify risk factors for failure will be severely reduced.

AIMS

In arthroplasty registers, the aims most commonly are to survey joint replacement surgery, to compare the quality of different prostheses, cements, and operative techniques, and to detect inferior implants and procedures as early as possible. In general, the aims of medical registers might be to assess and compare results of the different devices or treatments that are in use, and the most appropriate outcome or response measure must be defined accordingly.

OUTCOMES

Revision surgery and prosthesis survival are usually chosen as the outcome or response in arthroplasty registers. With baseline data on the primary operations and data from the revisions, the survival of different implant components can be assessed and the possible causes for revisions established. Further, if sufficient data are registered on age, gender, diagnosis, operative techniques, use of antibiotic prophylaxis, and other patient-, surgeon- or hospital-related risk factors, the impact of these risk factors on the revision rates can also be investigated.

Revision surgery is often the only outcome that is reported to most arthroplasty registers, but quality of life measures, mortality, level of pain, satisfaction and function, or X-radiography findings after different time intervals might also be chosen as outcomes.

Comments

As the decision to revise the patient may depend on many factors, it can be questioned if revision is an adequate outcome variable. The proportion of patients who have their prostheses still in place gives no information on clinical and radiographic outcome or the patient's satisfaction (Fender *et al.* 1999). However, parameters such as quality of life measures, pain, function and X-radiography findings might be more suitable only in smaller studies that are continuing for limited time periods. We consider it impossible to get all the surgeons in a country to control every one of their patients and report the clinical and radiographic findings to the register. Furthermore, if revision surgery is not used as outcome, then the choice of level for the definition of a

clinical failure is a problem. Söderman *et al.* (2000) evaluated revision as an end-point in the Swedish hip register by analysing the clinical and radiographic outcome of 1113 randomly selected patients from the register. These authors concluded that the failure end-point in the register (revision) was valid and very exact. The general experience is that in large permanent register studies on joint arthroplasty, revision surgery is the only practical end-point.

PATIENT IDENTIFICATION AND FOLLOW-UP

In the Scandinavian arthroplasty registers, the surgeon reports the patient's national personal identification (ID) numbers for identification of the patient and the surgery (Paavolainen *et al.* 1991; Knutson *et al.* 1994; Herberts and Malchau 1997, 2000; Puolakka *et al.* 1999; Robertsson *et al.* 1999; Lucht 2000). In some countries, such as Norway, the surgeon needs the patient's consent to be allowed to send data with this information to most central registries, and the registries must treat data with patients ID confidentially. By use of the ID numbers, the information on outcomes (revisions) can be linked to the baseline information (primary operation) even if the outcome is discovered or treated at another hospital than the primary operation. With such a system, in which all hospitals and all surgeons are participating and where data on patients' deaths or emigration are available, the follow-up of patients will be nearly complete.

In countries without national ID numbers or in regional registries, other systems for follow-up, such as questionnaires to the surgeons or patients, must be established.

SELECTION OF A MINIMAL SET OF NECESSARY DATA

The recording of data should be based on individual reports for each patient. A register should comprise both baseline data (e.g. primary operations) and the outcome response *(*e.g. revision) at follow-up. The aims of the study must be decided upon early in the planning process, and based on these aims decisions can be made about the minimal necessary set of well-defined data to be collected.

RECORDED IMPLANT DATA

In an arthroplasty register, the date of the operation (primary or revision) and information such as diagnosis or reasons for reoperation, type of revision, approach, use of bone transplant, prostheses, cement, and antibiotic prophylaxis, are necessary. The Norwegian Arthroplasty Register collect data on the proximal (e.g. cup), distal (e.g. stem), and intermediate (e.g. head) prosthesis components separately and on a catalogue number level. In this way, results for the different implant designs, can be calculated separately, both for proximal and distal components. To ensure accurate information on the implant, the surgeons may use stickers with catalogue numbers of the implants supplied by the manufacturers.

COLLECTION OF DATA

As register studies usually cover longer time periods and contain larger numbers of surgeons and patients than most other study approaches, a few principles should be emphasized at this point:

- Correct and complete reporting are most easily achieved if the reporting is performed by the surgeon immediately after the operation has been performed, or when the studied response has occurred.

- It is important to use short and simple forms, since the level of dedication may vary among the participants (Figs. 5.1 and 5.2).

- As cases with incomplete information usually cannot be included in the statistical analyses, only information that is essential and easily available for the reporting surgeons should be asked for.

We are of the opinion that, at present, the reporting to registers is most practical by the use of paper forms. In some registries, such as the Swedish hip registry (Herberts and Malchau 2000), the data are reported by e-mail. Due to regulations on data security in Norway, it is not permitted to send data that contain patient information by e-mail.

DATA ANALYSIS

In order to handle the large amounts of data in a register study, a statistical program package is needed. The statistical packages most commonly used by the authors are the SPSS (SPSS, Inc., Chicago, IL, USA) and the S-PLUS (Statistical Sciences, Inc., Seattle, WA, USA), although others are both available and suitable (e.g. SAS, SAS Institute, Cary, NC, USA).

Descriptive statistical data analyses must be carried out, and follow-up times and demographic data for the different compared treatment groups should be given. Survival analyses have most commonly been used in arthroplasty registers, but they are applicable also to other fields of orthopaedic surgery, especially in studies where groups of patients with certain treatments are followed until an outcome (response) such as healing or a complication.

Survival analyses

The different methods for calculation of survival have in common that they analyse the length of time to a response (death, failure). The possibility to include data from patients in which the response has not yet occurred distinguishes survival analyses from other statistical methods (Benedetti *et al.* 1990). Such data are called 'incomplete' or 'censored', and they may arise from loss to follow-up, death, or no response (failure) before the end of the study. The survival function is the probability that, for any specific survival time, a subject will survive at least for that long or longer.

Two methods for estimating the survivor functions are common. In the actuarial life-table method (Cutler and Edere 1958), the time-to-response is

THE NORWEGIAN ARTHROPLASTY REGISTER
TOTAL HIP REPLACEMENTS
Patient ID and date of birth:
....

Hospital: ....

Previous operation in index hip:
0 No
1 Osteosynthesis for prox. femur fracture
2 Hemiprosthesis
3 Osteotomy
4 Arthrodesis
5 Total hip prosthesis
Type: ....
Year: ....
Number of prostheses in index hip: ....
6 Other operations:
....
....

Date of operation: ....

Index operation is:
1 Primary operation
2 Revision

Hip:
1 Right
2 Left
3 Right, prosthesis in left hip
4 Left, prosthesis in right hip

Diagnosis (primary operation):
1 Idiophatic coxarthrosis
2 Rheumatoid arthritis
3 Sequelae after hip fracture
4 Sequelae after dysplasia
5 Sequelae after dysplasia with dislocation
6 Sequelae after slipped capital femoral
    epiphysis or Perthes disease
7 Ankylosing spondylitis
8 Other: ....

Reasons for revision (one or more):
1 Loosening of acetabular component
2 Loosening of femoral component
3 Dislocation
4 Deep infection
5 Fracture of femur
6 Pain
7 Osteolysis in acetabulum
8 Osteolysis in proximal femur
9 Other: ....

Type of revision (one or more):
1 Change of femoral component
2 Change of acetabular component
3 Change of all components
4 Other:
  – Removal of component (e.g. Girdlestone)
    Which parts: ....
    – Exchange of PE liner
    – Exchange of caput
    – Other: ....

Approach:
1 Anterior
2 Anterolateral
3 Lateral
4 Posterolateral

Osteotomy of greater trochanter:
0 No   1 Yes

Bone transplantation:
0 No
1 In acetabulum
2 In femur
3 Bone impaction in acetabulum
4 Bone impaction in femur (a.m. Ling/Gie)

Acetabulum:
Name/type: ....
Catalogue number: ....
Hydroxyapatite coated: 0 No   1 Yes
1 Cement with antibiotic.
Name: ....
2 Cement without antibiotic.
Name: ....
3 Uncemented

Femur:
Name/type: ....
Catalogue number: ....
Hydroxyapatite coated: 0 No   1 Yes
1 Cement with antibiotic.
Name: ....
2 Cement without antibiotic.
Name: ....
3 Uncemented

Caput:
1 Fixed caput
2 Modular system
Name/type:
....
Catalogue number: ....
Diameter (mm): ....

Systemic antibiotic prophylaxis:
0 No   1 Yes
Name: ....
Dosage: ....
Duration (days): ....

Operating theatre:
1 'Green house'
2 With laminar air flow
3 Without laminar airflow

Duration of operation:
Skin to skin (min.):

Peroperative complication:
0 No
1 Yes. Type: ....

Surgeon (who has filled in the form):

....
(Surgeon's name is not registered)

Figure 5.1 English translation of the form (from 1994) used for the reporting of hip replacements to the Norwegian Arthroplasty Register. Reprinted with permission from J. Michael Ryan Publishing, Inc.

grouped into time intervals. For each time interval, the life table records the number of patients still in the study at the beginning of the interval, and the number of responses and censored observations. From these numbers the survival at the beginning of each interval is estimated. This method has been applied in orthopaedic surgery as described by Dobbs (1980). For register studies, the product-limit or Kaplan-Meier method might be more appropriate (Kaplan and Meier 1958). The advantage of this is that it provides results which are independent of the choice of time intervals, as the survival is estimated at every response (failure) time. Another method is the Cox model, which is a multiple regression analysis of survival times (Cox 1972). With Cox regression it is possible to estimate relative failure risks with adjustment for multiple variables.

By linking information on the revisions (response) to the primary operations by use of the patient ID numbers, the time to response is found, and survival of the implants or treatments can be assessed. If sufficient data are collected, survival of the different prosthesis components (stem, polyethylene insert, head, and cup) with end-points such as *all revisions* or revision from aseptic loosening, dislocation, infection, fracture, osteolysis, or pain can be estimated.

KAPLAN-MEIER METHOD

The Kaplan-Meier method is most commonly applied to estimate the prosthesis survival and to

---

THE NORWEGIAN ARTHROPLASTY REGISTER
KNEES AND OTHER JOINTS (not hips)
Patient ID and date of birth:

....

Hospital: ....

Patient's weight: ....
Localisation:

I Knee	5 Elbow
2 Ankle	6 Wrist
3 Toe Joints:	7 Finger joints: ....
4 Shoulder	8 Others ....
I Right	**2 Left**

Previous operation in index joint:

0 No	4 Prosthesis
I Osteosynthesis	5 Synovectomy
2 Osteotomy	6 Other: ....
3 Arthrodesis	
If Prosthesis. Type: .... Year	

Date of operation: ....

Index operation is: I Primary op.   2 Revision

Diagnosis (primary operation):
I Idiophatic arthrosis
2 Rheumatoid arthritis
3 Sequelae after fracture
4 Ankylosing spondylitis
5 Sequelae, ligament tear
6 Sequelae, menisceal tear
7 Acute fracture
8 Sequela, infection
9 Other ....

Reasons for revision (one or more):

I Loose prox. Comp.	7 Malalignment
2 Loose distal comp.	8 Deep infection
3 Loose patella comp.	9 Fracture
4 Dislocated patella	I0 Pain
5 Dislocation	I I Defect polyethylene
6 Instability	I2 Other ....

KNEE
Prosthesis type:

I Tricondylar	3 Unicondylar
2 Bicondylar	4 Patellofemoral

Femoral component:
Name/size: ....
Catalogue no: ....
Stem/Stabilized/Wedge: ....
I Cement with antibiotic.
Name: ....
2 Cement without antibiotic.
Name: ....
3 Uncemented

Tibial component:
Name/size:

....

Catalogue number:

....

Stem/Stabilized/Wedge:..........................
I Cement with antibiotic.
Name: ....
2 Cement without antibiotic.
Name: ....
3 Uncemented

Patella component:
Name/type: ....
Catalogue number: ....
Metal-back 0 No   I Yes
I Cement with antibiotic.
Name: ....
2 Cement without antibiotic.
Name: ....
3 Uncemented

Figure 5.2 English translation of the form used for the reporting of arthroplasties in joints other than the hip, to the Norwegian Arthroplasty Register. Reprinted with permission from J. Michael Ryan Publishing, Inc.

Type of revision (one or more):
1 Change of distal component
2 Change of proximal component
3 Change of all components
4 Change of patella component
5 Change of polyethylene: ....
6 Removal.
Components: ....
7 Insert of patella component
8 Other:

....

Structural bone transplant: 0 No
1 Autograft   2 Allograft   3 Bone impaction prox.
4 Bone impaction distal   5 Other: ....

Systemic Antibiotic prophylaxis:
0 No   1 Yes:
Type .... Combinations ....
Dosage .... Duration, days ....

Duration of operation: ....
Peroperative complication:
0 No   1 Yes:

Type: ....

Cruciate ligaments
1 Anterior, intact before operation   0 No   1 Yes
2 Anterior, intact after operation   0 No   1 Yes
3 Posterior, intact before operation   0 No   1 Yes
4 Posterior, intact after operation   0 No   1 Yes

OTHER JOINTS:
Prosthesis type:
1 Total   2 Hemi   3 One-component prosthesis

Proximal component:
Name/size:

....

Catalogue number:

....

1 Cement with antibiotic.
Name: ....
2 Cement without antibiotic.
Name: ....
3 Uncemented

Distal component:
Name/size:

....

Catalogue number:

....

1 Cement with antibiotic.
Name: ....
2 Cement without antibiotic.
Name: ....
3 Uncemented

Intermediate component (e.g. caput humeri):
Name/size:

....

Catalogue number:

....

Surgeon (who has filled in the form):

....

(Surgeon's name is not registered)

Figure 5.2 English translation of the form used for the reporting of arthroplasties in joints other than the hip, to the Norwegian Arthroplasty Register. – *continued*

construct survival plots, with different end-points as described above. By using the log-rank test, the statistical significance of differences can be assessed. However, the Kaplan-Meier method does not provide any possibilities to adjust for confounding factors.

COX MULTIPLE REGRESSION

With the Cox model, relative risks for revision can be assessed with adjustment for differences in the compared treatment groups concerning age, gender, diagnosis and other confounding factors. The impact on the results of the confounding factors

(age, gender, diagnosis and others) can be assessed, and corresponding Cox-adjusted survival curves can be constructed.

HOMOGENEOUS SUBGROUPS

Another way to handle prognostic differences in subgroups of patient materials, is to limit the inclusion of patients in the analyses to certain patient groups (e.g. to only one gender, or most commonly, to certain age groups within a diagnostic group). A combination, where the Cox model is applied on a homogenous group of patients, is often the best solution.

PATIENTS' DEATHS

Data on deceased patients are needed in register studies. In survival analyses, intact implants in dead (or emigrated) patients are followed from the primary operation until the date of death (or emigration) when the follow-up of these patients are stopped, and their follow-up times are included as censored observations. The patients' dates of death can be obtained from national population registries. In countries without such registries or if national ID numbers are not available, other methods must be found to collect the data on deaths, as these are needed to perform most survival analyses.

In the Swedish registry a Poisson regression model has sometimes been used (Malchau *et al.* 1993). With that model, the patients' individual baseline data and dates of deaths are not strictly necessary, but if these data are not included then the possibility to adjust for confounding factors will be either lost or reduced.

STATISTICAL EXPERTISE

As very few orthopaedic surgeons are competent to perform and fully understand the assumptions of more advanced statistical analyses than the Kaplan-Meier method, there has to be a continuous close working relationship between orthopaedic surgeons and medical statisticians. This cooperation should be established right from the start, as the medical statisticians will provide important advice when the registry is planned. Preferably, the orthopaedic surgeons and statisticians should plan and run studies together. It is also important that the orthopaedic surgeons participate in the statistical work, as the knowledge they have about the recorded data and about orthopaedic surgery is needed in the process of statistical analysis.

Examples

It has been possible to find and document inferior results of prostheses and cements based on data from the Norwegian Arthroplasty Register. Early identification of inferior results of several brands of threaded cups and smooth uncemented stems were documented with about 200 implants of each brand registered during the first three-year period that the register was functioning (Havelin *et al.* 1995b, c). The inferior results of the Boneloc cement, which was used in most European countries between 1991 and 1995, was documented after this cement had been in use for three years (Havelin *et al.* 1995a). During the 1970s, before the register was started, about 6000 Christiansen prostheses (Sudmann *et al.* 1983) and 2200 double-cup prostheses were used in this country before results from randomized trials could document their inferior results.

CEMENTED VERSUS UNCEMENTED POROUS-COATED ACETABULAR CUPS

A comparison of cemented cups and uncemented hemispheric porous-coated acetabular cups registered in the Norwegian Arthroplasty register from 1987–2000 will be used as an example.

Methods

Patients who had received one of the six most commonly used brands of cemented all-polyethylene cups and all cases with uncemented hemispheric porous-coated cups were selected. Demographic data on the patients are listed in Table 5.1, which demonstrates the skewed distribution of patients in the two groups. Survival analyses by the Kaplan-Meier method, with all cup revisions (exchange or removal of cup or exchange of the polyethylene liner) as end-point, were performed to estimate the revision probability at 10 years and to construct survival curves. Cox regression was used to assess the relative risk for revision in the total material and in patients under the age of 60 years, with adjustment for age, gender and diagnosis. Cox-adjusted survival curves, and 10-year revision probabilities with cup design as strata factor was also assessed.

Results

The main finding was that the cemented cups performed better than the uncemented hemispheric porous-coated cups (Fig. 5.3a, b, c; Table 5.2). The difference was less pronounced after adjustment in

Table 5.1: Patient characteristics by cup design

Characteristics	All patients		Aged <60 years	
	Cemented all-polyethylene	Uncemented porous-coated	Cemented all-polyethylene	Uncemented porous-coated
No. of primary operations	40 503	3972	2986	2354
No. of revisions	852	166	132	118
Mean follow-up (years)	5.4	4.2	6.1	4.8
Males (%)	28	38	35	41
Mean age (years) (min–max)	72 (16–100)	57 (14–91)	54 (16–59)	49 (14–59)
Primary coxarthrosis (%)	73	53	46	37

the Cox model, and when the analyses were performed on patients under the age of 60 years, which is the age-group that ordinarily receives uncemented porous-coated cups.

Comments

The uneven distribution of diagnosis, age and gender – as seen in the two study groups – had an influence on the results. These differences were taken care of by selecting a more homogenous subgroups of patients and by adjustment in the Cox model (see Table 5.2 and Fig. 5.3). We consider the results from the Cox model, on patients under the age of 60 years, to be most valid. As seen in Fig. 5.3, the curves follow each other until about six years of follow-up, but thereafter they diverge. The risk ratios could have been assessed separately for the time periods 0 to 6 years and 6 to 13 years. A larger difference than that shown in Table 5.2 would then have been found during the last period.

STATISTICAL CONSIDERATIONS

The ideal approach to evaluate the performance of implants and techniques would be to carry out RCTs. Properly conducted large randomized trials would eliminate any systematic differences between the different treatment groups that might lead to confounded results. However, randomized studies are rarely performed in orthopaedic surgery for several reasons. They are difficult to organize, are expensive, require a large workload, and take a long time using a consistent technique. This applies especially to fields such as arthroplasty surgery where the results in general are good. Since differences among treatments are small, large numbers of patients and long follow-up are needed to be able to detect statistically significant differences.

A randomized trial can only address one or two primary research questions. As long as results from clinical trials are not mandatory before new implants or treatments can be freely used, the number of trials will remain limited.

As results from clinical trials with satisfactory long follow-up periods do not exist for the majority of joint replacement devices, one alternative is to use register studies. With this approach, results for practically all different implant- or treatment modifications reported to the register can be assessed with minimal workload for the reporting surgeons. Because of the huge numbers in a national register, it is commonly possible to find significant results earlier than in randomized studies. The results from register studies will also reflect the outcome for the average surgeon rather than for specialized centres. With arthroplasty registers, it has been possible to identify inferior results of some implants after only

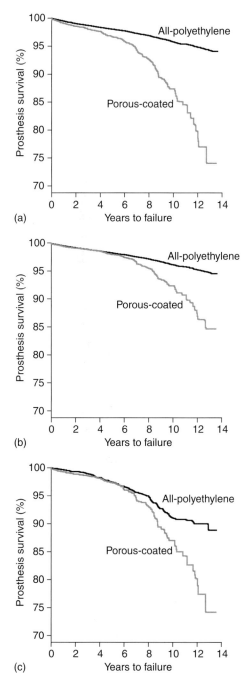

(a)

(b)

(c)

Figure 5.3 Survival of cemented all-polyethylene cups and uncemented porous-coated cups. The uncemented porous-coated cups were inferior to the cemented Charnley cups. End-point (response) is revision of the cup (exchange or removal of the whole cup or of the plastic liner). (a) Kaplan-Meier analysis with all patients included. (b) Cox model with adjustment for age, gender and diagnosis, all patients included. (c) Cox model with adjustment for age, gender and diagnosis, only on patients under the age of 60 years.

three years if the differences are large, but to find and document small differences, larger numbers of patients and longer observation usually are needed. It must be borne in mind that register-based studies are observational, and confounding issues must therefore be carefully scrutinized and accounted for. Analytic approaches to handle confounding include adjustment by multiple regression (the Cox model) and by limiting analyses to homogenous subgroups. As confounding by unknown risk factors is possible in register studies, small differences among treatments with good results must not be overestimated, and changes in clinical practice should not be based on marginal results.

Results from observational register-based studies may be less conclusive than those of RCTs. However, when Benson and Hartz (2000) and Concato *et al.* (2000) compared the results of observational studies with those of randomized trials, they found little evidence for the results of well-designed observational studies being qualitatively different from those of randomized trials.

We recommend that a register study should include individual data not only from patients with complications (e.g. revisions), but also from all the patients with the studied diagnosis or treatment. Only in this way can information such as the patients' age, gender, diagnosis and other confounding factors be recorded and adjusted for through multiple regression methods and by selecting homogenous subgroups.

When presenting survival results, 95 per cent confidence limits should be given; these can be presented in tables or as 95 per cent confidence lines on curves. There is no general agreement upon whether lines representing 95 per cent confidence limits should be given on the survival curves, and it is also unclear which method should be preferred if confidence lines are constructed. Confidence lines on survival curves gives a good visual impression of the result and of the numbers of patients left towards the end of the time period. However, as confidence lines are constructed by point-wise calculations, results can be statistically significantly different even if their confidence lines are overlapping each other, and if analyses involve more than two treatment groups

Table 5.2: Survival probabilities by Kaplan-Meier (K-M) and Cox regression with end-point defined as any revision of the acetabular component (exchange or removal of cup or exchange of polyethylene liner)

| Cup design | All patients | | | | | | | | | | <60 years | | |
| | K-M[1] | | Cox-unadjusted | | | Cox-adjusted[2] | | | | | Cox-adjusted[2] | | |
	10-yr (%)	95% CI	RR	95% CI	P	10-yr (%)	95% CI	RR	95% CI	P	RR	95% CI	P
Cemented all-polyethylene	96.0	95.7–96.3	I			96.1	96.4–96.7	I			I		
Uncemented porous-coated	88	86–91	2.6	2.2–3.1	<0.001	92.3	90.5–94.1	1.6	1.3–3.1	<0.001	1.6	1.2–2.1	0.001

[1] Survival probabilities at 10 years based on the Kaplan-Meier method.
[2] Revision risk ratios (RR) for cup design based on a Cox regression model with adjustment for potential confounding by gender, age at primary operation (<50, 50–59, 60–69, 70–79, ≥80 years) and diagnosis (primary coxarthrosis, other). Survival probabilities at 10 years estimated with cup design as strata factor.

confidence lines or bands may be confusing. There-fore, we prefer to give *P*-values and 95 per cent confidence limits in tables rather than show confi-dence lines on curves.

COMPLETENESS

In Norway, the arthroplasty registry receives reports from more than 95 per cent of operations (Havelin *et al.* 2000). This good compliance is partly due to the high level of motivation among the orthopaedic surgeons based on the background of the prosthetic catastrophes seen in the years before the register was established. Continuous feedback to the surgeons and a simple reporting system are other important factors for the compliance not declining.

Reporting system

The reporting of each case on a paper form is prob-ably the simplest system for the participating surgeons, though other reporting systems may be considered.

Feedback to the reporting surgeons

Most register studies are dependent on the partici-pation from large groups of orthopaedic surgeons, also those that normally are not dedicated to scien-tific work. Feedback is therefore important to main-tain the surgeons interest in the project and thereby a good compliance.

All contributors should receive an annual report and, if possible, each hospital or surgeon should be given their own production statistics and survival results, which they can compare with the national result and with the results of other hospitals (given anonymously). Production numbers in the hospitals can be compared with the corresponding numbers in the register, and missing cases can be reported to the register. Further, those who are running a register study must regularly give updates on results at meet-ings, conferences, courses, and in scientific articles.

DATA PROTECTION

When starting a registry it must first be decided how the individual surgeons' and hospitals' results will be handled. A complete registration of all joint replacement operations is important in our system, and since some surgeons in Norway did not want to participate unless they were guaranteed anonym-ity, it was decided not to register the identity of the surgeons. The main aim of the register was decided as being quality control of the implants and sur-gical techniques, while the quality of surgeons would be monitored locally in the hospitals.

Results at hospital level are treated confidentially in the Norwegian register, whereas in the Swedish and Finnish hip registries they are made public.

In some countries it is feared that the health authorities will take control over registers in order to regulate orthopaedic surgery, and this concern among orthopaedic surgeons appears to have caused difficulties for the establishment of registers. In order to obtain continuous, complete and correct reporting, and to analyse the data correctly, the health authorities depend on the orthopaedic sur-geons. Experience gained from existing registers indicates that the health authorities wish for reg-isters to serve as tools for continuous surveillance and quality control rather than as a means of regulating the surgeons' practice. In Norway, the Arthroplasty Register is owned by the Orthopaedic Association, and only summary data and summary results are released to the authorities, who respect this practice.

STAFF AND BUDGET

From Norway's population of 4.4 million people, reports are obtained annually from about 7500 operations, and the registry now (in 2001) contains approximately 90 000 cases. At the present time, the staff consists of one secretary, and one position for an orthopaedic surgeon, which is split between three doctors. There is also one statistician who prepares the annual reports and produces scientific publications, in addition to counselling orthopaedic surgeons with their statistical work. The register also has one research fellow who is financed externally, and regular (weekly) meetings are held with a professor at the Section for medical statistics at the University of Bergen.

Funding

Funding has been a major problem in establishing most joint replacement registries. The health authorities usually have a great interest in register studies, but experience shows that it takes time to obtain financial support from this source. At the present time (2001), the Government covers practically all expenses for the Norwegian Arthroplasty Register, which is about 1.4 million NOK or 175 000 Euro annually. The cost per hip replacement is approximately 22 Euro. By comparison, in Trent (England), data available from the register shows the cost for total hip replacement to be approximately £50 (Fender *et al.* 1996).

If the financial resources cannot be obtained from an independent source, then one possibility is to allow each hospital to pay a fee per registered implant. Some registries also obtain financial support from industry sources, although in such cases it is preferable that many or all manufacturers are involved, rather than the register being financed by one company. As case registries most often will assess the results of implants or treatment systems provided by industrial companies, it is preferable that implant registries remain economically independent from the industry.

CONCLUSION

In fields where too few randomized studies are performed, register studies might be the most practical solution to the problem of data acquisition. Registers may function as tools in surveillance and quality control, and the register data provide a good basis for research. The present authors' experience is that, by the use of a register it is possible to detect inferior implants before they are used in large numbers of patients.

REFERENCES

Benedetti, J., Young, K., and Young, L. (1990): Life Tables and Survivor Functions. In: Dixon, W. J. (ed.), *BMDP Statistical Software Manual*. Berkeley, California, USA: University of California Press, pp. 729–69.

Benson, K., and Hartz, A. J. (2000): A comparison of observational studies and randomized, controlled trials. *N Engl J Med* **342**, 1878–86.

Concato, J., Shah, N., and Horwitz, R. I. (2000): Randomized, controlled trials, observational studies, and the hierarchy of research designs. *N Engl J Med* **342**, 1887–92.

Cox, D. (1972): Regression models and life tables (with discussion). *J Roy Statist Soc B* **34**, 187–220.

Cutler, J. S., and Edere, F. (1958): Maximum utilization of the life-table method in analyzing survival. *J Chron Dis* **8**, 699–713.

Dobbs, H. S. (1980): Survival of total hip replacement. *J Bone Joint Surg Br* **62B**, 168–73.

Fender, D., Harper, W. M., and Gregg, P. J. (1996): Need for a national arthroplasty register. Funding is important. *Br Med J* **313**, 1007.

Fender, D., Harper, W. M., and Gregg, P. J. (1999): Outcome of Charnley total hip replacement across a single health region in England: the results at five years from a regional hip register. *J Bone Joint Surg Br* **81**, 577–81.

Havelin, L. I., Espehaug, B., Vollset, S. E., and Engesæter, L. B. (1995a): The effect of cement type on early revision of Charnley total hip prostheses. A review of 8,579 primary arthroplasties from the Norwegian Arthroplasty Register. *J Bone Joint Surg Am* **77-A**, 1543–50.

Havelin, L. I., Espehaug, B., Vollset, S. E., and Engesæter, L. B. (1995b): Early aseptic loosening of uncemented femoral components in primary total hip replacement. A review based on the Norwegian Arthroplasty Register. *J Bone Joint Surg Br* **77-B**, 11–17.

Havelin, L. I., Vollset, S. E., and Engesæter, L. B. (1995c): Revision for aseptic loosening of uncemented cups in 4,352 primary total hip prostheses. A report from the Norwegian Arthroplasty Register. *Acta Orthop Scand* **66**, 494–500.

Havelin, L. I., Engesæter, L. B., Espehaug, B., Furnes, O., Lie, S. A., and Vollset, S. E. (2000): The Norwegian Arthroplasty Register: 11 years and 73,000 arthroplasties. *Acta Orthop Scand* **71**, 337–53.

Herberts, P., and Malchau, H. (1997): How outcome studies have changed total hip arthroplasty practices in Sweden. *Clin Orthop* **344**, 44–60.

Herberts, P., and Malchau, H. (2000): Long-term registration has improved the quality of hip replacement: a review of the Swedish THR Register comparing 160,000 cases. *Acta Orthop Scand* **71**, 111–21.

Kaplan, E. L., and Meier, P. (1958): Nonparametric estimation from incomplete observations. *J Am Statist Assoc* **53**, 457–81.

Knutson, K., Lewold, S., Robertson, O., and Lidgren, L. (1994): The Swedish knee arthroplasty register. A nation-wide study of 30,003 knees 1976–1992. *Acta Orthop Scand* **65**, 375–86.

Lucht, U. (2000): The Danish Hip Arthroplasty Register. *Acta Orthop Scand* **71**, 433–9.

Malchau, H., Herberts, P., and Ahnfelt, L. (1993): Prognosis of total hip replacement in Sweden. Follow-up of 92,675 operations performed 1978–1990. *Acta Orthop Scand* **64**, 497–506.

Paavolainen, P., Hämäläinen, M., Mustonen, H., and Slätis, P. (1991): Registration of arthroplasties in Finland. A nation-wide prospective project. *Acta Orthop Scand* **62**, 27–30.

Puolakka, T. J., Pajamaki, K. J., Pulkkinen, P. O., and Nevalainen, J. K. (1999): Poor survival of cementless Biomet total hip: a report on 1,047 hips from the Finnish Arthroplasty Register. *Acta Orthop Scand* **70**, 425–9.

Robertsson, O., Dunbar, M. J., Knutson, K., Lewold, S., and Lidgren, L. (1999): The Swedish Knee Arthroplasty Register: 25 years experience. *Bull Hosp Joint Dis* **58**, 133–8.

Söderman, P., Malchau, H., and Herberts, P. (2000): Outcome after total hip arthroplasty: Part I. General health evaluation in relation to definition of failure in the Swedish National Total Hip Arthroplasty register. *Acta Orthop Scand* **71**, 354–9.

Sudmann, E., Havelin, L. I., Lunde, O. D., and Rait, M. (1983): The Charnley versus the Christiansen total hip arthroplasty. *Acta Orthop Scand* **54**, 545–52.

6

Measures of health status, health-related quality of life and patient satisfaction

Raymond Fitzpatrick

INTRODUCTION

This chapter is concerned with patient-assessed measures; that is to say, questionnaires or similar instruments completed by the patient rather than by the health professional. These measures are increasingly used to assess patients' needs for and outcomes of treatment, and a remarkable proliferation of such instruments has occurred during the past 20 years. The health professional has problems of choosing between the enormous array of instruments, even within a single field such as orthopaedics and trauma. This chapter is intended to be an introductory guide to the principles that should inform choice of a patient-assessed instrument. More detailed guides exist which describe both the range of available instruments and the principles of measurement involved in their use (Bowling 1995; Fitzpatrick *et al.* 1998). Three broad types of instrument are considered that are measures of: (i) health or functional status; (ii) health-related quality of life; and (iii) patient satisfaction. In practice, distinctions between these categories are difficult to maintain, and so instruments may contain items addressing all three areas.

Patient-assessed measures have emerged to serve a number of different purposes. First, they can be used to assess levels of need in populations or groups of patients attending healthcare. Thus, a health status measure can be used to assess the varying levels of pain and disability amongst patients on surgical waiting lists, or to assess the prevalence of pain and disability in the community that might benefit from surgical intervention. The second purpose is to assess outcomes of interventions in groups of patients. This may either be in the context of observational studies; for example, an audit of outcomes for patients of a specific group of surgeons, or in the context of a randomized controlled trial (RCT) of alternative interventions. The third main type of use of patient assessed instruments is as an aid or adjunct to individual patient care, to determine need and to assess progress of interventions at the level of the individual patient. To date, regular use of such instruments at the level of the individual patient is far less common, and it is the first two applications, with groups of patients, that are more widespread.

The main rationale for the use of patient-assessed instruments is that they provide evidence that is distinct from that provided by clinical assessment. In a number of studies in other fields of medicine and surgery, it has been shown that patients and doctors significantly disagree about health status (Sprangers and Aaronson 1992). Such disagreements have also been observed in orthopaedics; for example, with surgeons rating outcomes of knee surgery quite differently from their patients (Bullens *et al.* 2001). At a practical level it is also becoming increasingly clear that self-completed questionnaires may provide a more feasible as well as more valid method of tracking outcomes, given the need, for example for large numbers of participating centres with long-term follow-up to provide clear evidence for surgical trials.

The most essential properties of any health status measure are that it be reliable, valid, and sensitive to change. How such properties are assessed in health status measures are considered in turn.

RELIABILITY

Reliability is concerned with the amount of random and systematic measurement error to be found in an instrument, and is assessed in terms of reproducibility and internal consistency. Reproducibility evaluates whether an instrument yields the same results on repeated applications, when respondents have not changed on the domain being measured. This is assessed by test-retest reliability. The degree of agreement is examined between scores at a first assessment and when reassessed. Respondents can, if necessary, be asked whether a change has occurred in the domain, and those answering positively excluded from the test of reproducibility. Commonly reproducibility is expressed in terms of a correlation coefficient between scores, but it is equally important to assess whether a shift in the distribution of scores has occurred. The reproducibility of the Oxford Knee Score was tested by asking 66 patients to complete the instrument on two occasions, 24 hours apart (Dawson *et al.* 1998). The correlation coefficient between scores was very high, $r = 0.92$. Equally importantly, there was no significant change in the distribution of scores as examined by t-test.

Internal consistency can be tested when there are several items (forming a scale), rather than a single item, to measure constructs. This practice is based on a basic principle of measurement that several related observations will produce a more reliable estimate than one. For this to be true, the items of a scale need to measure aspects of only one attribute (known as 'homogeneous'). Internal consistency can be measured by 'split-half reliability', the degree of agreement of two halves of the items in the scale. Most commonly internal consistency is measured by means of Cronbach's alpha, essentially the average level of agreement of all possible split-half tests for a set of items (Cronbach 1951). The range of Cronbach's alpha is from 0.0 to 1.0, with values between 0.70 and 0.90 considered optimal.

VALIDITY

The validity of instrument is an assessment of the extent to which it measures what it purports to measure. It is rarely, if ever, possible to identify a 'gold standard' against which to assess health status instruments. Thus, 'criterion' validity is not feasible. Instead, face and content validity are used to examine whether items appear to address the important issues in a construct. Such judgements can be made by patients and clinicians. Appropriate patients should have been involved in the development of items.

Construct validity is a more quantitative form of assessment of validity. The construct, for example, disability, intended to be measured by an instrument, is expected to have a set of quantitative relationships with other constructs, such as age, disease status and recent use of healthcare facilities. No single correlation provides sufficient support for construct validity; a cumulative pattern of evidence is required.

The Arthritis Impact Measurement Scale (AIMS), described below, was developed as an instrument to assess health status in the rheumatic diseases (Meenan 1982). One aspect of the assessment of the construct validity of AIMS was to examine patterns of cor-relations with clinical rating scales. For example, scales of AIMS concerned with lower-limb function correlated more with clinical ratings of walking time than measures of grip strength. Conversely, the scale of AIMS concerned with dexterity was more correlated with grip strength than the clinical assessment of walking time. The AIMS pain scale correlated best with the number of joints affected. These associations, which were broadly consistent with those expected, were further tested in a range of patient groups with differing clinical and demographic characteristics. It was the overall pattern of correlations that contributed to the evidence for construct validity.

SENSITIVITY TO CHANGE

It is essential that health status instruments are sensitive to changes over time within individuals, when used in clinical trials or any other form of evaluative research. It is possible for an instrument to be reliable and valid but insensitive to changes over time. Methods for the assessment of sensitivity to change are more diverse and less standardized than for other desirable properties. Approaches may be distinguished by whether they rely on statistical or external evidence (Husted *et al.* 2000). Statistical evidence of sensitivity to change, is change identified by the instrument. This can be examined by means of an effect size (mean change in a score divided by standard deviation in baseline score) or standardized response mean (mean change in a score divided by standard deviation in change score). The assumption behind such statistical approaches is that those instruments most sensitive to change are those with the largest effect size. Instruments are tested in patient groups where it is assumed that substantial change is truly occurring. Patients undergoing hip or knee replacement surgery, because they normally experience substantial improvement over time following surgery are appropriate for such statistical approaches.

Alternative approaches rely on external evidence by, for example, correlating change scores in a health status instrument with changes over time in other variables such as disease severity or examining change scores in an instrument for groups of patients who differ in their own or their clinicians' retrospective judgements as to whether they have experienced change. The advantage of this external evidence over statistical methods is that there exists some external bench-mark or criterion. Statistical methods rely on the strong assumption that greater effect sizes are alone evidence of greater sensitivity to change. Increasingly the two approaches are combined. Thus, in a series of patients undergoing revision hip replacement surgery, patients completed assessments before and one year after surgery (Dawson *et al.* 2001). The relative sensitivity to change of the specific instrument (Oxford Hip Score; OHS) and a generic instrument (EQ-5D) were compared by calculating the effect sizes for the two instruments amongst patients who judged retrospectively their pain to have improved. Effect sizes were greater in the more specific instrument, indicating a greater sensitivity to change. A quite separate external criterion was also used. It was postulated that the greater the number of previous revision replacement operations, the less favourable should be patients' health status change scores. The OHS proved more sensitive to change over time between groups of patients distinguished in this way than was the generic instrument.

OTHER DESIRABLE PROPERTIES

There are other features that one would expect to find in optimal health status measures. Instruments should be acceptable to patients and feasible to use in the context of clinical practice. Examples are the time taken to complete an instrument, and the degree of difficulty involved in the task. These can affect the completeness of data obtained. The Health Assessment Questionnaire, an instrument widely used to assess health status in arthritis, typically requires only 3 minutes to complete. This is considerably less time than most instruments (Wolfe *et al.* 1988). The method of administration of an instrument can influence time to complete. Patients in a general medical clinic were randomly assigned to complete the Short Form (SF)-36, either by interview or by self-completion (Weinberger *et al.* 1996). The latter approach required 3 minutes longer (on average 13 minutes) to complete. Feasibility refers to the amount of staff effort and cost required to collect and process information. There is a spectrum of feasibility from shorter and simpler self-complete questionnaires to instruments involving complex interviews and scoring systems.

Instruments also need to produce interpretable results. Numerical scores need to have some meaning for decision-makers. Generic health status measures, because of their general applicability, can be completed by representative samples of the general population. Results of such community surveys provide normative bench-marks with which the results in a specific trial using such measures can be compared. An alternative approach is to relate scores to other data that are more readily interpretable. Thus, an estimate can be made of the change scores on a health status instrument associated with life events, such as becoming unemployed. The difference in scores between primary care and hospital patients can be compared to give more meaning to numerical scores. Another way of anchoring numerical scores is to relate changed scores to so-called 'transition questions'. These are questions which ask respondents to say whether they are 'better', 'worse' or 'stable' compared to a previous assessment. In this way, scores typically associated with a patient's judgement of improvement or deterioration can be specified.

HEALTH OR FUNCTIONAL STATUS

The distinction between health or functional status instruments and health-related quality of life scales is particularly difficult. There is a continuum between instruments that focus narrowly on core aspects of symptoms and physical function to those that include a broader range of dimensions of health-related quality of life, such as emotional and social functioning.

An example of a functional status instrument commonly used in the rheumatological disorders is the Health Assessment Questionnaire (HAQ) (Fries *et al.* 1982). The core of this instrument is a disability index comprising 20 items to assess activities of daily living that might be affected by arthritis: dressing and grooming, rising from a chair or bed, eating, walking, hygiene, reach, grip, and outside activity. Items are answered on a four-point scale from 'without difficulty' to 'unable to do'. The scores are averaged to produce a single index. The scheme has been extensively validated, and there is substantial agreement with observers' ratings of function, with clinical and laboratory measures of disease severity and other measures of patient-assessed health status. It is also predictive of longer term outcome in rheumatoid arthritis (RA). There is good evidence for its acceptability and feasibility. It requires less than 5 minutes to complete, and it is widely used in clinical trials, especially of RA. One problem identified in the HAQ is a potential floor effect, whereby patients with poor scores seem unable to report further deterioration if re-assessed several years later.

While the HAQ has largely been used for patients with RA, the Western Ontario and McMaster Universities Osteoarthritis (WOMAC) index is intended for use in osteoarthritis (OA) (Bellamy *et al.* 1988). It assesses three dimensions of health status: pain (five items), stiffness (two items), and function (17 items). Answers are on a five-point scale from 'none' to 'extreme'. It has sometimes been used with a continuous visual analogue scale, and has been the subject of extensive evaluation for its measurement properties. Patients assessed before and after total hip replacement surgery with WOMAC correlated with independent observers' ratings of stride and walking abilities (Boardman *et al.* 2000). The HAQ has also been shown to be sensitive to changes over time arising from medical or surgical interventions for OA.

For some purposes it may be essential to have more condition-specific instruments in orthopaedics and trauma. For example, in order to evaluate outcomes of hip replacement surgery, it is desirable to have health status instruments that are sensitive to change in health status in relation to the operated hip. Many older patients may have co-morbidity: problems of pain and function arising from a range of other health problems not relevant to hip replacement surgery. The OHS was developed and validated specifically for use in assessing pain and function following hip replacement surgery (Dawson *et al.* 1996). It comprises 12 items, each with five response categories reflecting different levels of severity, and is summed to a single score. It was shown to produce different levels of post-surgical improvement according to the number of previous replacement operations that patients had undergone for the operated hip. This is consistent with clinical expectations. If a hip is revised, it is less likely to have a satisfactory outcome (Dawson *et al.* 2001). Similar region-specific measures have been developed and validated against clinical scales for use in orthopaedic surgery for knee and shoulder.

HEALTH-RELATED QUALITY OF LIFE

Instruments may assess a broader range of consequences of health: the more they do so, the more it is appropriate to consider them measures of health-related quality of life. Some instruments purport to measure broader consequences of health but remain disease-specific. A good example is an instrument for use in arthritis, the AIMS (Meenan 1982). This consists of 45 items over nine dimensions: mobility; physical activity; activities of daily living; dexterity; household activities; pain; depression; anxiety; and social activities. The separate scales are not intended to be summed, although factor analyses have suggested that the nine scales may reduce down to five underlying dimensions: upper-extremity function; lower-extremity function; mood; symptoms; and social function. The instrument has been extensively examined for relationships with clinical measures (grip strength, joint counts, clinical ratings of disease severity) and has also been shown to be sensitive to change over time in drug trials.

The advantage of disease-specific instruments such as AIMS is that it is supposed to contain items highly relevant and specific for use in trials and evaluations of interventions for the disease in question, with minimal redundancy of content. However, there are disadvantages. A questionnaire designed for patients with arthritis normally cannot be completed by respondents free of arthritis. It is inappropriate for administration to the general community to produce normative and comparative data. It is also not possible to compare outcomes of treatments for different health problems; so consistency cannot be used to compare cost effectiveness.

GENERIC HEALTH STATUS MEASURES

To address limitations of disease-specific instruments, a number of so-called 'generic health status instruments' have been developed. These are intended to be applicable across the widest range of health problems and healthcare interventions. Three generic health status instruments have been applied to the context of orthopaedics: the Sickness Impact Profile; the Nottingham Health Profile; and the SF-36. These differ somewhat in their content and distinctive focus.

The Sickness Impact Profile (SIP) consists of 136 items in the form of statements describing behaviour in relation to illness to which the respondent gives 'yes' or 'no' answers (Bergner et al. 1981). Positive answers have a weighted score derived from prior studies of the severity of items. Items contribute to one of 12 dimensions: walking; body care and movement; mobility; work; sleeping and rest; eating; housework; recreation; emotions; social interaction; alertness; and communication. Scores in the first three dimensions may be summed to produce a physical scale. The last four scales may be summed to produce a psychosocial scale. Unlike many generic instruments, all items may also be summed to produce a total score. Patients completing the SIP before and six months after total hip replacement surgery experienced significant improvements in both physical and psychosocial domains (Knutsson and Engberg 1999).

The SIP was one of the first generic instruments to be developed, and it is now considered too long (it may require up to 30 minutes to complete) for regular use in clinical contexts. The Nottingham Health Profile (NHP) was also developed as a generic measure (Hunt et al. 1985). Like the SIP, its response categories are simply 'yes' or 'no'. Positively answered items receiving a weighted score. There are only 38 items which contribute to six scales: physical mobility; pain; emotional reactions; energy; sleep; and social isolation. Nilsson and colleagues (Nilsson et al. 1994) investigated patients five years after total hip replacement surgery, and found evidence of poorer outcomes in some patients with radiographic loosening. These patients were not detected by surgeon-assessed Charnley hip scores, but did have significantly poorer NHP scores.

The most widely used generic instrument is the SF-36 (Ware and Sherbourne 1992). This comprises 36 items measuring eight dimensions of health status: physical functioning; role limitations due to physical problems; role limitations due to emotional problems; social functioning; mental health; energy/vitality; pain; and general perceptions of health. It is also increasingly reported as two summary scales assessing physical and mental health. It has been extensively tested for use in orthopaedic surgical outcome assessment. For example, Jones et al. (2000) assessed patients receiving either knee or hip replacement surgery before and six months after surgery. They showed that, whilst patients experienced very substantial improvements in pain and physical function, changes to psychosocial function were much smaller. Improvements were greater for patients receiving hip compared with knee replacement surgery.

INDIVIDUALIZED MEASURES

One criticism levelled against all of the approaches reviewed so far is that patients' views and experiences are assessed by means of standardized items predetermined by researchers. Patients receiving orthopaedic surgery may have concerns that are not addressed by such instruments (Wright et al. 1994). To respond to such challenges, a number of instruments have begun to appear that have in common that they are designed for patients to identify their own concerns rather than respond to predetermined categories. One of the earliest of so-called 'individualized' instruments to appear was the Schedule for the Evaluation of Individual Quality of Life (SEIQoL) (O'Boyle et al. 1992). This system requires detailed interviewing in order to persuade patients to identify their five most important personal concerns with regard to quality of life and then rate them. When applied to patients undergoing total hip replacement surgery, the SEIQoL appeared to be less sensitive to change over time than more conventional measures (O'Boyle et al. 1992).

Another individualized instrument, the McMaster-Toronto Arthritis (MACTAR) Patient Preference Disability Questionnaire – in this case asking respondents to identify three aspects of life adversely affected by arthritis – has been used specifically to assess outcomes of hip replacement surgery (Laupacis et al. 1993).

Instruments such as SEIQoL and MACTAR are very similar in format to the utility measures used by health economists. The main similarity is that both individualized and utility measures normally require interviews because complex judgements are required of the respondent. The utility measure is different in that it is intended to obtain a single overall preference or value from respondents regarding their health. Utility measures have occasionally been used in the assessment of outcome of orthopaedic surgery, but it is not clear from such studies what advantages they have over simpler methods (Laupacis et al. 1993).

PATIENT SATISFACTION

A quite different focus in patient assessed measures is provided by examining patient satisfaction. Instead of asking patients about aspects of their health status, questions focus upon their judgements of the success, acceptability and value of healthcare received. Most commonly, studies of patient satisfaction have focused upon non-clinical aspects of care. These include courtesy and communication from health professionals, and the accessibility and convenience of services (Fitzpatrick 1991). However, in the field of orthopaedics questionnaires have proved particularly helpful in obtaining evidence of patients' views about the outcomes of their surgery. For example, Kay et al. (1983) carried out a survey of patients approximately one year after total hip replacement surgery and found that 90 per cent of patients were satisfied with the outcome of their surgery; the remainder were either dissatisfied or uncertain. An indication of the validity of the results was provided by the higher rate of dissatisfaction in patients undergoing revision surgery. A follow-up study of patients on the Swedish Knee Arthroplasty Register asked patients to rate their satisfaction with their knee surgery on a single four-point scale from 'very satisfied' to 'dissatisfied' (Robertsson and Dunbar 2001). Overall, 81 per cent of patients were satisfied, with dissatisfaction being higher in patients undergoing revision surgery. Patient satisfaction was found to be higher in those patients with more favourable scores for pain and physical function on a range of health status measures. Importantly, the response rate of patients to the patient satisfaction questionnaire was 95 per cent, whereas responses to health status questionnaires such as SF-36 and NHP were considerably lower. This suggests a specific advantage in terms of acceptability of the shorter and simpler questions about satisfaction.

It is striking that less effort has been invested in standardizing and validating patient satisfaction questionnaires than has occurred with health status measures, within and outside the field of orthopaedics. Yet it is apparent that simple questions concerning satisfaction with outcome may well provide an ideal compromise between the more detailed information provided by health status measures and the need for high response rates to avoid bias in evaluation of outcome.

COMPARATIVE EVALUATION OF MEASURES

There is now such a large array of candidate measures from which to choose in order to assess patients' perceptions of health outcomes, that the most important priority now is for comparative assessment of instruments. Comparative evaluation is most effectively carried out by patients within a study completing study instruments at specific times. These studies should be prospective, so that performance of instruments can be evaluated with minimal bias from differences due to patients, settings or other factors.

Several studies have shown that patient-assessed outcome measures are more sensitive than conventional clinically completed scales in measuring changes over time in patients undergoing orthopaedic surgery. For example, Nilsdotter et al. (2001) found both the WOMAC and SF-36 to be more responsive than a clinician-completed scale to changes after total hip replacement surgery.

A simple example of a direct comparative study of patient assessed measures was provided by Stucki et al. (1995), who asked patients before and three months after total hip replacement surgery to complete both the SF-36 and the SIP. The SIP was found to be less appropriate to the patient group because in 10 out of 12 scales the median score was zero (that is, no problem), compared to only one of the SF-36 scales. As importantly, the effect size for change scores for SF-36 was greater, interpreted by the investigators as evidence of increased sensitivity to change of SF-36.

In a more ambitious comparative study (Dunbar et al. 2001), four generic and three disease-specific instruments were administered to 3600 patients randomly selected from the Swedish Knee Arthroplasty Registry. Instruments were assessed against a number of criteria: response rate, completion rate, time required to complete, reliability, and validity. From the simple scoring used to rank instruments, the SF-12 (based on SF-36) emerged as the best generic measure and Oxford Knee Score as the best disease-specific measure.

To date, there are few general truths established from the growing body of comparative evaluation of patient-assessed measures in orthopaedics. There seems little evidence that longer and more detailed instruments are more sensitive to important changes, whereas they usually prove less acceptable to patients because of length. There would appear to be enormous scope for accurate assessment of outcomes from quite short and simple patient-assessed outcome measures of complementary constructs of health status, health-related quality of life and patient satisfaction. Such measures are increasingly recognized as having a unique and important contribution to make to the evaluation of orthopaedic and trauma surgery.

REFERENCES

Bellamy, N., Buchanan, W., Goldsmith, C., et al. (1988): Validation study of WOMAC: a health status instrument for measuring clinically important patient relevant outcomes to antirheumatic drug therapy in patients with osteoarthritis of the hip or knee. J Rheumatol 15, 1833–40.

Bergner, M., Bobbitt, R., Carter, W., and Gilson, B. (1981): The Sickness Impact Profile: development and final revision of a health status measure. Med Care 1, 787–805.

Boardman, D. L., Dorey, F., Thomas, B. J., and Lieberman, J. R. (2000): The accuracy of assessing total hip arthroplasty outcomes: a prospective correlation study of walking ability and 2 validated measurement devices. J Arthroplasty 15, 200–4.

Bowling, A. (1995): *Measuring Disease*. Open University Press, Buckingham.

Bullens, P. H., van Loon, C. J., de Waal Malefijt, M. C., Laan, R. F., and Veth, R. P. (2001): Patient satisfaction after total knee arthroplasty: a comparison between subjective and objective outcome assessments. *J Arthroplasty* **16**, 740–7.

Cronbach, L. (1951): Coefficient alpha and the internal structure of tests. *Psychometrika* **16**, 297–334.

Dawson, J., Fitzpatrick, R., Carr, A., and Murray, D. (1996): Questionnaire on the perceptions of patients about total hip replacement. *J Bone Joint Surg* **78-B**, 185–90.

Dawson, J., Fitzpatrick, R., Frost, S., Gundle, R., McLardy-Smith, P., and Murray, D. (2001): Evidence for the validity of a patient-based instrument for assessment of outcome after revision hip replacement. *J Bone Joint Surg Br* **83**, 1125–9.

Dawson, J., Fitzpatrick, R., Murray, D., and Carr, A. (1998): Questionnaire on the perceptions of patients about total knee replacement. *J Bone Joint Surg Br* **80**, 63–9.

Dunbar, M. J., Robertsson, O., Ryd, L., and Lidgren, L. (2001): Appropriate questionnaires for knee arthroplasty. Results of a survey of 3600 patients from the Swedish Knee Arthroplasty Registry. *J Bone Joint Surg Br* **83-B**, 339–44.

Fitzpatrick, R. (1991): Surveys of patient satisfaction I – important general considerations. *Br Med J* **302**, 887–9.

Fitzpatrick, R., Davey, C., Buxton, M., and Jones, D. (1998): Evaluating patient-based outcome measures for use in clinical trials. *Health Technol Assessment* **2**, 1–74.

Fries, J., Spitz, P., and Young, D. (1982): The dimensions of health outcomes: the Health Assessment Questionnaire, disability and pain scales. *J Rheumatol* **9**, 789–93.

Hunt, S., McEwan, J., and McKenna, S. (1985): Measuring health status: a new tool for clinicians and epidemiologists. *J Roy Coll Gen Pract* **35**, 185–8.

Husted, J. A., Cook, R. J., Farewell, V. T., and Gladman, D. D. (2000): Methods for assessing responsiveness: a critical review and recommendations. *J Clin Epidemiol* **53**, 459–68.

Jones, C. A., Voaklander, D. C., Johnston, D. W., and Suarez-Almazor, M. E. (2000): Health related quality of life outcomes after total hip and knee arthroplasties in a community based population. *J Rheumatol* **27**, 1745–52.

Kay, A., Davidson, B. E. B., and Wagstaff, S. (1983): Hip arthroplasty: patient satisfaction. *Br J Rheumatol* **22**, 243–9.

Knutsson, S., and Engberg, I. B. (1999): An evaluation of patients' quality of life before, 6 weeks and 6 months after total hip replacement surgery. *J Adv Nurs* **30**, 1349–59.

Laupacis, A., Bourne, R., Rorabeck, C., Feeny, D., Wong, C., Tugwell, P., Leslie, K., and Bullas, R. (1993): The effect of elective total hip replacement on health-related quality of life. *J Bone Joint Surg Am* **75-A**, 1619–26.

Meenan, R. F. (1982): The AIMS approach to health status measurement: conceptual background and measurement properties. *J Rheumatol* **9**, 785–8.

Nilsdotter, A. K., Roos, E. M., Westerlund, J. P., Roos, H. P., and Lohmander, L. S. (2001): Comparative responsiveness of measures of pain and function after total hip replacement. *Arthritis Rheum* **45**, 258–62.

Nilsson, L., Franzen, H., Carlsson, A., and Onnerfalt, R. (1994): Early radiographic loosening impairs the function of a total hip replacement. *J Bone Joint Surg* **76-B**, 235–9.

O'Boyle, C., McGee, H., Hickey, A., O'Malley, K., and Joyce, C. (1992): Individual quality of life in patients undergoing hip replacement. *Lancet* **339**, 1088–91.

Robertsson, O., and Dunbar, M. (2001): Patient satisfaction compared with general health and disease-specific questionnaires in knee arthroplasty patients. *J Arthroplasty* **16**, 476–82.

Sprangers, M., and Aaronson, N. (1992): The role of health care providers and significant others in evaluating the quality of life of patients with chronic disease: a review. *J Clin Epidemiol* **45**, 743–60.

Stucki, G., Liang, M. H., Phillips, C., and Katz, J. N. (1995): The Short Form-36 is preferable to the

SIP as a generic health status measure in patients undergoing elective total hip arthroplasty. *Arthritis Care Res* **8**, 174–81.

Ware, J., and Sherbourne, C. (1992): The MOS 36-item short form health survey (SF-36). 1 Conceptual framework and item selection. *Med Care* **30**, 473–83.

Weinberger, M., Oddone, E., Samsa, G., and Landsman, P. (1996): Are health-related quality of life measures affected by the mode of administration? *J Clin Epidemiol* **49**, 135–40.

Wolfe, F., Kleinheksel, S., Cathey, M., Hawley, D., Spitz, P., and Fries, J. (1988): The clinical value of the Stanford Health Assessment Questionnaire Functional Disability Index in patients with rheumatoid arthritis. *J Rheumatol* **15**, 480–8.

Wright, J., Rudicel, S., and Feinstein, A. (1994): Ask patients what they want. *J Bone Joint Surg* **76-B**, 229–34.

7

The measures of pain

Henry J. McQuay

"It would be wonderfully helpful to have objective signs of subjective change; but it seems unlikely that many such aids will be readily available in any precise way for years to come."

Beecher (1959)

Pain is a personal experience, and consequently is difficult to define. It includes both the sensory input and any modulation by physiological, psychological and environmental factors. Not surprisingly, there are no objective measures – there is no way to measure pain directly by sampling blood or urine or by performing neurophysiological tests. Measurement of pain must therefore rely on recording the patient's report. The assumption is often made that because the measurement is subjective it must be of little value. The reality is that if the measurements are made properly, then remarkably sensitive and consistent results can be obtained. There are contexts, however, when it is not possible to measure pain at all, or when reports are likely to be unreliable. These include impaired consciousness, young children, psychiatric pathology, severe anxiety, unwillingness to cooperate, and inability to understand the measurements. Such problems are deliberately avoided in trials, but are all too common in the clinical setting.

MEASUREMENT SCALES (RESEARCH)

Most analgesic studies include measurements of pain intensity and/or pain relief, and the commonest tools used are categorical and visual analogue scales.

Whose pain is it?

Judgement of the patient rather than by the carer is the ideal. Carers over-estimate the pain relief compared with the patient's version (Rundshagen *et al.* 1999).

Categorical scales

Categorical scales use words to describe the magnitude of the pain or pain relief, and were the earliest-used measure of pain (Keele 1948). The patient picks the most appropriate word to describe the pain, with most research groups using four categories (none, mild, moderate, and severe). Scales to measure pain relief were developed later; the most common of these is the five-category scale (none, slight, moderate, good or lots, and complete) (Fig. 7.1).

Pain intensity	
severe	3
moderate	2
mild	1
none	0

Pain relief	
complete	4
good	3
moderate	2
slight	1
none	0

Figure 7.1 Categorical verbal rating scales.

Pain intensity scale

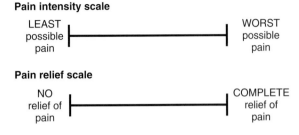

Figure 7.2 Visual analogue scales for pain intensity and pain relief.

For analysis numbers are given to the verbal categories (for pain intensity, none = 0, mild = 1, moderate = 2 and severe = 3; and for relief none = 0, slight = 1, moderate = 2, good or lots = 3 and complete = 4). Data from different subjects are then combined to produce means (rarely medians) and measures of dispersion (usually standard errors of means). The validity of converting categories into numerical scores was checked by comparison with concurrent visual analogue scale measurements (Fig. 7.2). A good correlation was found, especially between pain relief scales using cross-modality matching techniques (Scott and Huskisson 1976; Wallenstein et al. 1980; Littman et al. 1985). Results are usually reported as continuous data, mean or median pain relief or intensity. Few studies present results as discrete data, giving the number of participants who report a certain level of pain intensity or relief at any given assessment point. The main advantages of the categorical scales are that they are quick and simple. The small number of descriptors may force the scorer to choose a particular category when none describes the pain satisfactorily.

Visual analogue scales

Visual analogue scales (VAS), which are lines with the left-hand end labelled 'no relief of pain' and the right-hand end labelled 'complete relief of pain', seem to overcome this limitation. Patients mark the line at the point which corresponds to their pain. The scores are obtained by measuring the distance between the no relief end and the patient's mark, usually in millimetres. The main advantages of VAS are

that they are simple and quick to score, avoid imprecise descriptive terms, and also provide many points from which to choose. However, more concentration and coordination are needed, and this can be difficult post-operatively or in patients with neurological disorders.

Pain relief versus pain intensity

Pain relief scales are perceived as more convenient than pain intensity scales, probably because patients have the same baseline relief (zero), whereas they could start with different baseline intensity (usually moderate or severe). Relief scale results are then easier to compare, and may also be more sensitive than intensity scales (Sriwatanakul et al. 1982; Littman et al. 1985). A theoretical drawback of relief scales is that the patient has to remember what the pain was like to begin with.

Numerical rating scales (Likert)

Numerical rating scales (NRS), also called Likert or ordinal scales, are analogous to the VAS in that they are generally 100 mm long and have the same anchor points, but the answers are constrained to the 11 or 7 possible responses, rather than freely ranging across the line. NRS are considered both valid and sensitive with a significant correlation to other measures of pain intensity (Jensen and McFarland 1993) and are said to be easier for some patients to use. They have been used widely in recent trials of anticonvulsants in neuropathic pain (Farrar et al. 2001).

Global rating scales

Global rating scales are designed to measure overall treatment performance. For research and clinical purposes, we use a modified global scale which is primarily categorical. The patient is asked the question, 'How effective was the treatment?', using five categories (poor, fair, good, very good, and excellent).

For analysis, numerical values of 0 to 5 are given to each category. Although these judgements probably include adverse effects, they can be the most sensitive discriminant between treatments. The global measure can provide results similar to those obtained with the categorical pain relief scale (Collins *et al.* 2001). This system is easier to use, because it is carried out just once at the end of the study, rather than at multiple times, as with the categorical pain relief scale.

WOMAC

The Western Ontario and McMaster Universities (WOMAC) osteoarthritis index may be an important tool for orthopaedic use (Bellamy *et al.* 1988). It is a disease-specific, self-administered, health status measure, which asks about clinically important symptoms in the areas of pain, stiffness and physical function, classically in patients with osteoarthritis (OA) of the hip and/or knee. The index has 24 questions (five pain, two stiffness and 17 physical function), and can be completed in less than 5 minutes. It has been used widely in recent drug studies in arthritis (e.g. Peloso *et al.* 2000).

Binary scales

One of the oldest scales was the binary question, 'Is your pain half gone?' The advantage of this is that it has a clearer clinical meaning than a 10-mm shift on a VAS. The disadvantage – for the small trial-intensive measure pundits at least – is that all the potential intermediate information (1 to 49% or greater than 50%) is discarded.

Analgesic consumption and time-to-next analgesic (TNA)

Another strategy for measuring pain depends on the pattern of analgesic consumption. After any given intervention, the number of doses of analgesic requested by the patient (analgesic consumption) and the time between the intervention and the first request of an analgesic dose (time-to-next analgesic; TNA), can provide indirect estimates of the efficacy of such an intervention. Although too crude to substitute for conventional subjective scales for pain measurement, these methods can work effectively, for instance to assess the efficacy of spinal opiates (Moore *et al.* 1984) or to show the effects of pre-medication and local anaesthetic blocks on post-operative orthopaedic pain (McQuay *et al.* 1988). The main drawback is that the sensitivity of these measurements can be affected by other factors, for instance the timing at which drugs are dispensed by the nurses on the ward. The use of patient-controlled analgesia (PCA) is an obvious alternative way to avoid results biased by schedules for drug administration and to obtain more accurate data on drug consumption, but the variability in the amount of drug requested by patients from the PCA is large, and PCA has not superseded the classic rating scales for precise pain measurement.

What change on the scales is clinically meaningful?

One point about scales is that we rarely know how much movement on a particular scale equates to a clinically meaningful change. One example of where scale change and clinical importance were tested comes from McMaster. These authors used seven-point Likert scales measuring dyspnoea, fatigue and emotional function in patients with chronic heart and lung disease to determine how much change constituted a minimal clinically important difference (MCID). The answer was that the MCID was a mean change in score of approximately 0.5 per item on the seven-point scale (Jaeschke *et al.* 1989). For the numerical rating scales, a 30 per cent reduction in pain was a clinically important difference (Farrar *et al.* 2001).

Analysis of scale results: summary measures

In the research context, pain is usually assessed before the intervention is made, and thereafter on multiple occasions. Ideally, the area under the time–analgesic effect curve for the intensity (sum of pain intensity differences; SPID) or relief (total pain relief; TOTPAR) measures is derived:

$$\text{SPID} = \sum_{t=1}^{n} \text{PID}_t \quad \text{TOTPAR} = \sum_{t=1}^{n} \text{PR}_t$$

where at the tth assessment point, $(t = 0, 1, 2, \dots n)$ P_t and PR_t are pain intensity and pain relief measured at that point, respectively; P_0 is pain intensity at $t = 0$; and PID_t is the pain intensity difference calculated as $(P_0 - P_t)$.

These summary measures reflect the cumulative response to the intervention. Their disadvantage is that they do not provide information about the onset and peak of the analgesic effect. If onset or peak are important, then knowledge is necessary of the time to maximum pain relief (or reduction in pain intensity) or time for pain to return to baseline.

MEASURING PAIN IN CLINICAL PRACTICE

Pain charts used as part of normal practice will improve quality of care (Gould *et al.* 1992; Rawal and Berggren 1994). The increasing trend in North America is for pain to be regarded as the fifth vital sign, to be recorded at the same times as the other vital signs, and the fact of a chart is probably more important than its form. An example of this is the Burford chart (Burford Nursing Development Unit 1984), of which special scales are available for children (McGrath *et al.* 1993). The chart which patients can use at home is shown in Fig. 7.3. However, the numerical rating scales mentioned above are most popular for clinical purposes in North America.

Name.. **Oxford Pain Chart** Treatment Week.....................

Please fill in this chart each evening before going to bed. Record your pain intensity and the amount of pain relief. If you have had any side-effects please note them in the side-effects box.

	Date								
Pain intensity How bad has your pain been today?	severe								
	moderate								
	mild								
	none								
Pain relief How much pain relief have the tablets given today?	complete								
	good								
	moderate								
	slight								
	none								
Side effects Has the treatment upset you in any way?									

How effective was the treatment this week? *poor fair good very good excellent* Please circle your choice

Figure 7.3 The Oxford pain chart.

Questionnaires

The main criticism levelled at the various pain scales is that they concentrate on just one dimension and ignore the quality of pain. Measuring just the one dimension, '... is like specifying the visual world in terms of light flux only, without regard to pattern, color, texture and many other dimensions of the visual experience.' (Melzack and Torgerson 1971). One method of pain measurement that overcomes this problem is the McGill Pain Questionnaire (MPQ). In this method, the 78 descriptors are divided into 20 subgroups to reflect three dimensions of pain: sensory (10 word sets), affective (five sets) and evaluative (one group) (Melzack 1975). Patients select the most relevant words from the groups, choosing only one word from those groups that are appropriate, and skip inappropriate sets. This questionnaire can yield three major measures. The first is the Pain Rating Index (PRI), which is based on the sum of the scale values of all the words chosen either in a given category (sensory, affective or evaluative) or for all categories. The second is a 'ranked score' that is the sum of all the rank values within each group of words chosen and can be computed for the total questionnaire or for each of the dimensions. The third measure is the 'total number of words chosen'. The rank score is the most commonly used measure due to its simplicity and sensitivity. The multidimensional approach and the discriminatory value of the MPQ come at some disadvantage, however. The questionnaire is complex and more time-consuming to administer (5–20 minutes) than either VAS or categorical scales. Hence, it may be unsuitable for very sick patients. The time involved in the assessments has limited its application in the acute pain setting, where the (faster) uni-dimensional scales have proven very efficient.

CHOOSING A SCALE AND A DIMENSION

The choice of a particular scale and dimension (intensity or relief) should reflect the objective (why are we measuring the pain?) producing maximal sensitivity in the clinical context in which the measurement will take place. When the objective is to measure the *state* of pain – as, for example, part of the initial assessment of a patient – then pain intensity scales are more appropriate than pain relief scales. Ideally, the MPQ should be administered. If the main goal of the measurements is to analyse the *clinical response* of pain to treatment, both pain intensity and pain relief scales are appropriate. For this purpose, a number of charts have been developed, such as the Oxford Pain Chart (see Fig. 7.3). This was designed for daily assessments of single pains, but can be easily adapted for more frequent measurement of single or multiple pains.

When the intention is to assess the *efficacy* of an intervention or to compare two or more treatments for research purposes, both relief and intensity are appropriate, and both dimensions should be included. In research, precision is important and so it is advisable to measure each dimension with multiple scales (categorical and visual analogue) at each assessment point. The reason is that if the patient provides measurements on one or more scales which are clearly incompatible with the readings for the same dimension on another scale, the observer has the opportunity to re-question at this sample time and therefore reduce the noise in the assessments.

Selecting the most appropriate dimensions and scales does not guarantee maximal sensitivity and accuracy. Some other practical aspects must be considered, and some questions should be answered to obtain the best results. Who should do the assessments? Again, the answer depends on the context and objectives of the measurements. During in-patient and out-patient analgesic studies, the person in charge of the assessments should be a research nurse. Unfortunately, many groups that conduct clinical analgesic trials do not include a research nurse, mainly due to financial constraints. In such cases, the assessments are performed by other members of the team, usually doctors. To obtain maximal reliability and accuracy from the results, only one person should be responsible for pain measurement during any study. If the measurement of pain is to be made for clinical and/or audit purposes in the ward, it is clear that the best option is the use of pain charts as mentioned above. Those charts should be administered by the ward nurses and become part of the routine of nursing care, just as with other measurements (blood pressure, temperature, etc.).

Asking patients to fill in diaries at home is increasingly popular, both as a clinical audit and also as a research method. Although initially self-report in pain patients was thought to produce inconsistent results (Beecher 1957, 1959), if the patients receive adequate instructions then the diaries can be very accurate (Follick *et al.* 1984). We have used diaries successfully coupled with self-medication in both acute and chronic analgesic studies.

Intermittent, multiple-site pain

This is an aspect of pain measurement which can be crucial. If every patient had a single and constant pain, then the assessments could be oriented at recording the whole painful experience, and general questions such as: 'How much pain are you having now?', or 'How much relief have you achieved?' would suffice. However, in reality patients usually complain of more than one pain, and the various pains can also change with different circumstances. They can be constant or intermittent, occur at rest or on movement, be evoked by light touch or deep pressure, etc. Perhaps more importantly, the same patient can have several pains each with a different character (nociceptive, neuropathic or idiopathic); these different pains may respond differently to the same intervention. Consequently, assessing just 'the pain' without considering number, character, time patterns or triggering events could lead to inconsistent results and therefore to misleading conclusions. Multiple pains must be evaluated separately; the same conditions must be reproduced at each assessment time.

CURRENT OR TYPICAL PAIN ASSESSMENTS?

It must be clear whether the patient is talking about *current* or *typical* pain, and the same criteria should apply throughout the study period. If *current*, the patient must report what he/she is feeling at the moment of the assessment. If *typical*, then the report should be a summary of their experience during a definite period of time. Current pain assessments are more widely used because they reflect instant conditions independent of memory. Typical pain assessments are not as precise and punctual as current, but may produce more accurate results under certain conditions, such as when assessing intermittent pains or analgesic effects which could be shorter than the assessment periods. These two modalities of assessment are not exclusive and can be used simultaneously.

CONCLUSION

Pain is common to most orthopaedic conditions, and its measurement necessarily depends on the patient's report as there are no objective measures available. The available scales and methods can produce remarkably cheap, quick, sensitive and reproducible results.

Most of the information available is derived from research conducted in the acute setting where techniques have been developed and refined. However, the measurement of pain within the clinical context has been sadly neglected, and very few investigations have been conducted in this area. Logic dictates that every health professional should know how to measure pain reliably, and that pain should be assessed systematically as part of the study and management of a patient with a painful disorder. The measurement of pain is the only way to ensure that patients are receiving the quality of service that they expect and we think we are providing.

REFERENCES

Beecher, H. K. (1957): The measurement of pain. *Pharmacol Rev* **9**, 59–210.

Beecher, H. K. (1959): *Measurement of Subjective Responses: Quantitative effects of drugs.* Oxford University Press, New York.

Bellamy, N., Buchanan, W. W., Goldsmith, C. H., Campbell, J., and Stitt, L. W. (1988): Validation study of WOMAC: a health status instrument for measuring clinically important patient relevant outcomes to antirheumatic drug therapy in patients with osteoarthritis of the hip or knee. *J Rheumatol* **15**, 1833–40.

Burford Nursing Development Unit (1984): Nurses and pain. *Nursing Times* **18**, 94.

Collins, S. L., Edwards, J., Moore, R. A., Smith, L. A., and McQuay, H. J. (2001): Seeking a simple measure of analgesia for mega-trials: is a single global assessment good enough? *Pain* **91**, 189–94.

Farrar, J. T., Young, J. P., LaMoreaux, L., Werth, J. L., and Poole, R. M. (2001): Clinical importance of changes in chronic pain intensity measured on an 11-point numerical pain rating scale. *Pain* **94**, 149–58.

Follick, M. J., Ahern, D. K., and Laser-Wolston, N. (1984): Evaluation of a daily activity diary for chronic pain patients. *Pain* **19**, 373–82.

Gould, T. H., Crosby, D. L., Harmer, M., Lloyd, S. M., Lunn, J. N., Rees, G. A. D., Roberts, D. E., and Webster, J. A. (1992): Policy for controlling pain after surgery: effect of sequential changes in management. *Br Med J* **305**, 1187–93.

Jaeschke, R., Singer, J., and Guyatt, G. H. (1989): Measurement of health status: ascertaining the minimal clinically important difference. *Controlled Clinical Trials* **10**, 407–15.

Jensen, M. P., and McFarland, C. A. (1993): Increasing the reliability and validity of pain intensity measurement in chronic pain patients. *Pain* **55**, 195–203.

Keele, K. D. (1948): The pain chart. *Lancet* **2**, 6–8.

Littman, G. S., Walker, B. R., and Schneider, B. E. (1985): Reassessment of verbal and visual analogue ratings in analgesic studies. *Clin Pharm Ther* **38**, 16–23.

McGrath, P. J., Ritchie, J. A., Unruh, A. M., Carroll, D., and Bowsher, D. (1993): *Paediatric Pain.* Butterworth Heinemann, Oxford.

McQuay, H. J., Carroll, D., and Moore, R. A. (1988): Postoperative orthopaedic pain – the effect of opiate premedication and local anaesthetic blocks. *Pain* **33**, 291–5.

Melzack, R. (1975): The McGill pain questionnaire: major properties and scoring methods. *Pain* **1**, 277–99.

Melzack, R., and Torgerson, W. (1971): On the language of pain. *Anesthesiology* **34**, 50–9.

Moore, R. A., Paterson, G. M., Bullingham, R. E., Allen, M. C., Baldwin, D., and McQuay, H. J. (1984): Controlled comparison of intrathecal cinchocaine with intrathecal cinchocaine and morphine. Clinical effects and plasma morphine concentrations. *Br J Anaesth* **56**, 837–41.

Peloso, P. M., Bellamy, N., Bensen, W., Thomson, G. T., Harsanyi, Z., Babul, N., and Darke, A. C. (2000): Double blind randomized placebo control trial of controlled release codeine in the treatment of osteoarthritis of the hip or knee. *J Rheumatol* **27**, 764–71.

Rawal, N., and Berggren, L. (1994): Organization of acute pain services: a low-cost model. *Pain* **57**, 117–23.

Rundshagen, I., Schnabel, K., Standl, S., and Schulte am Esch, J. (1999): Patients' vs. nurses' assessments of postoperative pain and anxiety during patient- or nurse-controlled analgesia. *Br J Anaesth* **82**, 374–8.

Scott, J., and Huskisson, E. C. (1976): Graphic representation of pain. *Pain* **2**, 175–84.

Sriwatanakul, K., Kelvie, W., and Lasagna, L. (1982): The quantification of pain: an analysis of words used to describe pain and analgesia in clinical trials. *Clin Pharm Ther* **32**, 141–8.

Wallenstein, S. L., Heidrich, I. G., Kaiko, R., and Houde, R. W. (1980): Clinical evaluation of mild analgesics: the measurement of clinical pain. *Br J Clin Pharmacol* **10**, 319S–327S.

8

Trauma severity indices

Julian P. Cooper

INTRODUCTION

It would be reasonable to ask why assessments of injury severity, which might appear to be classifications, have a place in a volume on outcome measures. The question of what actually defines a severe injury requires outcome to be considered, however. We need to assess the effect of the injury on the patient rather than solely the details of the injury itself. A severe injury is an injury with a poor outcome such as death, prolonged hospital stay, significant long-term pain – the list could continue with any of the poor trauma outcomes mentioned in this book. This does not necessarily correlate with comminution of a bone, estimated blood loss, capillary refill or any of the many variables that are measured in the assessment of the trauma victim. When we diagnose a severe injury, we are effectively saying to our patient that we believe a poor outcome is likely. Trauma severity indices exist to bridge the gap between assessment and prognosis where many complex variables interact.

Measures of injury severity have also become linked with the audit of trauma management to the extent that the measures themselves become modified in the light of outcome. A perfect classification should guide management and predict outcome. Well-documented deficiencies in trauma care noted in the past (Royal College of Surgeons of England 1988) highlighted the concept of preventable death – the prediction of mortality may be made possible by the use of trauma severity indices. Comparison of observed outcome with predicted mortality provides one measure of performance.

What can severity indices be used for?

AUDIT AND PLANNING OF TRAUMA SERVICES

The huge variation in patterns of injury is a prime reason for trying to develop objective measures of severity so that trauma care can be compared between institutions and resources allocated appropriately. Within and between institutions, variation in outcome may well be related to different case-mix. Take, for example, two hospitals A and B. If hospital A receives a high proportion of penetrating trauma and hospital B relatively more blunt trauma, then differences in outcome are likely to be owed to case-mix. Any index of severity would need to be able to take this into account so that unjustified comparisons are not made. The initial presentation of the Abbreviated Injury Scale, for example, did not include codes for penetrating trauma, which made scoring impossible for such injuries.

RESEARCH

Case-mix similarly affects research; in orthopaedics – and particularly in orthopaedic trauma – it is notoriously difficult to set up randomized controlled trials (RCTs). Case-mix differences need to be controlled for, and severity indices may provide a method of stratifying data. When reporting series of polytrauma patients, the use of a severity index as a cut-off will allow clear definition of which patients the study applies to. Severity indices could potentially be used to define subsets of trauma patients who might benefit from a particular treatment.

COMMUNICATION

When describing injury patterns, a 'shorthand' way of describing the severity of injury may be convenient. Measures such as the Glasgow Coma Scale (Teasdale and Jennett 1974) or most fracture classifications provide this type of information. When talking about a patient, stating that a patient has a Glasgow Coma Scale of 8 or has a Schatzker VI tibial plateau fracture instantly conveys an impression of the severity of that individual injury to anyone with experience of the particular field. The essence of such measures is in their simplicity. The Glasgow Coma Scale is very easy to calculate, and most useful fracture classifications are simple, easily memorable and should convey an instant picture of a typical pattern of injury.

Generalized trauma scores, on the other hand (e.g. the Injury Severity Score) require a detailed knowledge of the underlying injury rating (the Abbreviated Injury Scale, AIS) and some calculation on top of this to derive the score. This means that communication is not intuitive for this and other scores.

DEFINITION

Outcome from polytrauma has usually been defined in terms of mortality. Many of the indices used to measure severity of trauma have been designed to assess the probability of death for a particular injury pattern. In recent years, alternative end-points have been considered, such as the development of multiple organ failure (MOF) (Balogh *et al.* 2000) or long-term disability (Michaels *et al.* 2001).

THE ASSESSMENT OF SCORING SYSTEMS

There are two main aspects to the performance of scoring systems. First, there is the power of discrimination between outcome groups. Second, there is the calibration of the score prediction – in other words, how well do the calculated probabilities fit the observed frequencies of a particular outcome? Beyond this the score must be reliable and easy to apply.

Power of discrimination

Traditionally, diagnostic tests have been assessed in terms of measures such as *misclassification rate*, *sensitivity*, the ability to detect true positive cases and *specificity* the ability to exclude true negative cases. If a severity score is assessed in this manner there is an important loss of information, which owes to the selection of an arbitrary cut-off point in the score creating binary data. The ideal situation would be to select a cut-off point, which maximizes both sensitivity and specificity.

The method used to achieve this is known as Receiver Operating Characteristic (ROC) curve analysis. This technique was initially developed for selecting the appropriate threshold for sensitivity of radar equipment with different operators. The method is best performed on a computer and is available in many statistical packages. The data are organized into two sets: those scores where the outcome is present; and those scores where it is absent. Sensitivity and specificity are then calculated using a cut-off point at each score in the range of sample values. So, for example, if the Injury Severity Score (see p. 73) is being assessed, 45 unique scores are possible (including 0 and 75). Up to 45 pairs of sensitivity and specificity must be calculated from the scores in the trauma database and then plotted as a curve with sensitivity as ordinate and (1 – sensitivity) as abscissa. The optimum cut-off can be determined from the plot; in the usual form of the plot this will be where the gradient of the curve is 1, maximizing sensitivity and specificity. The area under the curve can be measured using a statistical software package, and provides a measure of discrimination of the score. The 95 per cent confidence intervals for the area permit comparisons to be made with other curves. Figure 8.1 shows three theoretical curves. The curve on the left illustrates the situation where there is complete discrimination; in other words, there is a definite cut-off above which all patients

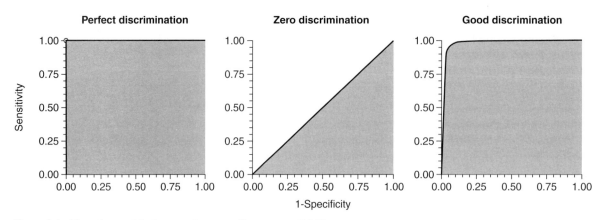

Figure 8.1 Three forms of the Receiver Operating Characteristic (ROC) curve.

die, and below which all patients survive. The area under the curve is 1 (the maximum possible) in this idealized situation. The centre curve depicts the situation when there is no discrimination. There is no cut-off that discriminates, and the area under the curve is 0.5 – the minimum possible. The plot on the right illustrates a more realistic situation where there is good discrimination – the area under the curve approaches 1.

Calibration

Logistic regression is a technique for the analysis of dependence of a binary outcome on one or more predictor variables. In the assessment of trauma scoring systems, the binary outcome is usually the state of being dead or alive, and the predictor variable the probability of death. Logistic regression is analogous to generalized linear regression, which analyses the corresponding analysis for normally distributed outcomes. When analysing the predictions of a trauma scoring system, the agreement between observed and predicted mortality rates across the range of the score is termed the 'calibration' of the score. A trauma severity index can be a mathematical model of the probability of death based on various anatomical and physiological parameters, and the calibration of this model measures how well the score represents reality.

A frequently quoted measure in the trauma severity index literature of calibration is the Hosmer-Lemeshow (H-L) statistic (Hosmer and Lemeshow 1989). The data are grouped into approximately ten deciles of risk, and the observed and expected number of deaths in each decile are compared by calculation of a χ^2 statistic. The lower the value of the H-L statistic, the closer the observed data fit the prediction. Unfortunately, there are at least three different methods by which the data can be grouped into deciles, as pointed out in a study comparing two measures of trauma severity (Hannan *et al.* 1995). The H-L statistic is also sensitive to the size of the dataset used to derive it – the larger the dataset, the larger the statistic. For this reason it is important to compare H-L statistics for scores based on the same underlying dataset.

SCORING SYSTEMS

Anatomical scoring systems

THE ABBREVIATED INJURY SCALE (AIS)

The AIS has received wide acceptance as a tool for describing the severity of a specific injury. The principle of this scale was established in 1971 (Committee on Medical Aspects of Automotive Safety 1971), and a manual rating a wide range of blunt injuries was published five years later. This manual is in its 1990 revision (Committee on

Injury Scaling 1990) and now includes penetrating trauma. Each injury has been classified by committee into a six-point scale. An injury with an AIS of 1 is classified as minor, while an unsurvivable injury receives a classification of 6. A critical injury, with a score of 5, is of the level of severity of complete abdominal aorta transection.

A number of criticisms can be levelled at such a system. The scoring is based on the consensus of a committee of experts in trauma, rather than directly upon patient outcome data (Osler *et al.* 1996). In any particular patient an injury may carry different significance, because of co-morbidity, or the presence of other injuries. Although the scale is ordered, it is not linear and hence simple combination of scores is not valid in the multiply injured patient. This latter problem led to the formulation of the Injury Severity Score (ISS) (Baker *et al.* 1974) (see below). In a theoretical study (Rutledge 1996) aimed at the ISS, but in fact criticising by implication the AIS and other scores based upon it, Rutledge suggested that AIS scores might be exaggerated by mismanagement of patients. An example given in the study was of a cervical spine fracture without cord injury (AIS = 2; ISS = 4) becoming as 'severe' as a patient with a well-managed complete cord injury (AIS = 5; ISS = 25) if the lesser injury had been missed and not immobilized. No patient-based studies have been published to confirm or refute this hypothetical problem, but this highlights a potential pitfall in interpretation of scores based upon AIS. Furthermore, scores might not be comparable between body regions: for example, an injury with a 'Head and Neck' score of 5 is likely to carry a worse prognosis than an 'Abdomen' score of 5.

Use of the AIS requires detailed examination of case records, and comparison with the current AIS manual to determine the appropriate score. This is time consuming and will not be possible in epidemiological studies where individual case records are not available. Many units record discharge diagnoses as International Classification of Disease diagnostic codes, and attempts have been made to map these to AIS body regions and scores (Mackenzie *et al.* 1989). This may allow calculation of AIS-based scores for population studies, but inaccuracies are

inevitable and performance shows generally poorer discrimination and calibration than conventionally scored measures (Sacco *et al.* 1999).

INJURY SEVERITY SCORE (ISS)

The ISS (Baker *et al.* 1974) was developed as a means by which AIS scores could be combined to provide a means of characterizing polytrauma and of examining the standard of care in trauma institutions. The ISS divides the body into six regions:

1. Head and neck

2. Face

3. Chest

4. Abdomen

5. Extremities including bony pelvis

6. Integument

To derive the ISS, the AIS scores for all injuries in the patient are first collected. The highest AIS scores in each region are then selected and, of these, the three most severe are combined to give the ISS by adding their squares. The AIS scores of all other injuries, however severe, are discarded. For example, a score of 4 for 'Head and Neck', 2 for 'Chest', 5 for 'Abdomen' and 3 for 'Extremities' would equate to an ISS of:

$$4^2 + 5^2 + 3^2 = 50$$

For this reason, a patient with a pelvic ring fracture and several long bone fractures will receive the same Extremities contribution to their overall ISS as a patient with the worst of these individual injuries and no others within that body region. Of course, if a patient has worse injuries in three other body regions, then these extremity scores will also be discarded. By convention, any patient with an AIS of 6 in any single body region receives a total score of 75, irrespective of their other injuries.

Apart from the loss of information and potential predictive value inherent in discarding data, there is a further potential problem with the ISS owing to the lack of consistency of AIS scores across different body regions. This may lead to inappropriate weighting of the ISS when injuries with equal scores but discrepant potential outcomes are combined.

Despite these criticisms the ISS has been widely accepted for many years. It has been shown to correlate with mortality (Baker and O'Neill 1976; Bull 1977), but more recent investigations have suggested that other measures, such as NISS (Osler et al. 1997) and ICISS (Rutledge et al. 1998) (see below), model outcome better than the original ISS. The ISS remains important as the anatomical component of the TRISS (Trauma and Injury Severity Score) methodology, a widely used system for prediction of mortality.

THE ANATOMIC PROFILE AND MODIFIED ANATOMIC PROFILE

Addressing the limitations of the ISS has been attempted by formulation of a different AIS-based score. The Anatomic Profile (AP) (Copes et al. 1990) was developed to provide a more logical summary of a patient's injuries by providing a description of the injury with numbers in three categories:

A. Injuries to head or central nervous system (brain/spinal cord) with AIS 3 to 6.

B. Injuries to thorax or front of neck with AIS 3 to 6.

C. All other injuries with AIS 3 to 6.

For recording purposes, all other injuries can be included in a fourth group (D). Within each category, all injuries fulfilling the severity criteria are combined as the square-root of the sum of squares of the AIS values. The division into these groups recognizes the worse prognosis of central nervous system injury and thoracic trauma in a more meaningful manner than the body regions of the ISS. In combining these figures into an overall score, different weights derived from logistic regression can be applied to the three categories. As each category makes use of the AIS of each serious (AIS >2) injury in the derivation of the score there is less information loss with this method.

Few published studies have utilized the AP on its own, although it forms part of the ASCOT (A Severity Characterization of Trauma) score (Champion et al. 1990a) described below. The group who introduced the AP have more recently changed its formulation to introduce the modified Anatomic Profile (Sacco et al. 1999) (mAP). This is a four-value score, which includes the original three categories as calculated before but now also includes a fourth component, the maximum AIS across all body regions. This appears to improve predictive power (Sacco et al. 1999), but at the cost of increased complexity. Another, much simpler, AIS-based score which seems to perform almost as well as the mAP is described in the next section.

THE NEW INJURY SEVERITY SCORE

One of the major concerns about the ISS has been the possible underestimation of a patient's injury severity, because only the most severe injury in a region can potentially contribute to the overall ISS. A simple modification of derivation of the ISS, to circumvent this problem, was developed by Osler and co-workers in 1997 (Osler et al. 1997). Termed the New Injury Severity Score (NISS), the new score abandons the concept of body regions and instead is calculated as the sum of squares of the worst three AIS-coded injuries. A number of studies have indicated superior predictive performance for this modification over traditional ISS (Brennerman et al. 1997; Osler et al. 1997; Sacco et al. 1999; Balogh et al. 2000), ICISS (Sacco et al. 1999), Anatomic Profile (Sacco et al. 1999), and similar performance to the modified Anatomic Profile (Sacco et al. 1999). This relative good performance and simplicity of calculation have led to suggestions that NISS should replace ISS as the AIS-based trauma severity score (Osler and Bedrick 1999). Further potential for improvement exists (Brennerman et al. 1997). In spite of this, ISS is in wide current usage – which makes change unappealing.

THE INTERNATIONAL CLASSIFICATION INJURY SEVERITY SCORE (ICISS)

The reliance of the AIS, and hence ISS, on consensus-based rather than data-based ratings of injury severity has been considered flawed by Osler and coworkers (Osler et al. 1996). They have derived a new trauma severity index based on injury diagnoses from the International Classification of Disease 9th Revision (ICD-9). The key difference from the AIS/ISS axis is that each injury is rated with a Survival Risk Ratio (SRR) based on data in a trauma registry rather than with a score determined by committee. The SRR is determined for each ICD-9 diagnosis code from the trauma registry as follows:

$$SRR = \frac{\text{Number of patients in registry surviving with this diagnosis code}}{\text{Total number of patients in registry with this diagnosis code}}$$

The ICISS is then calculated by multiplying the SRRs for each of a patient's injuries together as follows:

$$ICISS = \prod_{j=1}^{j=n} SRR_j$$

n = total number of injuries
SRR_j = SRR of injury j

This method of calculation was originally used for the RESP (Revised Estimated Survival Probability) index described in 1982 (Levy *et al.* 1982). The RESP index was also based on the International Classification of Disease of the day, but had survival probabilities assigned rather than derived from data. The ICISS should also not be confused with AIS and ISS ratings based on mapping (Mackenzie *et al.* 1989) the AIS definitions to ICD codes.

ICISS can also be used to predict outcome and resource utilization (Osler *et al.* 1998; Rutledge and Osler 1998) for disease in general, by extension of the underlying registry data to include all ICD diagnoses. Somewhat confusingly, the abbreviation ICISS (for ICD-9-based *Illness* Severity Score) is used to refer to this broader severity index as well as the trauma-based score.

The ICISS has been found to outperform ISS (Rutledge *et al.* 1998; Sacco *et al.* 1999) and TRISS (Rutledge *et al.* 1998) as a trauma severity score, but there are differences in calibration and performance according to which underlying trauma registry is used to derive the SRRs (Rutledge *et al.* 1998; Sacco *et al.* 1999), and other measures such as NISS have better published discrimination and calibration (Copes *et al.* 1990). The International Classification of Disease undergoes revision from time to time – currently the tenth revision. A comparison of ICD-9- and ICD-10-based ICISS scoring (Kim *et al.* 2000) found that changes in the way that intracranial injuries were classified in the newer ICD led to poorer predictive power in these patients, but that otherwise the methodology could migrate satisfactorily to ICD-10. Questions must be asked about how future revisions will affect outcome predictions and whether revisers will take illness or injury severity measurement into account when formulating further updates.

PHYSIOLOGICAL SCORING SYSTEMS

The prototype physiological score was the Glasgow Coma Scale (Teasdale and Jennett 1974); this was a simple, easily reproducible score which aided management, albeit in one system. The development of physiological indices of trauma severity started with measures of simple parameters in a similar way to the GCS.

The Trauma Score (TS) and Revised Trauma Score (RTS)

The TS (Champion *et al.* 1981) was one of the first useful physiological scores, and was used as a triage tool in the United States. Rapid assessment is possible as five simple parameters are measured:

1. GCS

2. Systolic blood pressure

3. Capillary return

4. Respiratory rate

5. Respiratory effort

The values of these variables are given weighted scores, which are combined to give an overall score. The Trauma Score ranges from 1 to 16, increasing with better prognosis. Capillary return and respiratory effort are difficult to assess in the field, particularly in the dark. The score was revised by its originators (Champion *et al.* 1989) as a result, dropping these two parameters and producing the Revised Trauma Score (RTS). More fundamentally, the score utilized weighting values derived from logistic regression analysis of the North American Major Trauma Outcome Study (Champion *et al.* 1990b) (MTOS) data. The use of large databases on outcomes has since become a characteristic of trauma scoring systems – values are mapped via a sigmoid probability function to give a Probability of Survival (P_s) from the score. The role of the RTS has become important, as it is one of the major components of the derivation of the TRISS methodology, an important combined severity assessment system.

THE ACUTE PHYSIOLOGY AND CHRONIC HEALTH EVALUATION (APACHE) SCORES

The APACHE scoring system was originally described in 1981 (Knaus *et al.* 1981), and has been revised successively to APACHE III. Its main role has been in the assessment and monitoring of patients on intensive care units (ICU). Victims of polytrauma are often treated on ICUs, and the scale has been used in assessment of injury severity. It is somewhat more complex than the RTS to calculate; APACHE III requires knowledge of 18 physiological parameters. One major difference from other measures is the 'Chronic Health' portion of the score, which takes into account co-morbidities. In trauma patients the presence of co-morbidities undoubtedly influences outcome (Sacco *et al.* 1993), but the incidence of these conditions is relatively low. Comparisons of APACHE II with TRISS (Wong *et al.* 1996), TS and ISS (Rutledge *et al.* 1993) have demonstrated that the APACHE system

is as good a predictor of ICU outcome as the other methods, but offers no great advantage in predicting individual patient outcome. At present, most published studies utilize one of the trauma indices rather than APACHE.

COMBINED SCORING SYSTEMS

The Trauma and Injury Severity Score (TRISS)

By combining physiological with anatomical assessments of injury severity, it is possible that outcome prediction might be improved. The TRISS methodology (Boyd *et al.* 1987) originally combined scores from the TS, ISS with a factor for age to provide an estimate of probability of survival (P_s). Presently, the RTS is used rather than the TS. These factors are combined to derive the P_s as follows:

$$P_s = \frac{1}{1 + e^{-b}}$$

The parameter b is calculated from the RTS, ISS and age using the following form of equation:

$$b = b_0 + b_1(\text{RTS}) + b_2(\text{ISS}) + b_3(\text{Age})$$

The individual coefficients b_0, b_1, ... b_3 are derived from logistic regression analysis of the trauma registry outcome data, and when combined into the equation for P_s produce a probability of survival figure which represents a population probability rather than the individual chance of survival. A P_s of 0.75 represents the chance that 75 per cent of patients presenting with these parameters will survive – *not* that an individual patient would have a 75 per cent chance of survival. The derivation of the coefficients depends on the relevance and quality of the underlying trauma registry. In particular there are significant differences in case-mix between the United Kingdom and the United States, such that use of American TRISS coefficients would lead to misleading estimates of P_s (Jones *et al.* 1995). These estimates are important, as one of the most common uses of trauma severity indices is in comparing the performance of institutions dealing with trauma – misleading predictions will lead to misleading performance estimates.

The US Major Trauma Outcome Study has used three statistics to describe the performance of an institution:

1. W: the number of excess survivors per 100 patients

$$W = \frac{S_{actual} - S_{predicted}}{N} \times 100$$

where S_{actual} = actual number of survivors; $S_{predicted}$ = predicted number of survivors (equivalent to the sum of P_s for all patients); and N = total number of patients.

2. Z: the standardized normal score for the W statistic:

$$Z = \frac{S_{actual} - S_{predicted}}{\sqrt{\sum_{j=1}^{N} P_{sj}(1 - P_{sj})}}$$

where P_{sj} = the value of P_s for the *j*th patient.

As it is normally distributed the Z statistic allows comparison with the standard data. $Z > 1.96$ or $Z < -1.96$ represents a significant deviation from the predicted performance at the 5 per cent level. Lack of statistical significance should not necessarily be taken as reassuring, as the sample size and variability may be such that a Type II error is made.

3. M: a statistic designed to express the comparability of the case-mix between the prediction data and the study data. This is calculated by dividing the range of P_s values into six ranges and recording the proportion of cases that occur in each P_s range for the prediction and study data. The proportions from each dataset in each range of P_s are then

compared and the minimum of each pair recorded and added together. Perfect comparability gives the value 1, while complete disparity gives zero.

The M statistic has been criticized (Hollis *et al.* 1995) for the fact that it does not say anything about the direction of the difference in case-mix variation. In fact, United Kingdom MTOS (now TARN; the Trauma Audit and Research Network) data differed from the US data to the extent that comparability was achieved only with exclusion of hip fractures. A new statistic, W_s, has been described (Hollis *et al.* 1995) which overcomes the problem of case-mix variation by dividing the P_s range into intervals as with the M statistic, but calculating a W score in each interval:

$$W_j = \frac{S_{actual\,j} - S_{predicted\,j}}{N_j} \times 100$$

where $S_{actual\,j}$ = actual number of survivors in interval; $S_{predicted\,j}$ = predicted number of survivors in interval; and N_j = number of patients in interval j.

By multiplying each W_j value by the proportion of the prediction data cases in the corresponding interval and adding the results from all intervals a new, standardized, W score is obtained. This is termed the W_s statistic. As case-mix is standardized to the prediction database the M statistic is obsolete. A Z_s value can be derived corresponding to the Z statistic. The W_s statistic is now used routinely to present the UK TARN results (Lecky *et al.* 2000).

A Severity Characterization of Trauma (ASCOT)

The Anatomic Profile (see above) was an attempt to get away from the limitations of the ISS as a measure of structural damage. This has been combined with physiological parameters and age, using weighting coefficients from MTOS data to give another combined prediction methodology called ASCOT (Champion *et al.* 1990a). The form of the

P_s variable is as for TRISS, but the parameter b is made up as follows:

$$b = b_1 + b_2\text{GCS} + b_3\text{SBP} + b_4\text{RR} \\ + b_5\text{A} + b_6\text{B} + b_7\text{C} + b_8(\text{Age})$$

The A, B and C parameters refer to the components of the Anatomic Profile (Copes *et al.* 1990), and hence the individualized coefficients derived from a trauma database should be able to model the influence of structural injury more closely than is possible with the single ISS component of TRISS. ASCOT has been compared with TRISS using MTOS- (Champion *et al.* 1996) and non-MTOS- (Hannan *et al.* 1995) derived coefficients and, broadly, ASCOT performed better. Despite its superior performance the question remains as to whether it is justified to change methodologies before an alternative to TRISS with considerably greater predictive power is developed.

PAEDIATRIC TRAUMA SEVERITY

The scores mentioned so far have been developed in adult patients. Attempts to apply physiological scores to children are prone to difficulties owing to varying normal ranges with age. The Pediatric Trauma Score (PTS) (Tepas *et al.* 1987) includes a parameter related to the weight of a child and utilizes ranges of systolic blood pressure appropriate to children. In comparing various trauma scoring systems, one study (Yian *et al.* 2000) has found that outcome was better correlated with TRISS and the Trauma Score rather than the specific PTS. It should be noted that this study only looked at orthopaedic polytrauma, and in general one should use caution when drawing conclusions about outcome predictions for a subset of the trauma population. The difficulties in the paediatric field are illustrated by a recent study, which could not demonstrate any superiority of the NISS over the ISS in children (Grisoni *et al.* 2001) for the prediction of mortality. The originator of the PTS has introduced a combined index for children, the Pediatric Risk Indicator (PRI) (Tepas *et al.* 1997), which includes ISS, GCS and the PTS in its derivation, and which may provide some improvement in performance.

NEW CONCEPTS

Artificial neural networks

From the foregoing discussion of trauma scoring it is apparent that many parameters need to be taken into account in developing a model of outcome in the trauma victim. Recently, several studies (Rutledge *et al.* 1998; DiRusso *et al.* 2000; Becalick and Coats 2001) have examined the use of Artificial Intelligence (AI) techniques to improve the modelling of many predictor variables. The AI technique of the artificial neural net (ANN) shows promise for developing a model with improved calibration. These mathematical techniques are designed to mimic the arrangement of interconnections in an animal nervous system. These systems can demonstrate high performance in otherwise unsatisfactory circumstances – working with incomplete data to produce useful output. These techniques may have many applications in medicine, but are currently in their infancy. One study in particular (DiRusso *et al.* 2000) showed extremely good calibration, and the area clearly shows promise.

CONCLUSION

There is currently a plethora of trauma severity indices and evidence about their relative efficacy. Many more have fallen by the wayside over the years. It is clear that improving outcome prediction, both in discrimination and in calibration is needed, but work towards this often appears uncoordinated. While TRISS remains the most widely used outcome prediction methodology, work examining alternatives to the ISS, such as ICISS or NISS, appears unlikely to result in ISS-based measures being supplanted.

REFERENCES

Baker, S. P., and O'Neill, B. (1976): The Injury Severity Score: an update. *J Trauma* **16**, 882–5.

Baker, S. P., O'Neill, B., Haddon, W., and Long, W. B. (1974): The Injury Severity Score: a method for describing patients with multiple injuries and evaluating emergency care. *J Trauma* **14**, 187–96.

Balogh, Z., Offner, P. J., Moore, E. E., and Biffl, W. L. (2000): NISS predicts postinjury multiple organ failure better than the ISS. *J Trauma* **48**, 624–8.

Becalick, D. C., and Coats, T. J. (2001): Comparison of artificial intelligence techniques with UKTRISS for estimating probability of survival after trauma. *J Trauma* **51**, 123–33.

Boyd, C. R., Tolson, M. A., and Copes, W. S. (1987): Evaluating trauma care: the TRISS method. *J Trauma* **27**, 370–8.

Brennerman, F. D., Boulanger, B. R., McLellan, B. A., and Redelmeier, D. A. (1997): Measuring injury severity: time for a change? *J Trauma* **43**, 393.

Bull, J. P. (1977): Measures of severity of injury. *Injury* **9**, 184–7.

Champion, H. R., Sacco, W. J., Carnazzo, A. J., Copes, W. S., and Fouty, W. J. (1981): Trauma Score. *Crit Care Med* **9**, 672–6.

Champion, H. R., Sacco, W. J., Copes, W. S., Gann, D. S., Genarelli, T. A., and Flanagan, M. E. (1989): A revision of the trauma score. *J Trauma* **29**, 623–9.

Champion, H. R., Copes, W. S., Sacco, W. J., Lawnick, M. M., Bain, L. W., Gann, D. S., Genarelli, T. A., Mackenzie, E., and Schwaitzberg, S. (1990a): A new characterization of injury severity. *J Trauma* **30**, 539–46.

Champion, H. R., Copes, W. S., Sacco, W. J., Lawnick, M. M., Keast, S. L., Bain, L. W., and Flanagan, M. E. (1990b): The Major Trauma Outcome Study: establishing national norms for trauma care. *J Trauma* **30**, 1356–65.

Champion, H. R., Copes, W. S., Sacco, W. J., Frey, C. F., Holcroft, J. W., Hoyt, D. B., and Weigelt, J. A. (1996): Improved predictions from A Severity Characterization of Trauma (ASCOT) over Trauma and Injury Severity Score (TRISS). *J Trauma* **40**, 42–9.

Committee on Injury Scaling (1990): *The Abbreviated Injury Scale–1990 Revision (AIS-90)*. Association for the Advancement of Automotive Medicine, Des Plaines, IL.

Committee on Medical Aspects of Automotive Safety (1971): Rating the severity of issue damage: I. The Abbreviated Scale. *JAMA* **215**, 277–80.

Copes, W. S., Champion, H. R., Sacco, W. J., Lawnick, M. M., Gann, D. S., Gennarelli, T., MacKenzie, E., and Schwaitzberg, S. (1990): Progress in characterizing anatomic injury. *J Trauma* **30**, 1200–7.

DiRusso, S., Sullivan, T., Holly, C., Cuff, S. N., and Savino, J. (2000): An artificial neural network as a model for prediction of survival in trauma patients: validation for a regional trauma area. *J Trauma* **49**, 212–13.

Grisoni, E., Stallion, A., Nance, M. L., Lelli, J. L., Garcia, V. F., and Marsh, E. (2001): The New Injury Severity Score and the evaluation of pediatric trauma. *J Trauma* **50**, 1106–10.

Hannan, E. L., Mendeloff, J., Farrell, L. S., Cayten, C. G., and Murphy, J. G. (1995): Validation of TRISS and ASCOT using a non-MTOS trauma registry. *J Trauma* **38**, 83–8.

Hollis, S., Yates, D. W., Woodford, M., and Foster, P. (1995): Standardized comparison of performance indicators in trauma: a new approach to case-mix variation. *J Trauma* **38**, 763–6.

Hosmer, D. W., and Lemeshow, S. (1989): *Applied Logistic Regression*. John Wiley & Sons, New York.

Jones, J. M., Redmond, A. D., and Templeton, J. (1995): Uses and abuses of statistical models for evaluating trauma care. *J Trauma* **38**, 89–93.

Kim, Y., Jung, K. Y., Kim, C. Y., Kim, Y. I., and Shin, Y. (2000): Validation of the International Classification of Diseases 10th edition-based Injury Severity Score (ICISS). *J Trauma* **48**, 280–5.

Knaus, W. A., Zimmerman, J. E., Wagner, D. P., Draper, E. A., and Lawrence, D. E. (1981): APACHE – acute physiology and chronic health evaluation: a physiologically based classification system. *Crit Care Med* **9**, 591–7.

Lecky, F., Woodford, M., Yates, D. W. (on behalf of the UK Trauma Audit and Research Network)

(2000): Trends in trauma care in England and Wales 1989–97. *Lancet* 355, 1771–5.

Levy, P. S., Goldberg, J., and Rothrock, J. (1982): The revised estimated survival probability index of trauma severity. *Public Health Rep* 97, 452–9.

Mackenzie, E. J., Steinwachs, D. M., and Shankar, B. (1989): Classifying trauma severity based on hospital discharge diagnoses: validation of an ICD-9CM to AIS-85 conversion table. *Med Care* 27, 412–22.

Michaels, A. J., Madey, S. M., Krieg, J. C., and Long, W. B. (2001): Traditional injury scoring underestimates the relative consequences of orthopaedic injury. *J Trauma* 50, 389–96.

Osler, T. M., and Bedrick, E. J. (1999): Comparison of alternative methods for assessing injury severity based on anatomic descriptors: Editorial comment. *J Trauma* 47, 446–7.

Osler, T., Rutledge, R., Deis, J., and Bedrick, E. (1996): ICISS: An International Classification of Disease-9 Based Injury Severity Score. *J Trauma* 41, 380–8.

Osler, T., Baker, S. P., and Long, W. (1997): A modification of the Injury Severity Score that improves accuracy and simplifies scoring. *J Trauma* 43, 922–6.

Osler, T. M., Rogers, F. B., Glance, L. G., Cohen, M., Rutledge, R., and Shackford, S. R. (1998): Predicting survival, length of stay, and cost in the Surgical Intensive Care Unit: APACHE II versus ICISS. *J Trauma* 45, 234–8.

Royal College of Surgeons of England (1988): *Report of the Working Party into the Management of Patients with Major Injuries*. Royal College of Surgeons of England, London.

Rutledge, R. (1996): The Injury Severity Score is unable to differentiate between poor care and severe injury. *J Trauma* 40, 944–50.

Rutledge, R., and Osler, T. (1998): The ICD-9-based Illness Severity Score: a new model that outperforms both DRG and APR-DRG as predictors of survival and resource utilization. *J Trauma* 45, 791–9.

Rutledge, R., Fakhry, S., Rutherford, E., Muakkassa, F., and Meyer, A. (1993): Comparison of Apache II, Trauma Score and Injury Severity Score as predictors of outcome in critically injured trauma patients. *Am J Surg* 166, 244–7.

Rutledge, R., Osler, T., Emery, S., and Kromhout-Schiro, S. (1998): The end of the Injury Severity Score (ISS) and the Trauma and Injury Severity Score (TRISS): ICISS, an International Classification of Diseases, Ninth Revision-Based Prediction Tool, outperforms both ISS and TRISS as predictors of trauma patient survival, hospital charges, and hospital length of stay. *J Trauma* 44, 41–9.

Sacco, W. J., Copes, W. S., Bain, L. W., Mackenzie, E. J., Frey, C. F., Hoyt, D. B., Weigelt, J. A., and Champion, H. R. (1993): Effect of preinjury illness on trauma patient survival outcome. *J Trauma* 35, 538–43.

Sacco, W. J., MacKenzie, E. J., Champion, H. R., Davis, E. G., and Buckman, R. F. (1999): Comparison of alternative methods for assessing injury severity based on anatomic descriptors. *J Trauma* 47, 441–6.

Teasdale, G., and Jennett, B. (1974): Assessment of coma and impaired consciousness. *Lancet* ii, 81–4.

Tepas, J. J. I., Mollitt, D. L., Talbert, J. L., and Bryant, M. (1987): The Pediatric Trauma Score as a predictor of injury severity in the injured child. *J Pediatr Surg* 22, 14–18.

Tepas, J. J. I., Veldenz, H. C., Discala, C., and Pieper, P. (1997): Pediatric Risk Indicator: an objective measurement of childhood injury severity. *J Trauma* 43, 258–62.

Wong, D. T., Barrow, P. M., Gomez, M., and McGuire, G. P. (1996): A comparison of the Physiology and Chronic Health Evaluation (APACHE) II score and the Trauma-Injury Severity Score (TRISS) for outcome assessment in intensive care unit trauma patients. *Crit Care Med* 24, 1642–8.

Yian, E. H., Gullahorn, L. J., and Loder, R. T. (2000): Scoring of pediatric orthopaedic polytrauma: correlations of different injury scoring systems and prognosis for hospital course. *J Pediatr Orthop* 20, 203–9.

9

Complications

Alasdair J. A. Santini and Simon P. Frostick

INTRODUCTION

Traditionally, morbidity and mortality meetings have been the cornerstones of peer review. The 'how' and 'when' of such meetings were discussed by Campbell (1988), who emphasized that these meetings are obligatory for the recognition of a hospital for surgical training by the Royal College of Surgeons. In this context, complications are viewed from the educational standpoint without regard for possible consequences upon outcome and quality of care. In morbidity and mortality meetings, complications are often used as a measure of a surgeon's competence – which some find a somewhat threatening scenario. However, with recent high-profile complications of surgery in various centres and in today's 'no-blame' environment, surgeons must be seen to be addressing their complications and taking appropriate counteraction.

An adverse event, such as a peri-operative complication, is likely to affect the ultimate outcome of any treatment regimen. Furthermore, complications may alter a patient's overall view of satisfaction and quality of care, especially if the complication has arisen directly as a result of a clinician's intervention. Complications are therefore only seen in a negative context. An attempt will be made in this chapter to address complications in a positive light where possible. They may be an important component for the comparison of different methods of treatment and in themselves may be used as a measure of outcome. In a clinical trial, the incidence of complications may be the only distinguishing feature between two treatment methods hence favouring one treatment. They may also be of sufficient frequency and severity

to end the trial. Complications are often used as a rough monitor of an individual's operating skills. However, this must be interpreted in the light of the type of surgery being undertaken, the severity of the disease, and the general health status of the patient. Complications can be used to educate peers and others allied health professionals. Finally, complications can also be used as 'end-points' or outcome measures in audit and clinical trials. From an economic standpoint, managers have become very interested in the whole concept of quality of care. The economics of the health service require that morbidity associated with any treatment be kept to a minimum. Many health service contracts now contain quality assurance measures and undoubtedly more will be required in the future.

A number of fundamental problems are apparent when considering complications. First, what is a complication? Second, what conditions actually should be regarded as complications and are these conditions accurately and consistently diagnosed? Third, should the conditions associated with a pre-existing non-orthopaedic disease be classified as a complication if they happen to occur during an orthopaedic admission? Fourth, how long after an orthopaedic procedure should a complication not be regarded as a complication of that particular procedure? Fifth – and not least – how does the health status of a patient affect the response to an adverse affect and how can the magnitude of a complication be assessed?

There are few scoring systems available for the assessment of complications. This chapter will endeavour to define what constitutes a complication. It will suggest ways of recording information about complications, discuss the severity of complications and touch on a number of specific complications.

DEFINITIONS

If accurate and universally accepted definitions of what does and does not constitute a 'complication' are not used, problems can occur. Clinicians may be reasonably happy with their own definitions but these may not be what other clinicians accept as a definition. Many define a complication as any event occurring during the course of treatment which results in some retardation or alteration of recovery from the norm. Thus, a complication may arise from a pre-existing disease in the patient or as a direct result of a treatment programme.

The other potential problem with terminology lies with the term 'complicated' rather than 'complication'. The general public may have a different view of a complicated illness than that of a clinician. A complex injury, in an orthopaedic setting, may be a communited or an intra-articular fracture. This may heal without significant problems – that is, there are no complications. Most people in the street, however, would regard this as being a complicated fracture. This problem is reflected in dictionary definitions. For example, *Butterworth's Medical Dictionary* (Second Edition) defines '*complications*' as:

1. 'The co-existence in a patient of two or more separate diseases'.
2. 'Any disease or condition that is co-existent with or modifies the course of the primary disease but need not be connected with it'.

and defines '*complicated*' as:

'Complex or involved; applied to a disease or injury with which another disease or injury has become associated so that the symptoms of the first are altered and the course changed'.

In addition, *Collins English Dictionary* (Third Edition) defines a '*complication*' as:

'A disease or disorder arising as a consequence of another disease'.

A further term that is gaining popularity, particularly in the North American literature, is 'co-morbiditor'. This is defined as a co-existent active medical or operative problem (Liang *et al.* 1991). A co-morbiditor may or may not modify the outcome of a procedure. In the context of this chapter, the term co-morbiditor will be used to refer to conditions such as diabetes or rheumatoid arthritis, which may increase the risk of complications associated with an orthopaedic procedure such as a wound infection. They may in themselves result in an adverse event because the condition has been modified as a result of the stress of an anaesthesia or orthopaedic procedure.

We will use the term 'complication' as a generic term for all adverse events in a treatment episode, and divide into those attributable to a pre-existing disease and those arising as a direct consequence of an orthopaedic intervention. Conventionally, complications have been divided into major and minor. Whilst clinicians may agree among themselves what is major and minor, this may not necessarily be in agreement with the patient – the very person who has the complication. The distinction between a major and minor complication is a very difficult one, and in general will depend on a number of factors such as the general health status of the patient, the severity of the complication itself and the ease of the diagnosis. Here, a 'major' complication is defined as any complication which causes a prolongation of admission, results in a further operative procedure or is potentially or actually life-threatening.

RECORDING COMPLICATIONS

The recording details of complications must be an easy process – it simply will not be undertaken accurately if this is not the case. In order to obtain an overall view and to allow proper audit, all complications must be recorded, however trivial. These may be assessed as a simple total of 'major' or 'minor' frequencies or details of specific events. A possible classification of complications and a form to record total occurrences is shown in Table 9.1.

Table 9.1: Suggested categories of complications

	Elective orthopaedics	Trauma
Life-threatening (pre-existing disease)		
Life-threatening (surgical)		
Major morbidity (pre-existing disease)		
Major morbidity (surgical)		
Minor morbidity (pre-existing disease)		
Minor morbidity (surgical)		

Table 9.2: American Society of Anesthesiologists' Classification of physical status. Any patients in any of the groups who are operated on in an emergency are deemed to be in a poorer state and are pre-fixed by the letter E

Class	Physical status
I	A healthy patient with no systemic disease process
II	Mild to moderate systemic disease process, which does not limit the patient's activities in any way
III	Severe systemic disturbance from any cause which imposes a definite functional limitation on the patient
IV	A severe systemic disease which is a constant threat to life
V	A moribund patient who is unlikely to survive 24 hours with or without surgery

Table 9.3: CEPOD classification for operations. Adapted from Buck et al. (1987)

Grouping	Timing of surgery
Emergency	Within 1 hour
Urgent	Usually within 24 hours
Scheduled	1 to 3 weeks
Elective	No specific time

An analysis of the overall health status of the patients should also be provided. Methods such as the SF-12 health survey give detailed accounts of patient's health, but an easier and more practical method is provided by the American Society of Anesthesiologists' (ASA) grading as shown in Table 9.2 although this is unreliable. This is a simple method, and gives a broad indication to the general status of the patients being treated. This can be coupled with a record of the Confidential Enquiry into Peri-Operative Deaths (CEPOD) categories (Buck *et al.* 1987), as shown in Table 9.3.

In orthopaedics and trauma, the complications that are of most interest are often the most difficult to diagnose. Wound infection and healing problems, thromboembolism and implant failure head the list of complications that, although not entirely specific to orthopaedics, tend to cause morbidity and diminish long-term outcome.

A specific audit method is sometimes used to examine complications. Occurrence screening (Bennett and Walshe 1990) is an audit method originating in the United States. In its widest application, the method examines all adverse events that enquire into all aspects of hospital care, including hotel services, treatment and complications. The proforma can be very detailed. The method is the most comprehensive

audit technique. We would suggest that occurrence screening is a useful method to use on an intermittent 'pulsed' basis. A specific problem (e.g. wound infection following surgery for fracture of the neck of femur) is defined. A questionnaire is developed specifically for the problem and is used over several randomly selected periods of time to record the incidence and severity of this event. It may then be used to determine if a change in practice has resulted in a reduction in infection rates. Whatever technique is used, the important factor is that audit is continually viewed to ensure complications are picked up and addressed.

SEVERITY

Recording the occurrence of a particular event may be fairly simple. It is, however, more difficult to establish its severity. Severity is not usually recorded although it will be an important factor in dictating outcome. It is also a subjective rather than object-ive outcome both with regard to the patient and the surgeon. The severity of a complication may be quite different to these two groups and may depend on four factors:

1. The existence of pre-existing major health problems and their treatment (e.g. immunosup-pression in patients with rheumatoid arthritis).

2. The physiological response to injury or disease (including those related to age).

3. Intrinsic features of the complication itself, such as the ease with which it is possible to diagnose the condition and the extent to which the complication effects an individual patient.

4. The incidence and severity of a complication may also be dependent upon the factors such as hospital type, staff available (including the experience and competence of the surgeon), the availability of equipment and population factors such as age distribution and social class.

THE EFFECTS OF EXISTING HEALTH PROBLEMS

In orthopaedics and trauma, like all surgical discip-lines, the consideration of co-morbidity and pre-existing diseases is very important in determining the outcome of the treatment. Based upon a disabil-ity evaluation, Ebrahim *et al.* (1991) demonstrated that disabled patients tended to rate ill health more adversely than able-bodied patients. They also rated death as being substantially better than a more severe state of ill health. Similarly, Barnett (1991) found that patients with overt symptoms perceived quality of life in chronic treatment differently from those without symptoms. Others (Greenfield *et al.* 1987)

found that age and co-morbid state both signifi-cantly, but independently, affected treatment pro-vided by physicians.

Concomitant disease is a predisposing factor for complications such as infection. One group (D'Ambrosia *et al.* 1976) showed that concomitant disease, such as rheumatoid arthritis, may predis-pose to post-operative infection in orthopaedic patients, while others (Poss *et al.* 1984) showed that rheumatoid arthritis and revision surgery predis-posed to an increase risk of infection. Other factors such as malnutrition are important in determining morbidity in orthopaedic and trauma patients. Jensen *et al.* (1982) reported that malnourished patients had a significantly greater incidence of post-operative complications following both total hip replacement and trauma than those who were normally nourished.

If we can have some assessment of pre-existing dis-ease, we may be able to predict the chances of mor-bidity and mortality for a particular patient. This can be categorized by means of one of many grading systems. Perhaps the best known is the American Society of Anesthesiologists (ASA 1963) grading sys-tem (see Table 9.2), which provides a broad measure of the general health of patients admitted with surgi-cal conditions. Numerous other more complex scor-ing systems assessing chronic ill-health are in regular use in many specialities. The Quality Adjusted Life Years (QALY) method (Williams 1985) was devel-oped to examine the cost benefits of particular dis-eases and their treatment. Mehrez and Gafni (1991) described an assessment called Healthy Years Equivalent (HYE), which is a reproducible assess-ment of chronic ill health, while others (Charlson *et al.* 1987a) used a weighted index based upon the number and seriousness of co-morbid disease to develop a prospectively applied evaluation of co-morbid conditions that may affect mortality. Finally, Brewster *et al.* (1989) described the Medical Illness Severity Grouping System, which allowed catego-rization of patients into one to five groups according to severity. All of these systems allow a score to be given to the patient to allow a better comparison of like with like when assessing complication rates and predicting morbidity and mortality.

PHYSIOLOGICAL RESPONSES TO SURGICAL AND TRAUMATIC INSULTS (See also Chapter 8)

Apart from the obvious causes of changes in physiology in response to surgery or trauma, such as hypovolaemia and decreased oxygen exchange in acute respiratory distress syndrome (ARDS), a number of factors have been shown to have an adverse effect. Luna *et al.* (1987) showed that the probability of survival following multiple trauma correlated well with the degree of hypothermia, age and blood transfusion requirements. Other factors that correlated with outcome were alcohol levels (Moore *et al.* 1991) and the resident's assessment of the stability of a disease (Charlson *et al.* 1987b).

Another group (Knaus *et al.* 1985) found a consistent relationship between the extent of the physiological derangement following trauma and the risk of death. This led them to develop the APACHE II scoring system for the assessment of physiological derangement (Knaus and Wagner 1985). The APACHE II system uses 12 routine physiological measurements, as well as the patient's age and previous health status to calculate the score. There are many other similar scoring systems such as the Revised Trauma Score (RTS) (Boyd *et al.* 1987); the Paediatric Trauma Score (PTS) (Tepas *et al.* 1988); the Simplified Acute Physiology Score (SAPS) (Le Gall *et al.* 1984) and the POSSUM system (Copeland *et al.* 1991). POSSUM was developed to determine a score of physiological and operative responses, which could predict morbidity and mortality. It was designed for patients in a general surgical setting. Recently Mohammed *et al.* (2002) have produced a variation on POSSUM for use in orthopaedic patients to account for the slight variation in factors that determine their outcome.

SEVERITY OF SPECIFIC COMPLICATIONS

In writing about medico-legal reporting, Jeffreys (1991) stated that complications such as deep vein thrombosis (DVT) and pulmonary embolism (PE), renal failure and infection after multiple trauma, could 'cause residual impairment and therefore have an effect on prognosis'. The recording that a patient has a DVT is in itself not a very useful piece of information. The mortality and morbidity associated with a DVT is determined, in the main, with the site and size of the thrombus rather than the fact that it exists. A mention in the case records that a patient had a wound infection provides no data concerning the outcome of that complication. Some determination of the extent of the wound infection needs to be made and information about the likely infection of any implant present recorded. The ability to determine this amount of detail about any complication presupposes that it is possible to consistently and to reproducibly make the diagnosis – this is often a far from easy task. Moreover, Ales and Charlson (1987) found that there is a tendency to report only the most severe and prognostically worse categories of disease and to miss the lesser episodes. If this is the case in reporting complications, then bias is introduced and the data about likely causes and course of many complications will be lost or, if presented, will be inaccurate. Therefore, detailed information about a complication is required, including the method of diagnosis. In the case of a DVT, the pick-up rate can alter depending on whether, for instance, a venogram or Doppler echo was used, as well as who undertook the investigation and evaluated the result.

SPECIFIC COMPLICATIONS

Wound infection

It is frequently stated in surgical review papers that there were a certain number of superficial and a certain number of deep wound infections; however the method by which the extent of the infection has been determined is not often stated. The concept of 'deep' and 'superficial' should really be avoided in orthopaedics as all wound infections must be assumed to be involving the deep layers of tissue, especially those around implants and fractures. Many publications (Benson and Hughes 1975; Nelson *et al.* 1980; Lidwell *et al.* 1982; Salvati *et al.* 1982; Gristina and Kolkin 1983) have demonstrated the serious problems of infection following total joint replacement, and have also discussed the contribution of prophylactic antibiotics, special theatres and appropriate clothing in reducing infections. Despite this, Wilson (1987) suggested that only about one-third of surgeons used antibiotic regimen of appropriate duration and timing in patients undergoing total hip replacement or other implant surgery.

It is uncommon for surgeons to 'score' wound problems and use these data as a possible predictor of outcome. Peel and Taylor (1991) suggested that all surgical specialities use the scoring system known as ASEPSIS (Wilson *et al.* 1986) for the assessment of wounds as shown in Table 9.4. This is a general scoring system; not all categories apply to everyday orthopaedic practice and some may be difficult to assess. Nevertheless, this type of system may be useful if adapted specifically to orthopaedic practice, providing there was full validation.

Thromboembolism

Thromboembolic complications are common in both elective and trauma orthopaedic practice. In total hip and knee replacement surgery, many studies have found the rate of DVT to be greater than 50 per cent. Similar figures have been produced for major fractures (Gillespie *et al.* 2000; Sagar *et al.* 1976).

There is continued debate in orthopaedic circles regarding acceptable prophylaxis regimens. However, measurable rates of DVT and PE still occur without changes on practice. This is because the outcome measures used in clinical trials, which are selected in order to let those trials achieve statistical significance, are not the same as the outcomes that concern the surgeon.

The principal outcome in thromboembolic disease is fatal PE. The reported prevalence of this is currently around one or two per 1000 operations (Murray *et al.* 1995), which is an order of magnitude less than previously held views. With these small numbers, there are few clinical trials in orthopaedic surgery that conclusively demonstrate a significant reduction of PE with any regimen of prophylaxis; such a trial has been calculated to require between 20 000 and 100 000 patients (Gillespie *et al.* 2000). The recent PEP trial recruited over 13 000 patients and concluded that compared with placebo, aspirin produced significant reductions in total thromboembolism, total PE, fatal PE and DVT. The absolute figures showed a reduction in total thromboembolism from 2.5 per cent to 1.6 per cent and fatal PE from 0.6 per cent to 0.3 per cent. This equates to treating 250 patients to prevent one death from a fatal PE (The Pulmonary Embolism Prevention (PEP) Trial 2000). The interpretation of the PEP trial results are open to criticism. The PEP trial did not show a reduction in total mortality which was the primary end-point according to the protocol. Further, there was a statistically significant increase in bleeding in the aspirin group. Finally, aspirin had no effect whatsoever in the lower-limb arthroplasty group.

Since it is difficult to study accurately the principal outcome, another outcome must be used and this tends to be the rate of DVT. This condition is a prerequisite for PE in the vast majority of cases, but not all DVTs predispose to PE. Minor calf vein thromboses are clinically insignificant and tend to disperse; thus, an outcome measure that emphasizes these is likely to be clinically inappropriate. Clinical detection of DVT is a useless outcome measure (Gallus *et al.* 1976). Some 50 per cent of legs that are symptomatic enough to warrant further investigation have no thrombosis, whilst a further 50 per cent of all thromboses are asymptomatic.

The options for investigation of DVTs are numerous. Many studies have used radio-labelled fibrinogen uptake (RFUT) as an initial outcome measure or selection criterion for venography. This is inappropriate for hip surgery, for two reasons. First, because the surgery itself increases uptake in the thigh; and second, because – unlike the situation in general surgery – the phenomenon of isolated proximal thrombosis is responsible for around

Table 9.4: ASEPSIS scoring for wound infections. Adapted from Peel and Taylor (1991)

Table A

Wound characteristic	Percentage of wounds					
	0	<20	20–39	40–59	60–79	>80
Serous exudate	0	1	2	3	4	5
Erythema	0	1	2	3	4	5
Purulent exudate	0	2	4	6	8	10
Separation of deep tissues	0	2	4	6	8	10

Table B

Criterion	Points
Additional treatments	
– Antibiotics	10
– Drainage of pus (LA)	5
– Débridement of wound (GA)	10
Serous discharge*	Daily 0–5 (from Table A)
Erythema*	Daily 0–5 (from Table A)
Purulent exudate*	Daily 0–10 (from Table A)
Separation of deep tissues*	Daily 0–10 (from Table A)
Isolation of bacteria	10
In-patient stay >14 days	5

*Given score only on five of first seven post-operative days

0–10	Satisfactory healing
11–20	Disturbance of healing
21–30	Minor wound infection
31–40	Moderate wound infection
>40	Severe wound infection

25 per cent of all thromboses (Stamatakis *et al.* 1977).

Ultrasonography in various forms has been utilized frequently in the detection of DVTs. Recent studies on real-time ultrasound have been most encouraging, showing excellent sensitivity and specificity for all but the smallest distal thromboses (Prandoni *et al.* 1990). Compression ultrasound is becoming the investigation of choice with a high reliability if repeated twice, seven days apart (Chunilal and Ginsberg 2000).

Venography is frequently described as the 'gold standard' for thrombosis detection (Bettman 1987). Its drawbacks are that it is invasive, expensive, mildly thrombogenic, and capable of causing allergic reactions. In clinical practice, venography is sometimes used routinely 7–14 days after high-risk surgery, but more frequently (in the UK) only when indicated by symptoms. Realistically, it cannot be used repeatedly and thus only gives a single-frame view of the venous system. Nevertheless, this investigation is at present the single most important measure in both thrombosis research and, to a certain extent, in clinical practice.

Traditionally, thromboprophylaxis has been used only for the in-patient stay following a surgical procedure. Among orthopaedic surgeons there has been an attitude that venous thromboembolism (VTE) is not a problem that they see, the reason being that many thromboembolic complications occur once the patient has been discharged from hospital. Recent data suggest that there is a significant new DVT rate occurring up to 35 days after surgery. This is an important observation as in-patient stay lengths are reducing every year. In the USA, many patients are discharged after lower-limb arthroplasty after only four days. The ACCP Guidelines specify a minimum of six days prophylaxis in all orthopaedic patients. In the UK, stay lengths for major lower-limb arthroplasty ranges from about 7 to 10 days, but this is likely to shorten considerably.

The argument against prolonged prophylaxis is identical to that used to argue against the use of chemical prophylaxis in-hospital – that is, the prevalence of clinical VTE events is low after lower-limb arthroplasty. This ignores the significance of 'subclinical' events that have been shown to be associated with major morbidity and mortality. Recently, however, data have been published reporting the late symptomatic DVT prevalence after lower-limb surgery. The late incidence of clinical DVT in a population of 19 586 patients undergoing total hip replacement (THR) was found to be 2.8 per cent, and for 24 059 patients undergoing total knee replacement (TKR) was 2.1 per cent, at three months after discharge (White *et al.* 1998). Dahl *et al.* (2000) have studied late clinical events in a group of patients that included those undergoing lower-limb joint arthroplasty. These authors report an annual incidence of DVT of 2.1 per cent with an average time for development of symptoms of 27 days after THR and 16 days after TKR. In addition, 50 per cent of the late DVTs after both THR and TKR are proximal. As far as TKR patients are concerned, this is a much higher proximal DVT rate than is found in clinical trials. The increase could be due to de-novo proximal DVT or an extension of an asymptomatic calf DVT.

One group (Oishi *et al.* 1994) studied 273 THR and TKR patients. Patients were examined with duplex ultrasound on the 4th postoperative day. Overall, there was a 9 per cent proximal DVT rate and a 15 per cent (41 patients) distal calf DVT rate. The patients with a calf DVT were re-examined on the 7th and 14th post-operative day, and seven proximal DVTs were detected by the 14th day. Unfractionated heparin (UH) was the drug of choice in a study by Manganelli *et al.* (1998). DVT was detected (by venography) in 16.3 per cent of patients after discharge, there were two symptomatic PEs. The authors state: 'The incidence of DVT was 21.4% in short- and 12.1% in long-term UH-treated patients. The incidence of only proximal DVT was 18.8% in short- and 3.0% in long-term UH-treated patients (p = 0.85). Prophylaxis with UH given up to postoperative day 30 appears more effective and safer in reducing the delayed thromboembolic risk compared to prophylaxis with UH given up to discharge only'.

Another group (Planes *et al.* 1996) performed venography in a group of THR patients at the time of discharge and then randomized them to either placebo or enoxaparin for a further 21 days. The authors showed that there was a late occurrence of DVT, and that if enoxaparin was continued then the risk of distal was significantly reduced. Interestingly, there was no difference between the groups for proximal DVT, with a prevalence in the enoxaparin group of 5.9 per cent and in the controls of 7.9 per cent. Berqvist and Jonsson (2000) also studied the use of continued prophylaxis with enoxaparin until day 30 after operation. Patients underwent venography between 19 and 23 days after discharge. These authors also showed that there was a continuing risk of VTE after discharge from hospital. If the enoxaparin was given for one month there was a significant reduction in VTE compared to those who only received the drug in-hospital.

Two other groups (Lassen *et al.* 1998; Dahl *et al.* 2000) have also shown that there is a significant occurrence of new DVTs up to 35 days after surgery, substantially after the normal period for in-hospital prophylaxis.

Colwell *et al.* (1999) compared enoxaparin and warfarin in a multicentre study of 3011 THR patients. The enoxaparin was given at 20 mg twice daily and started within 24 hours after surgery. Warfarin was given from as early as 48 hours pre-operatively and no later than 24 hours post-operatively. Both drugs were only given while the patients were in hospital. The patients were clinically assessed, and the symptomatic DVT rates were seen to be 3.6 per cent after enoxaparin and 3.7 per cent after warfarin. In-hospital the rates were: total 1.1 per cent (0.3% enoxaparin; 1.1% warfarin; $p = 0.0083$). After discharge, the rates were: total 4 per cent (warfarin 2.6%, enoxaparin 3.4%; $p = NS$). There were four deaths due to PE (two in each group), and more clinically important bleeding complications occurred in the enoxaparin group. The authors concluded that enoxaparin gave better protection whilst in-hospital, but at three months there was no difference between the treatments. Comp *et al.* (2001) concluded that enoxaparin given for four weeks reduced the risk of VTE 'without compromising safety'.

The second phase of the North American Fragmin Trial (Hull *et al.* 2000) provides the most recent and very convincing evidence that dalteparin provides significantly better protection against DVT up to 35 days post-operatively as compared with warfarin given in-hospital only. In this study, there were no episodes of major bleeding in the prolonged phase. These authors showed that prolonged treatment of only 24–28 patients is required to prevent one out-of-hospital proximal DVT. The study by Hunter *et al.* (1995) also confirmed that there was a risk of death from PE after stopping in-hospital prophylaxis.

Pulmonary embolism is under-diagnosed in both routine clinical practice and at post-mortem examination (Sandler and Martin 1989). The main diagnostic test for PE is a ventilation/perfusion (V/Q_c) scan, but this is exclusively performed in symptomatic patients except in clinical trials. As most patients to whom PE proves fatal, die within 1–2 hours of the onset of symptoms (Havig 1977), this modality has a rather limited role in the prevention of fatal PE. The relationship between asymptomatic PE and subsequent lung function has not been elucidated.

The post-phlebitic limb, as an end-point requires careful definition, which normally includes oedema, varicosities, pigmentation and ulceration. There remains some doubt as to whether proximal valve failure or calf perforator incompetence is the more important predisposition to post-phlebitic changes. Although prevention of chronic venous disease is part of the rationale for thromboprophylaxis, there is no good evidence that asymptomatic thrombi are an important factor in its development (Francis *et al.* 1988). The same group reviewed a small number of patients who had undergone THR and TKR followed by a post-operative venogram; among 51 patients seen, many were found to have venous thrombi and significant evidence of venous insufficiency, though only one patient was reported as having a definite post-phlebitic syndrome. Prandoni *et al.* (1997) estimated that at five years after a proven DVT, some 29.8 per cent of the patients had developed a post-thrombotic syndrome. When others (Johnson *et al.* 1995) studied 78 patients with acute DVTs, the results showed that only 12 per cent of limbs returned to normal as determined by using duplex ultrasonography. A further 13 per cent of patients developed skin changes, but 41 per cent had definite features of post-thrombotic syndrome. Another group (Siragusa *et al.* 1997) studied patients who had undergone THR between two and four years previously. Those patients who had had a post-operative asymptomatic DVT (46.9%) were studied; 23.9 per cent of them had objective evidence of post-thrombotic syndrome, which was comparable with a prevalence of 3.8 per cent in control patients. Moreover, the authors showed that an asymptomatic proximal DVT was the most important risk factor. In a similar study, Ginsberg *et al.* (2000) suggested that post-thrombotic syndrome is extremely rare after either THR or TKR; there was no difference between proximal or distal DVT.

In summary, the most feared thromboembolic outcome is a fatal PE. Using fatal PE as the only endpoint to argue against the use of effective prophylaxis is both unreasonable and illogical. A considerable body of data obtained from studies of clinical endpoints, from clinical trials, and from basic science support the need for chemical prophylaxis to reduce the prevalence of all venous thromboembolic complications.

IMPLANT PROBLEMS

Dislocation of a total hip replacement, whether during the immediate post-operative period or at a later date, constitutes a complication of that type of surgery. Similarly, infection detected soon after surgery and that found months or years later is a complication of the original surgery. The need to revise the joint replacement for these reasons must be regarded as a late complication. However, the question remains as to whether the need to revise a total joint replacement for aseptic loosening be regarded as an operative complication, or whether it reflects the natural history of bone/cement/metal contact. If the loosening is due to poor implant design, rather than surgical technique, then it is a complication – but not for the surgeon. In this context, the time after surgery and the reason for the revision is important. Early (and the meaning of this needs careful definition) loosening due to poor cementing technique may be regarded as a complication, but otherwise loosening may be regarded as part of the natural history of this type of implant. The revision of an implant because of loosening is frequently used as an outcome measure in orthopaedics. Survival analysis of total hip and knee replacements usually depends upon the revision rate. However, the main problem is the ability to diagnose accurately any loosening prostheses. If revision rate is the outcome measure, this will mostly be based upon symptomatic loosening, with the real loosening rate probably being higher. The scoring systems available for assessing loosening are discussed in later chapters of this book.

FRACTURES

Outcome of treatment of fractures, like other orthopaedics conditions, will depend upon hospital and personnel factors, as well as factors related to the fracture itself. Severe fractures, open fractures and multiple trauma are associated with high rates of complications including infection, delayed union and implant failure. A major problem for orthopaedic surgeons has been the comparison of treatments in ill-defined heterogeneous groups of fractures. An accepted classification, though complex, is the AO classification of fractures (Muller et al. 1987; Colton 1991). When applied correctly, it is possible to recognize the type of fracture being treated. Some injuries have their own specific grading systems in common use such as the Schatzker classification for tibial plateau fractures (Schatzker et al. 1979) or Gustillo and Anderson's classification for open tibial fractures (Gustillo and Anderson 1976). Further, an accurate definition of associated soft tissue damage is needed to accompany AO classifications. The AO Foundation has developed a method of coding soft tissue injuries including severity. Again, some specific classifications have been developed for particular fracture types, such as Tscherne's classification for tibial fractures (Tscherne and Gotten 1984). This is of great importance as limb trauma is a soft tissue injury with an underlying bony fracture. Complications following limb trauma are highly dependent on the state of the soft tissues. Even when classifications are used, there may still be disagreement amongst surgeons. Brumback and Jones (1994) asked a number of surgeons at an orthopaedic trauma association meeting to classify 12 open tibial fractures using the Gustillo and Anderson classification, having given them a clinical history, X-radiograms and an intra-operative view of the surgical débridement. There was only a 60 per cent agreement rate for the 12 fractures.

Patients with major trauma often have serious and sometimes fatal complications. This group of patients is an example of the interaction between the three areas discussed above under the title 'severity'. Very careful documentation is required in order to delineate what are avoidable and what are unavoidable complications in these patients.

CONCLUSIONS

Complications occur in all forms of surgery. In both orthopaedics and trauma, a number of complications such as DVT and PE, infection and implant problems can have a major effect on the short- and long-term outcome. However, there are very significant problems with recording accurately the incidence and severity of these adverse affects. For those wishing to record complications on computer, the present coding systems (ICD-9 and OPCS-40) are inadequate. A multi-disciplinary coding system for complications is urgently required.

REFERENCES

Ales, K. L., and Charlson, M. E. (1987): In search of the true inception cohort. *J Chron Dis Anaesthesiol* **40**, 881–5.

Barnett, D. B. (1991): Assessment of quality of life. *Am J Cardiol* **67**, 41C–44C.

Bennett, I., and Walshe, K. (1990): Occurrence screening as a method of audit. *Br Med J* **300**, 1238–51.

Benson, M. K. D., and Hughes, S. P. F. (1975): Infection following total hip replacement in a general hospital without special orthopaedic facilities. *Acta Orthop Scand* **146**, 968–78.

Berqvist, D., and Jonsson, B. (2000): Cost-effectiveness of prolonged out-of-hospital prophylaxis with low-molecular-weight heparin following total hip replacement. *Haemostasis* **30** (Suppl. 2), 130–5.

Bettman, M. A. (1987): Contrast venography of the leg: diagnostic efficacy, tolerance and complication rates with ionic and nonionic contrast material. *Radiology* **165**, 113–16.

Boyd, C. R., Tolson, M. A., and Copes, W. S. (1987): Evaluating trauma care. The TRISS method. *J Trauma* **27**, 370–8.

Brewster, A. C., Jordan, H. S., Young, J. A., and Throop, D. M. (1989): Analyzing in-hospital mortality and morbidity with adjustment for admission severity. *Social Health Systems* **1**, 49–61.

Brumback, R. J., and Jones, A. L. (1994): Inter-observer agreement in the classification of open fractures of the tibia. *J Bone Joint Surg* **76-A**, 1162–6.

Buck, N., Devlin, H. B., and Lunn, J.N. (1987): *The Report of the Confidential Enquiry into Perioperative Deaths*. Nuffield Provincial Hospitals Trust/King's Fund, London.

Campbell, W. (1988): Surgical morbidity and mortality meetings. *Ann Royal Coll Surg Engl* **70**, 363–5.

Charlson, M. E., Pompei, P., Ales, K., and MacKenzie, C. R. (1987a): A new method of classifying prognostic co-morbidity in longitudinal studies: development and validation. *Chronic Dis* **40**, 373–83.

Charlson, M. E., Sax, F. L., MacKenzie, C. R., Braham, R. L., Fields, S. D., and Douglas, R. G. (1987b): Morbidity during hospitalization: can we predict it? *Chronic Dis* **40**, 705–12.

Chunilal, S. D., and Ginsberg, J. S. (2000): Strategies for the diagnosis of deep vein thrombosis and pulmonary embolism. *Thromb Res* **97**, 33–48.

Colton, C. L. (1991): Telling the bones. *J Bone Joint Surg* **73-B**, 362–4.

Colwell, C. W., Jr, Collis, D. K., Paulson, R., McCutchen, J. W., Bigler, G. T., Lutz, S., and Hardwick, M. E. (1999): Comparison of enoxaparin and warfarin for the prevention of venous thromboembolic disease after total hip arthroplasty – evaluation during hospitalization and three months after discharge. *J Bone Joint Surg* **81-A**, 932–40.

Comp, P. C., Spiro, T. E., Friedman, R. J., Whitsett, T. L., Johnson, G. J., Gardiner, G. A., Jr, Landon, G. C., and Jove, M. (2001): Prolonged enoxaparin therapy to prevent venous thromboembolism after primary hip or knee replacement. Enoxaparin Clinical Trial Group. *J Bone Joint Surg Am* **83-A**, 336–45.

Copeland, G. P., Jones, D., and Waiters, M. (1991): POSSUM: a scoring system for surgical audit. *Br J Surg* **78**, 355–60.

D'Ambrosia, R. D., Shoji, H., and Heaten, R. (1976): Secondarily infected total joint replacements by hematogenous spread. *Bone Joint Surg* **58-A**, 450–3.

Dahl, O. E., Gudmundsen, T. E., and Haukeland, L. (2000): Late occurring clinical deep vein thrombosis in joint-operated patients. *Acta Orthop Scand* **71**, 47–50.

Ebrahim, S., Britts, S., and Wu, A. (1991): The valuation of states of ill-health: the impact of age and disability. *Age Ageing* **20**, 37–40.

Francis, C. W., Ricotta, J. J., Evarts, C., and Marder, V. J. (1988): Long-term clinical observations and venous functional abnormalities after asymptomatic venous thrombosis following total hip or knee arthroplasty. *Clin Orthop* **232**, 271–8.

Gallus, A. S., Hirsh, J., and Hull, R. (1976): Diagnosis of venous thromboembolism. *Semin Thromb Haemost* **2**, 203–31.

Gillespie, W., Murray, D., Gregg, P. J., and Warwick, D. (2000): Risk and benefits of prophylaxis against venous thromboembolism in orthopaedic surgery. *J Bone Joint Surg* **82-B**, 475–9.

Ginsberg, J. S., Turkstra, F., Buller, H. R., MacKinnon, B., Magier, D., and Hirsh, J. (2000): Postthrombotic syndrome after hip or knee arthroplasty: a cross-sectional study. *Arch Intern Med* **160**, 669–72.

Greenfield, S., Blanco, D. M., Elashoff, R. M., and Ganz, P. A. (1987): Patterns of care related to age of breast cancer patients. *Am Med Assoc* **257**, 2766–70.

Gristina, A. G., and Kolkin, J. (1983): Total joint replacement and sepsis. *Bone Joint Surg* **64-A**, 128–34.

Gustillo, R. B., and Anderson, J. T. (1976): Prevention of infection in the treatment of 1025 open fractures of long bones. *Bone Joint Surg* **58-A**, 453–8.

Havig, O. (1977): Deep vein thrombosis and pulmonary embolism. *Acta Chir Scand* **478**, 1–120.

Hull, R. D., Pineo, G. F., Francis, C., Bergqvist, D., Fellinius, C., Soderberg, K., Holmqvist, A., Mant, M., Dear, R., Baylis, B., Mah, A., and Brant, R. (2000): Low-molecular-weight heparin prophylaxis using dalteparin extended out-of-hospital vs. in-hospital warfarin/out-of-hospital placebo in hip arthroplasty patients: a double-blind, randomized comparison. North American Fragmin Trial Investigators. *Arch Intern Med* **160**, 2208–15.

Hunter, J. B., Gregson, R., and Frostick, S. P. (1995): *Dalteparin (Fragmin) for the Prevention of Fatal Pulmonary Embolus Following Joint Replacement*. British Orthopaedic Association Meeting, Nottingham, September 1994.

Jeffreys, E. (1991): *Prognosis in Musculoskeletal Injury*. Butterworth-Heinemann, Oxford.

Jensen, J. E., Jensen, T. G., Smith, T. K., Johnston, D. A., and Dudrick, S. J. (1982): Nutrition in orthopaedic surgery. *Bone Joint Surg* **64-A**, 1263–72.

Johnson, B. F., Manzo, R. A., Bereglin, R. O., and Strandness Jr, D. E. (1995): Relationship between changes in the deep venous system and the development of the postthrombotic syndrome after an acute episode of lower limb deep vein thrombosis: a one to six year follow up. *Vasc Surg* **21**, 307–12; discussion 313.

Knaus, W. A., Draper, E. A., Wagner, D. P., and Zimmerman, J. E. (1985): APACHE II: a severity of disease classification system. *Crit Care Med* **13**, 818–29.

Knaus, W. A., and Wagner, D. P. D. (1985): Relationship between acute physiologic derangement and risk of death. *Chronic Dis* **38**, 295–300.

Lassen, M. R., Borris, L. C., Anderson, B. S., and Group, D. P. P. S. (1998): Efficacy and safety of prolonged thromboprophylaxis with a low molecular weight heparin (dalteparin) after total hip arthroplasty in the Danish Prolonged Prophylaxis Study. *Thromb Res* **89**, 281–7.

Le Gall, J. R., Loirat, P., Alperovitch, A., Glaser, P., Granthil, C., Mathieu, D., Mercier, P., Thomas, D., and Villers, D. (1984): A simplified acute physiology score for ICU patients. *Crit Care Med* **12**, 975–7.

Liang, M. H., Katz, J. N., Philips, M. P. H., Sledge, C., W, L.-B., and Measures, A. A. (1991): The total hip arthroplasty outcome evaluation form of the American Academy of Orthopaedic Surgeons. *J Bone Joint Surg* **73-A**, 639–46.

Lidwell, O. M., Lowbury, E. J. C., Whyte, W., Blowers, R., Stanley, S. J., and Lowe, D. (1982): Effect of ultraclean air in operating rooms on deep sepsis in the joint after total hip and knee replacement. A randomised study. *Br Med J* **285**, 10–14.

Luna, G. K., Maier, R. V., Pavlin, E. G., Anardi, D., Copass, M. K., and Oreskovich, M. R. (1987): Incidence and effect of hypothermia in seriously injured patients. *Trauma* **27**, 1014–18.

Manganelli, M., Pazzagli, D., Punzi, G., Manca, M., Vignali, C., Palla, A., Troiani, R., and Rossi, G. (1998): Prolonged prophylaxis with unfractionated heparin is effective to reduce delayed deep vein thrombosis in total hip replacement. *Respiration* **65**, 369–74.

Mehrez, A., and Gafni, A. (1991): The healthy years equivalent. *Medical Decision Making* **11**, 140–6.

Mohammed, K., Copeland, G. S., and Frostick, S. P. (2002): An assessment of the POSSUM system in orthopaedic surgery. *J Bone Joint Surg Br* **84-B**, 735–9.

Moore, T. J., Wilson, J. R., and Hartman, M. (1991): Train versus pedestrian accidents. *Southern Med* **84**, 1097–8.

Muller, M. E., Nazarian, S., and Koch, P. (1987): *Classification AO des Fractures*. Springer-Verlag, Berlin.

Murray, D. W., Carr, A. J., and Bulstrode, C. J. K. (1995): Pharmacological prophylaxis and total hip replacement. *J Bone Joint Surg Br* **77-B**, 3–5.

Nelson, J. P., Glassbum, A. R., Talbott, R. D., and McElhinney, J. P. (1980): The effect of previous surgery, operating room environment and preventive antibiotics on postoperative infection following total hip arthroplasty. *Clin Orthop* **147**, 167–9.

Oishi, C. S., Grady-Benson, J. C., Otis, S. M., Colwell, C. W., Jr and Walker, R. H. (1994): The clinical course of distal deep venous thrombosis after total hip and total knee arthroplasty as determined with duplex ultrasonography. *J Bone Joint Surg* **76-A**, 1658–63.

Planes, A., Vochelle, C., Darmon, J. Y., Gaola, M., Bellaud, M., and Huet, Y. (1996): Risk of deep venous thrombosis after hospital discharge in patients having undergone total hip replacement: double blind randomised comparison of enoxaparin versus placebo. *Lancet* **348**, 224–8.

Poss, R., Thornhill, T. S., Ewald, F. C., Thomas, W. H., Batte, N. J., and Sledge, C. B. (1984): Factors influencing the incidence and outcome of infection following total joint arthroplasty. *Clin Orthop* **182**, 117–26.

Prandoni, P., Lensing, A. W., Poss, R., Thornhill, T. S., Ewald, F. C., Thomas, W. H., Batte, N. J., and Sledge, C. B. (1990): New developments in noninvasive diagnosis of deep vein thrombosis of the lower limbs. *Res Clin Lab* **20**, 11–17.

Prandoni, S., Villalta, P., Bagatella, P., Rossi, L., Machiori, A., Piccioli, A., Bernard, E., Girolami, B., Simioni, P., and Girolami, A. (1997): The clinical course of deep-vein thrombosis. Prospective long-term follow-up of 528 symptomatic patients. *Haematologia* **82**, 423–8.

Sagar, S., Stamatakis, J. D., Higgins, A. F., Nairne, D., Maffei, F. H., Thomas, D. P., and Kakkar, V. V. (1976): Efficacy of low-dose heparin in prevention of extensive deep-vein thromboses in patients undergoing hip replacement. *Lancet* **64A**, 1151–4.

Salvati, E. A., Robinson, R. P., Zeno, S. M., Kuslin, B. L., Brause, B. D., and Wilson, P. D. (1982): Infection rates after 3175 total hip and knee replacements performed with and without a horizontal unidirectional filtered air-flow system. *Bone Joint Surg* **1**, 525–35.

Sandler, D. A., and Martin, J. F. (1989): Autopsy proven pulmonary embolism in hospital patients: are we detecting enough deep vein thrombosis? *Roy Soc Med* **82**, 203–5.

Schatzker, J., McBroom, R., and Bruce, D. (1979): Tibial plateau fractures: the Toronto experience 1968–1975. *Clin Orthop* **138**, 94.

Siragusa, S., Beltrametti, C., Barone, M., Piovella, F., and Minerva, T. (1997): Clinical course and incidence of post-thrombophlebitic syndrome after profound asymptomatic deep vein thrombosis. Results of a transverse epidemiologic study. *Minerva Cardiol* **45**, 57–66.

Stamatakis, J. D., Kakkar, V. V., Sagar, S., Lawrence, D., Nairn, D., and Bentley, P. G. (1977): Femoral vein thrombosis and total hip replacement. *Br Med J* **2**, 223–5.

Peel, A. L., and Taylor, E. W. (1991): Surgical Infection Study Group. Proposed definitions for the audit of postoperative infection. A discussion paper. *Ann Royal Coll Surg Engl* **73**, 385–8.

Tepas, J. J., Ramenofsky, M. L., Mollitt, D. L., Gans, B. M., and DiScala, C. (1988): The pediatric trauma score as a predictor of injury severity: an objective assessment. *Trauma* **28**, 425–9.

The Pulmonary Embolism Prevention (PEP) Trial Collaborative Group (2000): Prevention of pulmonary embolism and deep venous thrombosis with low dose aspirin: Pulmonary Embolism Prevention (PEP) trial. *Lancet* **355**, 1295–302.

Tscherne, H., and Gotten, L. (1984): *Fractures with Soft Tissue Injuries*. Springer-Verlag, Berlin.

White, R. H., Romano, P. S., Zhou, H., Rodrigo, J., and Bargar, W. (1998): Incidence and time course of thromboembolic outcomes following total hip or knee arthroplasty. *Arch Intern Med* **158**, 1525–31.

Williams, A. (1985): Economics of coronary artery bypass grafting. *Br Med J* **291**, 326–9.

Wilson, A. P. R., Treasure, T., Sturridge, M. F., and Gruneburg, R. N. (1986): A scoring method (ASEPSIS) for postoperative wound infections for use in clinical trials of antibiotic prophylaxis. *Lancet* **1**, 311–13.

Wilson, N. (1987): A survey, in Scotland, of measures to prevent infection following orthopaedic surgery. *Hosp Infect* **9**, 235–42.

10

Outcome after blast, missile and gunshot wounds
Jonathan C. Clasper

INTRODUCTION

Despite extensive material having been published on the physics, pathophysiology and injury patterns from weapons, relatively few investigations have been conducted on the outcome of the injuries, and very few specific outcome measures have been identified. Most reports document the mortality and short-term morbidity, and particularly amputation rates, but few long-term studies exist. This is often due to difficulties in reviewing patients who are rapidly evacuated, may be prisoners of war, or who are frequently discharged from the armed forces (Spalding *et al.* 1991).

Military injuries differ considerably from civilian trauma. Some 90 per cent of all battle casualties are due to penetrating trauma, from gunshot or other fragments (Bellamy *et al.* 1999), and many of these are high-energy injuries. Even with the high levels of urban violence seen in American inner cities, penetrating trauma accounted for only 25 per cent of admissions to a level 1 trauma centre (author, personal experience), though the majority of these injuries were caused by knives or low-energy weapons. In addition to penetrating wounds, battle casualties may also be injured by the direct effects of explosions – particularly land mines – and standard civilian classifications are difficult to apply to these injuries.

This chapter will initially discuss the pathophysiology of weapon systems, and broadly consider the outcome to the indiviual from these weapons. Specific systems have been developed to classify military-type trauma, and these will be detailed below. In addition, civilian outcome measures – in particular, the Injury Severity Score (ISS) – have been used, and these will be discussed. Finally, the specific grading systems used by the British armed forces will be described.

PATHOPHYSIOLOGY OF MISSILE AND BLAST INJURIES

Missile injuries

In most wars, the majority of penetrating injuries are caused by fragments rather than bullet wounds. During the Gulf War, 90 per cent of the penetrating injuries seen in one British military hospital were caused by fragments (Spalding *et al.* 1991). These fragments may be from parts of a shell or grenade, or from objects packed around the explosive such as nails or ball-bearings. In addition, any object in the vicinity of the blast, which is 'blown up' and accelerated away from the site of the explosion can produce fragment wounds. It is, therefore, appropriate to consider both bullet and fragment injuries, together, as missile injuries.

Missiles cause direct damage to any structure through which they pass. However, energy may also be dissipated to the surrounding tissues, to produce indirect damage outside of the wound tract. The formation of a temporary cavity, behind the missile, is the most significant factor in tissue injury from indirect mechanisms. As the projectile passes through the tissue, energy is transferred to anything in contact with the projectile, and as a result of this energy transfer the tissue is accelerated away from the projectile. This results in the formation of a temporary cavity, as the inertia of the tissue results in continued displacement even after the projectile has passed through it. This is more likely to occur with high-energy wounds, especially (though not invariably) from high-velocity rifle bullets.

The outcome after missile injuries is related to the damage caused, either directly or indirectly, and so some missiles may cause death without actually striking a vital structure. The effect of indirect damage accounts for the increased mortality from high-velocity bullet wounds. In a report from Vietnam, bullets were responsible for 30 per cent of penetrating wounds, but caused 45 per cent of the deaths (WDMET 1970). It has been estimated that a casualty struck by a bullet, in a military conflict, has a 1 in 3 chance of dying (Bellamy *et al.* 1999). This compares to a 1 in 7 chance of dying if struck by shrapnel from a shell, and 1 in 20 if struck by a fragment from a grenade (Bellamy *et al.* 1999).

Overall, it has been estimated that approximately 20 per cent of personnel wounded during battle will die. Of the casualties killed during the Vietnam War, 90 per cent died on the battlefield, before any medical attention was given, and the majority of these died within 5 minutes of wounding (Bellamy *et al.* 1999). The most common causes of death were major haemorrhage (46%), usually from major vessels in the chest or abdomen, brain injury (21%), respiratory injury (4.5%), or a combination of these injuries (9%).

In battle, some 10 per cent of deaths were in casualties who survived to reach medical care, and again, the most common causes of death included brain injury and major haemorrhage.

Blast injuries

There are a number of mechanisms by which personnel may be injured following an explosion (Cooper *et al.* 1983). These include:

- Direct exposure to a high-pressure *blast wave* – this can cause severe injuries to gas-filled structures such as the lungs and ears, and occasionally also the bowel.

- *Blast wind* – the rapidly expanding gas accelerates objects in its path; this can blow the casualty over, and if the victim is close to the explosive, it may cause traumatic amputations. If the casualty is very close to the blast, then total disintegration of the body can occur.

- *Burns* – as a direct result of the explosive detonating.

- *Penetrating trauma* from fragments (missiles) – as noted earlier, from either the explosive device itself, or from any object accelerated by the blast wind.

- *Secondary effects* of the blast – fire, smoke, collapsing buildings, etc.

Despite the different mechanisms, most injuries in survivors of explosions are caused by penetrating trauma from fragments. Both the blast wave and blast wind are fatal close to the explosion, and this distance is dependent upon the size of the explosive force. The effects of the blast, however, fall rapidly with increasing distance from the point of detonation and there is, therefore, a very small zone where a casualty will survive the blast but sustain significant injuries directly due to the blast wave or wind.

In addition, burns may also be very severe if the casualty was close to the blast, but most of these patients will die from the other effects. In survivors, burns directly caused by an explosion are often superficial and confined to exposed areas (Cooper *et al.* 1983). If, however, the bomb was specifically designed as an incendiary device, or secondary fires have resulted, then burns may be a significant problem.

As a general rule, the outcome after an explosion is related to the proximity and size of the explosive force, and the effect of any penetrating trauma. The outcome after penetrating trauma is related to the structure injured either directly, or indirectly. Penetrating trauma to the head, chest or abdomen is much more likely to be fatal (33–50% mortality) than injuries to the extremities (0.5–2% mortality) (Owen-Smith 1981).

Landmine injuries

Landmines are explosive devices which are usually buried superficially in the ground and designed to be activated by direct contact or a trip wire. Broadly, two types can be considered: (i) anti-tank mines, with a large explosive charge designed to disable or destroy armoured vehicles; and (ii) anti-personnel devices that contain a much smaller charge and are designed to maim, rather than kill, an individual. It is believed that the injuries – particularly traumatic amputations – inflicted by anti-personnel mines will have a greater psychological effect than a sudden death.

Many victims of the larger anti-tank mines will die at the scene, and this is again related to the size of the explosive device force and the proximity of the victim. Among survivors who reach medical care, the mortality appears to be relatively low. Jacobs (1991) described 57 patients who were admitted to hospital in Namibia, most of whom had sustained lower-limb injuries. However, the injuries were less severe than those seen in patients who stood on anti-personnel devices, with a 28 per cent lower-limb amputation rate documented. Only three patients died, all of whom had sustained severe respiratory burns.

In contrast, the majority of victims of anti-personnel mines will survive. Coupland and Korver (1991) reported only six deaths among 757 patients (0.8%), while Chaloner (1996) reported only one death among 60 patients (1.7%) injured by anti-personnel mines in Angola. A retrospective analysis from the International Committee of the Red Cross, of 757 victims, has identified three patterns of injuries among survivors (Coupland and Korver 1991):

- Pattern 1 injuries occur when a buried mine is stepped on; here, severe limb injuries including traumatic amputations of the lower limbs are common, as well as genital injuries.

- With pattern 2 injuries, the device explodes near the victim; this may be due to a buried mine activated by another individual, or due to a pull-action mine that is placed above ground level and is activated by pulling on a wire connected to the device. Lower-limb injuries occur, but they are less severe than in pattern 1, with traumatic amputations less likely. Injuries to the head, chest and abdomen are common.

- Pattern 3 injuries occur when the device explodes whilst the victim is handling it. Severe facial and upper-limb injuries are common in this group.

Despite the low mortality rate, the morbidity after landmine injury is very high. As discussed above, severe lower-limb injuries (including traumatic amputations) can occur. Of 40 patients reported by Traverso *et al.* (1981), 90 per cent sustained traumatic amputations, most of which were below the knee. Two patients (5%) sustained bilateral traumatic amputations, and all 40 patients required definitive surgical amputations. Coupland and Korver (1991) reported 186 traumatic lower-limb amputations and five traumatic upper-limb amputations in 201 patients who had sustained pattern 1 injuries. In addition, most of the patients sustained injuries to the other limb, and 13 per cent of them sustained genital injuries. The majority of contralateral limb injuries were, however, salvageable.

Of the pattern 2 injuries, only 5 per cent of the patients required amputation, but with pattern 3 injuries 80 per cent of the victims sustained traumatic upper-limb amputations, and many of the survivors required a definitive surgical amputation for non-salvageable injuries.

Long-term outcome

Although there is considerable potential for psychological problems, as well as difficulties related to musculoskeletal injuries, many patients appear to have a good quality of life. Dougherty (1999) has reported a long-term follow-up of bilateral above-knee amputees from Vietnam, using the Short Form 36 Health Survey. The author concluded that the patients led relatively normal, productive lives within the context of their physical limitations.

OUTCOME MEASURES AFTER BLAST OR MISSILE INJURY

Specific military classifications

HOSTILE ACTION CASUALTY SYSTEM

Introduction

The Hostile Action Casualty System (HACS) was set up by Owen-Smith, the Professor of Military Surgery, during the late 1970s. It was designed to allow an analysis of military wounds – not only the cause and nature of the wounds, but also the treatment and outcome (Owen-Smith 1981). With the civil unrest in Northern Ireland, this system – together with the accurate forensic data that were available – allowed a detailed assessment to be made of the servicemen killed and wounded. The system is essentially a database, and allows accurate outcomes to be reported.

Description

A coding sheet was completed for all injured personnel; this detailed the specific details of the incident, the proximity of the serviceman to any explosion, and the nature of any protection worn (e.g. helmet or flak jacket). Regional details of the injuries, together with specific anatomical details were recorded, as was the treatment and outcome. The completed form was retained and the data analysed by the Professor of Military Surgery.

As well as allowing the outcome after specific injuries to be determined, the HACS allowed specific weapons such as high-velocity bullets or bombs to be studied.

The use of HACS

In his Hunterian lecture of 1980, Owen-Smith reported the results of almost 1600 servicemen injured by bullets or bombs in Northern Ireland. Almost 50 per cent of the injuries were caused by bullets, and this – as discussed previously – was higher than would be expected from most armed conflicts.

Owen-Smith classified the outcome based on the military employment standard (see Table 10.1). This included death, medical discharge from the services, medical downgrading, or a return to full duties.

He confirmed the worse prognosis associated with high-energy weapons, with a mortality of 31 per cent and medical discharge rate of approximately 17 per cent. This compares with a mortality of 3.5 per cent and discharge rate of 8.5 per cent for injuries from low-velocity weapons. The mortality rate from high-energy injuries to the brain was 100 per cent, and to the chest or abdomen was 50 per cent.

Owen-Smith reported that most of the fatalities from penetrating wounds were due to damage to vital structures in the head, chest or abdomen, and that the deaths were due to massive brain injury or haemorrhagic shock. This was confirmed in Vietnam, where a 96 per cent mortality rate from aortic injuries was reported (WDMET 1970).

Owen-Smith also reported the incidence of, and outcome following, blunt and penetrating injuries to specific abdominal structures. This information is listed in Table 10.1.

The overall mortality from abdominal injuries is high in this series, and lower death rates have been reported. In a report evaluating wound data and munitions effectiveness in Vietnam, an overall mortality rate of 9.2 per cent from abdominal injuries was reported (WDMET 1970). These differences may be due to the lower incidence of bullet wounds (when compared with other fragments) in the data obtained

Table 10.1: Outcome after injuries to specific abdominal structures (includes fatalities and survivors). Adapted from Owen-Smith (1981)

Site of injury	No. of injuries	Mortality (%)	Medical discharge (%)
Liver	60	78	8
Spleen	35	74	6
Stomach and duodenum	26	65	19
Pancreas	8	100	–
Small bowel	37	38	19
Large bowel	59	51	12
Genito-urinary	42	48	5
Major vessel	26	77	23

from Vietnam, and also the use of specific anti-personnel devices in Northern Ireland. Despite the lower mortality rates reported from Vietnam, there was still a more than 50 per cent mortality rate from injuries to the liver or major vessels.

Prognosis for survivors with abdominal injuries

The HACS data relates to the overall mortality, and does not provide any indication of the prognosis for survivors. Hardaway (1978) has documented the outcome of over 17 000 American soldiers admitted to military hospitals in Vietnam, and the mortality rate of these patients is shown in Table 10.2.

Use of the HACS in blast injuries

As accurate forensic data were available from Northern Ireland, the quantity of explosive used and the proximity of the casualty to a blast could be calculated. This information was used to analyse the outcome of 828 servicemen killed or wounded by explosion between 1970 and 1984 (Mellor and Cooper 1989). With the information given on the HACS forms, the authors were able to estimate the blast overpressure (or blast loading) to which the victim was exposed, and relate this to the injuries sustained. The relationship of blast loading to the distance and quantity of explosive is shown in Table 10.3, and these authors were able to demonstrate a

relationship between the degree of injury and the degree of blast loading (Table 10.4).

Discussion

The HACS was specifically set up as a database, and this has allowed the analysis to be conducted of all victims of military injuries. It has confirmed the increased mortality associated with high-velocity weapons, and demonstrated the relationship of

Table 10.3: Relationship of blast loading to distance and quantity of explosive. Adapted from Mellor and Cooper (1989)

Size of explosive (lb)	Distance from explosion		
	<10 feet	10–50 feet	>50 feet
2	Severe	Minor	Minor
2–6	Very severe	Minor	Minor
7–20	Very severe	Moderate	Minor
21–99	Very severe	Severe	Minor
>100	Very severe	Severe	Minor

Table 10.2: Mortality rates, in survivors, after injury to specific abdominal structures. Adapted from Hardaway (1978)

Site of injury	Mortality rate (%)
Large bowel	6.5
Small bowel	5.6
Liver	8.5
Stomach	7.3
Kidney	7.8
Spleen	4.5
Pancreas	5.7
All abdominal injuries	4.5
All wounds	1.8

Table 10.4: Degree of injury in relation to the estimated blast loading. Adapted from Mellor and Cooper (1989)

	Minor	Moderate	Severe	Very severe
Number of cases	255	135	200	238
Dead	5 (2.0)	28 (20.7)	38 (19.0)	145 (60.9)
Major injury	14 (5.5)	13 (9.6)	38 (19.0)	27 (11.4)
Moderate injury	23 (9.0)	16 (11.9)	35 (17.5)	15 (6.3)
Minor injury	213 (83.5)	78 (57.8)	89 (44.5)	51 (21.4)

Values in parentheses are percentages of the number of cases in that group.

serious injuries to the level of blast overpressure. As well as providing a source for planning medical resources and audit, the HACS can be used to investigate methods of protection from blast injury.

THE RED CROSS WOUND CLASSIFICATION

Introduction

This scoring system was introduced to allow the classification of wounds based on their appearance, rather than on any specific cause (Coupland 1993). The weapon used is often unknown by the surgeon treating the wound, and this is particularly true for surgeons working for the International Committee of the Red Cross (ICRC), where there may be a delay of several days between wounding and arrival at hospital. The classification was designed, not only to permit wound assessment, but also to allow surgical audit, and to attempt to determine the relationship of war wounds to experimental ballistic injuries (Coupland 1993).

Description

At initial assessment, either when the patient first reaches hospital, or at the initial operation, a number of aspects of the wound are recorded:

- **E:** The maximum diameter of the entry wound is measured in centimetres.

- **X:** The maximum diameter of the exit wound is measured in centimetres.

- **C:** The presence (C = 1) or absence (C = 0) of a cavity is determined depending upon the ability to insert two fingers into the wound prior to surgery.

- **F:** Any fracture is graded as: no fracture (F = 0), simple or insignificant fracture (F = 1) or clinically significant comminution (F = 2).

- **V:** The presence (V = 1) or absence (V = 0) of damage to vital structures, or vessels is noted.

- **M:** Any visible metallic fragments on radiographs are graded as: no fragments (M = 0), one fragment (M = 1) or multiple metallic fragments (M = 2).

Débridement, together with any other appropriate surgical procedures was carried out. The information recorded from each wound could then be further analysed, either at the hospital, or at the headquarters of the ICRC in Switzerland. This included grading the wounds based on the extent of soft tissue injury, and also subtyping them, based on any bone, or other vital structures damaged:

- Grade 1: E + X < 10 cm, with scores of C0 and F0 or F1 (low-energy transfer wounds).

- Grade 2: E + X < 10 cm, with scores of C1 or F2 (high-energy transfer wounds).

- Grade 3: E + X ⩾ 10 cm (massive wounds).

The types of wounds were subdivided based on injuries to other structures:

- Type ST: Soft tissue only, no fracture or vital structures injured.

- Type F: Fracture present, but no vital structures injured.

- Type V: No fracture present, but vital structures injured.

- Type VF: Fracture present, in addition to injury to vital structures.

Use of the Red Cross Wound Classification

There is little information available on the use of this classification, and in particular on the treatment or outcome of wounds based on it. Bowyer *et al.* (1993) used this classification to grade wounds seen at one of the British Field Hospitals during the Gulf War, and reported that approximately 50 per cent of the penetrating wounds were Grade 1, ST. This is of clinical relevance, as reports from American trauma centres (Knapp *et al.* 1996) and experimental studies (Hill and Watkins 1998) suggested that these wounds, and also selected Grade 2 wounds, may be treated non-operatively.

Discussion

The Red Cross Wound Classification is a valid attempt to classify wounds, and it may be useful as a prognostic indicator. However, there is little information available on its use as an outcome measure, and factors such as the site of wounding and any neurological injury are not recorded. It is known that open injuries to certain areas of the body (e.g. the distal tibia) are associated with a worse prognosis than other locations such as open injuries of the upper limb (Dellinger et al. 1988; Jacob and Murphy 1992). Despite the different outcomes, the wounds may have the same ICRC classification. In addition, neurological function has major implications on the outcome after a limb injury and, for some injuries, this may influence the decision of whether to amputate a limb, or not. The absence of neurological assessment from the ICRC classification has been noted previously (Bowyer et al. 1993).

Non-military classifications

INJURY SEVERITY SCORE

Introduction and description

A detailed description of the Injury Severity Score (ISS) is given in Chapter 8.

Use of the ISS

Beverland and Rutherford (1983) assessed the validity of the ISS on the outcome of 875 patients who sustained gunshot wounds in Northern Ireland (Beverland and Rutherford 1983). They reported an increasing mortality with increasing ISS, but reported that this relationship was not linear, and that a graph of mortality plotted against ISS was different from that plotted from the patients reported in the original description of the ISS (Baker et al. 1974). In the original description there is an exponential rise in mortality with an increasing ISS. This is perhaps not surprising, as with road traffic accidents (the most common source of patients for a civilian trauma centre), there are often associated injuries to other systems, and these may dramatically affect the overall survival rate. In contrast, many gunshot victims have a either single gunshot or single system injury, and it is this individual injury rather than multisystem factors which influences survival. Most fatalities (~70%) after gunshot wounds are due to massive

haemorrhage from the chest or abdomen, or severe head injuries. These would be associated with an ISS of 16–25. This can be seen on the graph plotted by Beverland and Rutherford (1983), where there is a dramatic increase in mortality between an ISS of 16 and 25, corresponding to a severe life-threatening injury to one system.

The ISS has also been applied to the victims of a terrorist bombing in Italy (Brismar and Bergenwald 1982), where it was noted that the majority (76%) of survivors had sustained only mild to moderate injuries (ISS <16), and that the mean ISS of the group was only 8. This was supported by the findings of Mellor and Cooper (1989), who noted that 90 per cent of fatalities from explosions occurred before, or very soon after arrival at hospital. Of the fatalities occurring after initial resuscitation, approximately 50 per cent were due to severe head injuries, which would not have been amenable to treatment and would have been graded with an ISS of at least 16. These findings would suggest that most patients who survive explosions are not severely injured, and have a relatively low ISS. As discussed earlier, this is due to the rapid reduction in the effect of the blast wave and wind with increasing distance from the explosion.

Discussion

Although the ISS has been used in the assessment of casualties with blast and missile injuries, this is not comparable with its use in casualties after blunt trauma following road traffic accidents. This has been discussed in depth by Ryan et al. (1990), who noted the increasing effect on mortality when more than one abdominal organ is injured from a military injury. There is a 15 per cent increase in mortality for each organ injured, despite no change occurring in the corresponding ISS.

Current outcome measures used by the British Armed Forces

INTRODUCTION

All personnel serving with the British Forces have a medical examination prior to and shortly after enlisting. This grading is reassessed at set intervals, and any injury or other medical problem suffered by the serviceman, may result in temporary or permanent 'downgrading'. This applies to military as well as civilian medical conditions, and can be used to assess the outcome after any medical problem.

DESCRIPTION

British Army

Soldiers are graded using the PULHEEMS system, where each letter, with the exception of P, represents a region of the body or organ. The specific details are given in Table 10.5. The capital letter P denotes an overall physical capacity and is graded from 2 to 8, based on the score for the ULHEEMS letters (P0 can be used as a temporary grading prior to a definitive grade being made). In general, the P grade will be the same as the lowest individual grade awarded. In addition, an employment standard is added to the P (e.g. P2FE, P7HO), and this indicates in which zone the soldier may serve. Further details are given in Table 10.6 and in the First Edition of this book.

Royal Navy

A similar PULHEEMS system is used as in the Army, but the employment standards reflect the need to assess an individual's ability to serve on a ship, either at sea, or in the dockyard (Table 10.7).

Royal Air Force

All personnel serving with the Royal Air Force are given a numerical grading based on their fitness for flying duties (A), ground duties (G), and also on the zone of duty where they may serve (Z) (Table 10.8).

USE OF THE ARMED FORCES SYSTEMS

These systems are in day-to-day use, and all service personnel have a physical grade. The grading is not universally accepted by medical journals, and so there is little published on its use as an outcome measure. As noted above, the final medical grade including medical discharges has been reported from Northern Ireland (Owen-Smith 1981), and in addition the PULHEEMS grade has been used as an outcome measure after anterior cruciate reconstruction (Bowyer and Matthews 1991).

Table 10.5: Details of the coding used by the British Army

Letter – System denoted	Grades used
U – upper limb	U2, 3, 7, 8
L – lower limb, including back	L2, 3, 7, 8
H – hearing	H1, 2, 3, 4, 8
E – eyesight	E1–8
M – mental capacity (neurological)	M2, 3, 7, 8
S – emotional stability (psychiatric)	S2, 3, 6, 7, 8

Table 10.6: PULHEEMS employment standards

Physical capacity and employment standards	Comments
P2FE	Forwards Everywhere – fit for full combatant duty anywhere in the world
P3LE	Lines of communication Everywhere – fit for service in all areas except primary combatant zones
P7BE	Bases Everywhere – employable only in base areas, but anywhere in the world
P7HO	Home Only – only employable in base areas close to suitable medical facilities – includes Northern Ireland and Germany unless specifically excluded
P8	Unfit for any military service

Medical grades, and in particularly medical discharge, have also been reported for Royal Naval personnel following retinal detachment (Low and Jeffrey 1992) and ureteroscopy (Spalding 1989).

COMMENTS

Despite the everyday use of these systems, they are very rarely reported in the medical literature, and when used, are usually confined to the journals of

Table 10.7: Royal Navy employment grades

Grading	Comments
P0	Temporary holding category
P2	Fit for all duties
P3R	Fit for sea on ships with medical facilities – restriction to be stated
P7A	Not fit for sea, but employable ashore, or on a ship in harbour in own trade
P7B	Employable ashore in own trade
P7C	Restricted duties within own trade ashore or on a ship in harbour
P7D	Restricted duties within own trade, ashore only
P8	Unfit for Naval service

Table 10.8: Royal Air Force medical grading

A1 – Full flying duties

A3 – Limited flying duties – restriction to be stated, e.g. co-pilot only

A4 – Fit to fly as a passenger only

A5 – Unfit to fly

G1 – Full ground duties

G3 – Limited ground duties – only in own trade

G4 – Limited in own trade – restriction to be stated

Z1 – Fit for service anywhere

Z2 – Fit for service anywhere except low-temperature zones

Z3 – Fit for service anywhere except high-temperature zones

Z4 – Fit for service temperate climates only

Z5 – Fit for service in UK only

the medical services themselves. This is due to both difficulties in publication using these systems, but particularly due to the lack of specific criteria for determining fitness, and the potential discrepancies between different grades for different ranks or employments. For example, the overall fitness of a paratrooper is likely to be different from that of an orthopaedic surgeon, despite the same grading of P2FE. The system does, however, provide a common language, within the military, which allows medical personnel to communicate with front-line commanders, to give an indication of an individual's medical fitness.

REFERENCES

Baker, S. P., O'Neill, B., Haddon, W., and Long, W. B. (1974): The Injury Severity Score, a method of describing patients with multiple injuries and evaluating emergency care. *Trauma* **14**, 187–96.

Bellamy, R., Champion, H., Mahoney, P., and Roberts, P. (1999): Introduction and epidemiology. In N. Rich (ed.), *Definitive Surgical Trauma Skills: Course manual.* The Royal College of Surgeons of England, London, pp. 1–5.

Beverland, D. E., and Rutherford, W. H. (1983): An assessment of the validity of the Injury Severity Score when applied to gunshot wounds. *Injury* **15**, 19–22.

Bowyer, G. W., and Matthews, S. J. (1991): Anterior cruciate ligament reconstruction using the Gore-tex ligament. *R Army Med Corps* **137**, 69–75.

Bowyer, G. W., Stewart, M. P. M., and Ryan, J. M. (1993): Gulf War wounds: Application of the Red Cross Wound Classification. *Injury* **24**, 597–600.

Brismar, B., and Bergenwald, L. (1982): The terrorist bomb explosion in Bologna, Italy, 1980: an analysis of the effects and injuries sustained. *Trauma* **22**, 216–20.

Chaloner, E. J. (1996): The incidence of landmine injuries in Kuito, Angola. *R Coll Surg Edinb*, **41**, 398–400.

Cooper, G. J., Maynard, R. L., Cross, N. L., and Hill, J. F. (1983): Casualties from terrorist bombings. *J Trauma* **23**, 955–67.

Coupland, R. M. (1993): *Appendix 1 – The Red Cross Wound Classification. War Wounds of Limbs. Surgical Management.* Butterworth Heinemann, Oxford, pp. 92–4.

Coupland, R. M., and Korver, A. (1991): Injuries from antipersonnel mines: the experience of the International Committee of the Red Cross. *Br Med J* 303, 1509–12.

Dellinger, E. P., Wertz, M. J., Grympa, M., Droppert, B., and Anderson, P. A. (1988): Risk of infection after open fractures of the arm or leg. *Arch Surg* 123, 1320–7.

Dougherty, P. J. (1999): Long-term follow-up of bilateral above-the-knee amputees from the Vietnam War. *J Bone Joint Surg Am* 81-A, 1384–90.

Hardaway, R. M. (1978): Vietnam wound analysis. *J Trauma* 18, 635–43.

Hill, P. F., and Watkins, P. E. (1998): The delayed treatment of ballistic fractures with antibiotics. Transactions of the 44th Annual Meeting of the Orthopaedic Research Society, pp. 282.

Jacob, E., and Murphy, K. P. (1992): A retrospective analysis of open fractures sustained by U.S. personnel during Operation Just Cause. *Mil Med* 157, 552–6.

Jacobs, L. G. H. (1991): The landmine foot: its description and management. *Injury* 22, 463–6.

Knapp, T. P., Patzakis, M. J., Lee, J., Seipel, P. R., Andollah, K., and Reisch, R. B. (1996): Comparison of intravenous and oral antibiotic therapy in the treatment of fractures caused by low-velocity gunshots. *J Bone Joint Surg Am* 38-A, 1167–71.

Low, C. D., and Jeffrey, M. N. (1992): Rhegmatogenous retinal detachment in Royal Naval personnel: a retrospective study. *R Nav Med Serv* 78, 151–8.

Mellor, S. G., and Cooper, G. J. (1989): Analysis of 828 servicemen killed or injured by explosion in Northern Ireland 1970–84. The Hostile Action Casualty System. *Br J Surg* 76, 1006–10.

Owen-Smith, M. S. (1981): Hunterian Lecture 1980. A computerised data retrieval system for the wounds of war: The Northern Ireland casualties. *R Army Med Corps* 127, 31–54.

Ryan, J. M., Sibson, J., and Howell, G. (1990): Assessing injury severity during general war: will the military triage system meet future needs? *R Army Med Corps* 136, 27–35.

Spalding, T. J. (1989): Experiences with uteroscopy. *R Nav Med Serv* 75, 95–7.

Spalding, T. J. W., Stewart, M. P. M., Tulloch, D. N., and Stephens, K. M. (1991): Penetrating missile injuries in the Gulf War 1991. *Br J Surg* 78, 1102–4.

Traverso, L. W., Johnson, D. E., Fleming, A., and Wongrukmitr, B. (1981): Combat casualties in Northern Thailand: emphasis on land mine injuries and levels of amputation. *Mil Med* 146, 682–5.

WDMET (1970): *Evaluation of Wound Data and Munitions Effectiveness in Vietnam*. Joint Technical Coordinating Group for Munitions Effectiveness Washington, DC (Confidential Document).

11

Deformity and cosmesis
T. N. Theologis

INTRODUCTION

Definition

'Beauty is in the eyes of the beholder' – that is, the perception of human body aesthetics can vary among different individuals and societies. Deformity of the human body can be the source of cosmetic concern. What is acceptable deformity, from the aesthetic point of view, is again subjective and dependent on the perceptions of the observer. Interest in human body aesthetics has existed throughout the history of organized societies. The modern term 'cosmetic' originates from the Roman public baths where slaves called 'cosmetae' undertook hair dying and the application of make-up. The term *cosmetae* evolved from the Greek word '*cosmetikos*' (arranging, putting in order) (Blanco-Davila 2000).

The aim of this chapter is to define the role of cosmesis in decision making, and as an outcome measure in orthopaedic surgery.

Quantification of cosmesis

Although body aesthetics vary in different individuals and societies, some basic principles may be universal. It may be possible to quantify a 'common feeling' on what degree of body deformity is acceptable from the cosmetic point of view. The hypothesis that a number of randomly selected individuals can represent the general population and give their opinion on body cosmesis has been tested in subjects with adolescent idiopathic scoliosis (Theologis 1991).

Photographs of 100 adolescent idiopathic scoliosis patients were examined by 10 non-medical judges. Each one of the judges gave a Cosmetic Spinal Score (CSS) for each patient's back, and the CSS obtained for each patient was compared with an ISIS scan (Integrated Shape Investigation System, Oxford Metrics) – an optical scanner that represents the surface topography of the back. The CSS correlated well with one of the ISIS parameters expressing the size of the rib prominence on the patient's back. This was shown to be the single major underlying factor that consistently influenced the judges. Furthermore, an equation was developed based on two of the ISIS parameters, which could predict the CSS with sufficient reproducibility. The practical value of this equation is that the cosmetic appearance of a patient's back could be calculated from ISIS parameters with reasonable approximation. This provides the surgeon with a single figure that gives an impression of the severity of the cosmetic deformity.

Theoretically, a similar process could be applied to various other musculoskeletal deformities, and methods of quantifying cosmesis could be developed. The study showed that the routine methods of measuring deformity do not necessarily express or quantify cosmesis. In the case of idiopathic scoliosis, the routine clinical measure of deformity is the Cobb angle (Cobb 1948). The above study showed that the judges were concerned with the size of the rib hump rather than the magnitude of the spinal curve in the coronal plane, as measured by the Cobb angle.

These two measurements are not necessarily related. The need for the development of outcome measures that are specific to cosmesis, but not necessarily to clinical measurements of body deformity, is apparent.

The orthopaedic surgeon is often asked to give his or her opinion on the treatment of musculoskeletal deformity that mainly, or entirely, causes cosmetic concerns. The surgeon's perception of the cosmetic deformity will rely entirely on his or her background, culture and training, but this may be different from the patient's background. There are often cases in which the patient insists on asking for treatment when there is no significant cosmetic deformity to the eyes of the surgeon (or vice-versa). When the cosmetic deformity involves children or adolescents, patient and family disagreement is not unusual. In these cases, the surgeon could be guided by objective cosmetic scores, forming his/her own opinion on the cosmetic deformity and its management.

COSMESIS AS AN INDICATION FOR ORTHOPAEDIC TREATMENT

Indications for orthopaedic treatment

Orthopaedic treatment aims at relieving pain, restoring function of the musculoskeletal system, and the correction of deformity. This is reflected in the numbers of patients who undergo joint replacement surgery and fracture fixation operations. The need for treatment of painful bone and joint conditions and the need to restore function of the musculoskeletal system are self-evident. This is not necessarily the case with musculoskeletal deformity. There are cases where the treatment of deformity is justified by the prevention of long-term disability. Angular or rotational post-traumatic bone deformity may require correction to prevent the onset of arthritis in adjacent joints. Asymptomatic hip dysplasia may be treated to prevent early osteoarthritis. Leg-length discrepancy is treated to prevent back problems and long-limb knee problems.

Musculoskeletal deformity can be the source of cosmetic concerns and indications for treatment even in the absence of any other long-term implications. This issue is not sufficiently covered in the orthopaedic literature, and is rarely acknowledged. Major operations are often performed to correct skeletal deformity for no other reason than the improvement of body appearance, but these are seldom labelled as 'cosmetic operations'. There are certainly important socioeconomic and funding considerations involved in management decisions in these cases. It can be argued that correction of cosmetic deformities is justified on the basis of the psychological impact of impaired cosmesis and its socioeconomic implications on the patient (see below).

The role of cosmesis in patient presentation and clinical decision making

CHILDREN

Paediatric orthopaedic clinics are frequently attended by parents who are concerned about their children's development. An 'abnormal' walking pattern, flat feet, bow legs or knock knees are common sources of concern (Wenger and Rang 1993).

Toeing-in or toeing-out are some of the most common gait deviations in children. *Toeing-out* is a common postural deviation in toddlers that tends to subside by the age of 18 months. In older children it may be due to external tibial torsion. *Toeing-in* is usually due to persistent femoral anteversion or metatarsus adductus. The assessment of these torsional deviations is based on clinical examination when underlying neurological abnormality should be excluded. The use of various jigs for the measurement of torsion as well as the use of ultrasound or computed tomography (CT)/magnetic resonance imaging (MRI) scanning have been suggested (Jacob *et al.* 1980; Moulton and Upadhyay 1982; Staheli *et al.* 1985). Clinical examination, however, is sufficient in the vast majority of cases. The clinical measurement of femoral anteversion was shown to be reliable (Ruwe *et al.* 1992). The natural history of these torsional deviations is benign, and 80 per cent improve to normal levels by the age of eight years (Fabry *et al.* 1973).

Knee alignment in the coronal plain is varus for the first 18–24 months of life, progresses to an average of 10° of valgus from two to six years of age, and assumes the average normal value of 5–7° valgus by the age of seven years. Parents are often concerned about their children's knee alignment, though this is more common when the children start to walk (when varus becomes apparent) or when they go through their peak of valgus alignment at the age of three to four years. History, clinical evaluation and often a radiograph of the knees are necessary to exclude metabolic bone disease or bone dysplasia. Clinical measurement of varus knee alignment is performed by measuring the distance between the medial femoral condyles. Measurement of valgus knee alignment relies on measuring the intra-malleolar distance (Askin *et al.* 1997). Both measurements are affected by rotational variation in the positioning of the legs. Repeated measurements over time are likely to be affected by longitudinal growth of the lower limbs. A true antero-posterior radiograph of the whole length of the lower limbs is probably the most reliable method of measuring knee alignment. Furthermore, radiographs allow the measurement of the metaphyseal-diaphyseal angle at the upper end of the tibia (Drennan's angle; Wenger and Rang 1993) to differentiate between physiological tibia vara and Blount's disease.

The natural history of the development of the longitudinal arch of the foot is now well established (Staheli *et al.* 1987). Flexible flat feet in children under the age of six years should be considered normal. Flexibility should be tested by extending the great toe; elevation of the longitudinal arch of the foot is observed if the foot is flexible. Only symptomatic or rigid flat feet should be investigated further with radiographs or CT scanning.

Regular attenders of paediatric orthopaedic clinics include children with congenital limb deformities or deficiencies. Even in severe lower-limb longitudinal deficiencies, such as fibular hemimelia, cosmesis remains a consideration when treatment is planned

(Naudie *et al.* 1997). Some forms of cleft foot or syndactyly may come to surgical treatment for cosmetic reasons only, although function remains a consideration (Wood *et al.* 1997). Genetic syndromes, skeletal dysplasias and metabolic bone disease can lead to severe musculoskeletal deformity with cosmetic implications. Although the main aim of any orthopaedic treatment would be to alleviate any pain and improve function, some procedures focus on cosmetic aspects. Limb lengthening in dwarfism of various aetiologies, for example, remains a controversial area for this reason.

THE SPINE

Cosmesis is the primary indication for the surgical treatment of the majority of patients with adolescent idiopathic scoliosis (Theologis 1991). Quantification of the cosmetic effects of idiopathic scoliosis (Theologis *et al.* 1993) has been discussed at the beginning of this chapter. The details of assessing deformity and cosmesis of the spine have been discussed elsewhere (Theologis and Fairbank 1997).

More recently, a subjective assessment of cosmesis was performed on severely physically handicapped patients treated for neuromuscular or congenital scoliosis, with improvement of cosmesis being considered as one of the targets of treatment. According to the authors, subjective cosmetic improvement was observed and patients, as well as their 'caregivers', were pleased with the results (Askin *et al.* 1997).

Body surface deformity has been suggested to be a prognostic factor for progression of idiopathic scoliosis (Duval-Beaupere and Lamireau 1985; Theologis *et al.* 1997). Some more recent studies based on surface topography (Quantec Spinal Imaging System, QSIS) supported previous findings (Thometz *et al.* 2000).

NEUROMUSCULAR CONDITIONS

Although treatment in these conditions mainly aims at treating or preventing pain and improving function, cosmesis also plays a role. Cosmetic considerations are given to the treatment of spinal deformity (Askin *et al.* 1997) or correction of upper- or lower-limb deformities that would not improve function. Correction of the flexion deformity of the wrist and fingers in the hemiplegic non-functional hand is often carried out for cosmetic benefit only (Hargreaves *et al.* 2000).

Multi-level lower-limb surgery in diplegic cerebral palsy is mainly performed to improve the efficiency of gait and prolong or maintain the ability of the individual to ambulate. From the patient and family's point of view, however, one of the targets is often to improve the appearance of the child's walking for cosmetic reasons. In this particular field, three-dimensional instrumented gait analysis is a helpful pre-operative evaluation and patient selection tool as well as an objective outcome measure. Management plans and expectations from treatment can therefore be discussed pre-operatively and assessed post-operatively on an objective basis. Simulation of the proposed surgery on computer models is not far from realistic and this would offer parents and children a clearer picture of the expected improvement following treatment (Harrington *et al.* 1999).

THE HAND

Cosmesis is often considered in the management of hand deformities. Separation techniques for syndactyly have been assessed for this purpose based on subjective criteria (DeSmet *et al.* 1998). Similarly, cosmetic considerations are taken for reconstruction of amputated fingers (Koshima *et al.* 1998). Subjective evaluation of cosmesis using patient questionnaires was presented in a study comparing patients who had undergone replantation-revascularization or primary amputation for major hand injuries (Holmberg *et al.* 1996).

THE FOOT

The foot appears to be the source of frequent cosmetic concerns. Maintaining a comfortable foot in fashionable shoes of various shapes can also necessitate alterations in foot shape. Patients often present with prominences or callosities in various areas of the foot, suffering from a variable level of symptoms. Difficulty in fitting shoes is a common complaint.

This is certainly a cosmetic issue, since these patients will rarely accept the advice to wear shoes that would allow space for their deformity.

Cosmesis is considered in hallux valgus surgery (Rossi and Ferreira 1992), the treatment of the rheumatoid foot (Hanyu *et al.* 1997), correction of brachymetatarsia (Fox, 1998) and lengthening of a short great toe – an operation performed not only for cosmesis but also to relieve pain and callosities (Takakura *et al.* 1997).

COSMESIS FOLLOWING ORTHOPAEDIC TREATMENT

Assessment of cosmesis following orthopaedic treatment has not been widely explored in the literature. Patient satisfaction, however, depends partly on the aesthetic result of an orthopaedic intervention.

Trauma

Few investigators have assessed cosmesis following the surgical treatment of trauma. Press *et al.* (1997) compared the outcome of surgical and conservative treatment of grade III acromioclavicular dislocation. Amongst the parameters compared between the two groups was a subjective evaluation of cosmesis. The surgical group was found to have better results.

Percutaneous pinning of supracondylar fractures in children was found to have better subjective cosmetic results than open reduction and internal fixation (Ong and Low 1996). Multiple relaxing skin incisions for lower-extremity trauma and difficult wound closure were found to have satisfactory cosmetic results (DiStasio *et al.* 1993). None of the above studies used validated measures for cosmetic assessment.

In a study of the severity of post-traumatic stress disorder, patients with burns or digital amputations were assessed (Fukunishi 1999). The severity of their cosmetic disfigurement was found to relate well to the severity of their stress disorder. While the psychiatric assessment of these patients was thorough and well-designed, the assessment of their cosmetic impairment was based only on whether they had facial burns or extensive hand scarring. The need to establish validated outcome measures for cosmesis was again apparent in this study.

Reconstruction

Consideration has been given to the cosmetic results of limb salvage surgery for childhood sarcomas (Womer 1996). Modern limb salvage surgery has replaced amputation and was considered as a major cosmetic, functional and psychological improvement for the patients concerned. To the present author's knowledge, there are no validated outcome measures for cosmesis following limb salvage tumour surgery. This would be particularly helpful in controversial operations such as the Van Ness rotation-plasty or fusion of major joints.

Controversy also exists in the area of complex and multiple operations for limb lengthening or correction of congenital or acquired deformity. The socio-economic and psychological implications of such treatment have been explored, but little is written on the patients' or independent observers' views on the cosmetic outcome of such treatment (Naudie et al. 1997). It is not uncommon for the salvaged limb to be severely scarred and disfigured.

Amputation

Cosmetic considerations are given to the design of prosthetic appliances for amputees. The upper limb has been given particular attention, and cosmetic gloves to cover hand prostheses have been designed for this purpose (Herder et al. 1998). Visco-elastic or silicone-based materials to cover prostheses for below-knee amputees have also been designed for better cosmesis (Prince et al. 1998; Taylor 1995). Furthermore, cosmesis was considered as one of the rehabilitation goals in a recent study on the effectiveness of rehabilitation following amputation (Kent and Fyfe 1999). Assessment of cosmesis in this clinical area was also subjective and not based on validated outcome measures.

Scars

The cosmetic appearance of surgical incision scars has been addressed in the orthopaedic literature. Arthroscopic surgery has been popular in this field, particularly in areas where open surgery leads to wide scars. Patients who underwent arthroscopic ankle arthrodesis were satisfied with their cosmetic result (Corso and Zimmer 1995). Similarly, arthroscopic stabilization of the shoulder provided a satisfactory cosmetic result (Cash 1991). A T-shape incision for exposure of the distal radius and wrist had a cosmetic result that was found to be acceptable by the majority of patients involved (Dao et al. 2000).

The cosmetic result of laceration repair has also attracted attention. Quinn et al. (1995) developed a visual-analogue cosmetic score to measure the outcome of healed lacerations. These authors went on to validate the method using four plastic surgeons (each blinded one from another) to study photographs of healed lacerations on two occasions separated by three months. The inter-observer agreement on the two occasions was 0.71 and 0.75. The same authors used their validated tool in a comparison study between the use of tissue adhesive and suture repair of lacerations (Quinn et al. 1998).

Hollander et al. (1995) also developed a wound cosmesis score using a different approach. These authors devised a six- (equally weighted) item scale where the items concerned individual components contributing to the cosmesis of a wound. The scale was validated in a pilot study of 100 patients evaluated independently by two observers, and a good inter-observer agreement was found (kappa = 0.61). The same group of investigators published an important article on the development of outcome measures using the development of their wound cosmetic score as an example (Singer et al. 2000).

The above articles show that the development of cosmetic scores is feasible with the use of either continuous (analogue) or categorical scales, though these require validation by independent observers. To the present author's knowledge, these wound cosmetic scores – together with the CSS described above – are the only objective and validated cosmetic outcome measures in the medical literature.

THE PSYCHOLOGICAL IMPACT OF IMPAIRED COSMESIS

It has been shown that spinal deformity causes a significant psychological disturbance to the majority of the patients involved (Theologis 1991; Climent *et al.* 1995). Scoliosis patients have a disturbed body image and affected psychosocial function. Likewise, cosmetic deformity may have a significant impact on psychological well-being, social integration and skills.

Patients with spina bifida were also shown to be at greater risk of depressive mood, low self-worth and suicidal ideation. Physical appearance self-concept appeared to be responsible for depressed mood in these patients (Appleton *et al.* 1997). A different study involving young women with spina bifida or rheumatoid arthritis showed a higher incidence of clinical or sub-clinical eating disorders in this population (Gross *et al.* 2000).

In a study comparing personality patterns between children with cleft lip and palate and those with orthopaedic deformity, some further psychological effects of cosmetic deformity were shown. Namely, children with musculoskeletal deformity scored high on aggression, activity level and somatization (Richman and Harper 1979).

Body image disturbance was studied in a group of plastic and reconstructive surgery patients. A significant percentage of patients reported a level of dissatisfaction and preoccupation consistent with the psychiatric diagnosis of body dysmorphic disorder. The authors suggested that patients seeking plastic surgery, even for an objective deformity, should be screened for body image dissatisfaction (Sarwer *et al.* 1998).

In conclusion, the clinical relevance of assessing and treating cosmetic deformity is based on the psychological effects of such deformity. Disturbed body image in these patients appears to be responsible for a variety of psychological disturbances that lead to poor psychosocial performance. Social acceptance and integration may represent the targets of treating cosmetic orthopaedic deformities. In the era of prioritization and clinical governance dictating choices in the provision of health services, the need for evidence-based studies in this area is evident.

CONCLUSIONS

Although cosmesis is often taken into consideration when orthopaedic treatment is planned, the role of cosmesis as one of the indications for orthopaedic treatment is rarely acknowledged and has been rarely explored in the orthopaedic literature. Further consideration of cosmetic deformity as an indication for orthopaedic treatment would be justified on the basis of its effects on body image disturbance and its psychosocial implications.

Cosmetic results of orthopaedic treatment are often presented in the literature, but these are not based on validated outcome measures. A subjective impression of cosmetic outcome may be reflected on some of the patient-based satisfaction scores. The patients involved, however, may have a disturbed body image, and this would increase the chance of these individuals expressing dissatisfaction from treatment. The need for validated cosmetic outcome measures is, therefore, evident. A few studies have shown that the development of valid analogue or categorical scales for this purpose is feasible.

REFERENCES

Appleton, P. L., Ellis, N. C., Minchom, P. E., Lawson, V., Boll, V., and Jones, P. (1997): Depressive symptoms and self-concepts in young people with spina bifida. *J Pediatr Psychol* **22**, 707–22.

Askin, G. N., Hallett, R., Hare, N., and Webb, J. K. (1997): The outcome of scoliosis surgery in the severely handicapped child. *Spine* **22**, 44–50.

Blanco-Davila, F. (2000): Beauty and the Body: the origins of cosmetics. *Plast Reconstr Surg* **105**, 1196–204.

Cash, J. D. (1991): Recent advances and perspectives on arthroscopic stabilisation of the shoulder. *Clin Sports Med* **10**, 871–86.

Climent, J. M., Reig, A., Sanchez, J., and Roda, C. (1995): Construction and validation of a specific quality of life instrument for adolescents with spine deformities. *Spine* **20**, 2006–11.

Cobb, J. R. (1948): An outline for the study of scoliosis. *Am Acad Orthop Surg Instructional Course Lectures* **5**, 261–75.

Corso, S. J., and Zimmer, T. J. (1995): Technique and clinical evaluation of arthroscopic ankle arthrodesis. *Arthroscopy* **11**, 585–90.

Dao, K. D., Shin, A. Y., and Berger, R. A. (2000): T-incision for exposure of the distal radius and wrist. *J Hand Surg* **25-B**, 544–7.

DeSmet, L., Van Ransbeeck, H., and Deneef, G. (1998): Syndactyly release: results of the Flatt technique. *Acta Orthop Belg* **64**, 301–5.

DiStasio, A. J., Dugdale, T. W., and Deafenbauch, M. K. (1993): Multiple relaxing skin incisions in orthopaedic lower extremity trauma. *J Orthop Trauma* **7**, 270–4.

Duval-Beaupere, G., and Lamireau, T. H. (1985): Scoliosis of less than 30°: properties of the evolutivity (risk of progression). *Spine* **10**, 421–4.

Fabry, G., MacEwen, G. D., and Shands, A. R. (1973): Torsion of the femur. *J Bone Joint Surg* **55-A**, 1726–38.

Fox, I. M. (1998): Treatment of brachymetatarsia by the callus distraction method. *J Foot Ankle Surg* **37**, 391–5.

Fukunishi, I. (1999): Relationship of cosmetic disfigurement to the severity of post-traumatic stress disorder in burn injury or digital amputation. *Psychother Psychosom* **68**, 82–6.

Gross, S. M., Ireys, H. T., and Kinsman, S. L. (2000): Young women with physical disabilities: risk factors for symptoms of eating disorders. *J Dev Behav Pediatr* **21**, 87–96.

Hanyu, T., Yamazaki, H., Murasawa, A., and Toyama, C. (1997): Arthroplasty for rheumatoid forefoot deformities by a shortening oblique osteotomy. *Clin Orthop* **338**, 131–8.

Hargreaves, D. G., Warwick, D. J., and Tonkin, M. A. (2000): Changes in hand function following wrist arthrodesis in cerebral palsy. *J Hand Surg* **25-B**, 193–4.

Harrington, M. E., Stevens, K., Thompson, N., O'Connor, J. J., and Theologis, T. N. (1999): Magnetic resonance imaging to customise lower limb modelling in cerebral palsy. *Gait Posture* **10**, 84–5.

Herder, J. L., Cool, J. C. and Plettenburg, D. H. (1998): Methods of reducing energy dissipation in cosmetic gloves. *J Rehabil Res Dev* **35**, 201–9.

Hollander, J. E., Singer, A. J., Valentine, S., and Henry, M. C. (1995): The wound registry: development and validation. *Ann Emerg Med* **25**, 675–85.

Holmberg, J., Lindgren, B., and Jutemark, R. (1996): Replantation-revascularisation and primary amputation in major hand injuries. *J Hand Surg* **21-B**, 576–80.

Jacob, R. P., Haertel, M., and Stussi, E. (1980): Tibial torsion calculated by computerised tomography and compared to other methods of measurement. *J Bone Joint Surg* **62-B**, 238–42.

Kent, R., and Fyfe, N. (1999): Effectiveness of rehabilitation following amputation. *Clin Rehabil* **13**, 43–50.

Koshima, I., Inagawa, K., Sahara, K., Tsuda, K., and Moriguchi, T. (1998): Flow-through vascularised toe-joint transfer for reconstruction of segmental loss of an amputated finger. *J Reconstr Microsurg* **14**, 453–7.

Moulton, A., and Upadhyay, S. S. (1982): A direct method of measuring femoral anteversion using ultrasound. *J Bone Joint Surg* **64-B**, 469–72.

Naudie, D., Hamdy, R. C., Fassier, F., Morin, B., and Duhaime, M. (1997): Management of fibular hemimelia: amputation or limb lengthening. *J Bone Joint Surg* **79-B**, 58–65.

Ong, T. G., and Low, B. Y. (1996): Supracondylar humeral fractures: a review of the outcome of treatment. *Singapore Med J* **37**, 508–11.

Press, J., Zuckerman, J. D., Gallagher, M., and Cuomo, F. (1997): Treatment of grade III acromioclavicular separations. *Bull Hosp Joint Dis* **56**, 77–83.

Prince, F., Winter, D. A., Sjonnensen, G., Powell, C., and Wheeldon, R. K. (1998): Mechanical efficiency during gait of adults with transtibial amputation: a pilot study comparing the SACH, Seattle and Golden Ankle prosthetic feet. *J Rehabil Res Dev* **35**, 177–185.

Quinn, J. V., Drzewiecki, A. E., Stiell, I. G., *et al.* (1995): Appearance scales to measure cosmetic outcomes of healed lacerations. *Am J Emerg Med* **13**, 229–31.

Quinn, J. V., Wells, G., Sutcliffe, T., Jarmuske, M., Maw, J., Stiell, I., and Johns, P. (1998): Tissue adhesive versus suture wound repair at 1 year: randomized clinical trial correlating early, 3-month and 1 year cosmetic outcome. *Ann Emerg Med* **32**, 645–9.

Richman, L. C., and Harper, D. C. (1979): Self identified personality patterns of children with facial and orthopaedic disfigurement. *Cleft Palate J* **16**, 257–61.

Rossi, W. R., and Ferreira, J. C. (1992): Chevron osteotomy for hallux valgus. *Foot Ankle* **13**, 7.

Ruwe, P. A., Gage, J. R., Ozonoff, M. B., and DeLuca, P. A. (1992): Clinical determination of femoral anteversion. *J Bone Joint Surg Am* **74-A**, 820–30.

Sarwer, D. B., Whitake, R. L. A., Pertschuk, M. J., and Wadden, T. A. (1998): Body image concerns of reconstructive surgery patients: an under-recognised problem. *Ann Plast Surg* **40**, 403–7.

Singer, A. J., Thode, H. C., and Hollander, J. E. (2000): Research fundamentals: selection and development of clinical outcome measures. *Acad Emerg Med* **7**, 397–401.

Staheli, L. T., Corbett, M., Wyss, C., and King, H. (1985): Lower extremity rotational problems in children. Normal values to guide management. *J Bone Joint Surg* **67-A**, 39–47.

Staheli, L. T., Chew, D. E., and Corbett, M. (1987): The longitudinal arch. *J Bone Joint Surg* **69-A**, 426–8.

Takakura, Y., Tanaka, Y., Fujii, T., and Tamai, S. (1997): Lengthening of short great toes by callus distraction. *J Bone Joint Surg* **79-B**, 955–8.

Taylor, B. S. S. (1995): Clinical evaluation of the Franklin Applied Physics Cosmetic Cover for lower limb prostheses: a preliminary report. *J Rehabil Res Dev* **32**, 74–8.

Theologis, T. N. (1991): *Quantification of the Cosmetic Effects of Adolescent Idiopathic Scoliosis using the ISIS Scan*. M.Sc. Thesis, Oxford.

Theologis, T. N., and Fairbank, J. C. T. (1997): Deformity and cosmesis of the spine. In: Pynsent, P. B., Fairbank, J. C. T., and Carr, A. J. (eds), *Orthopaedic Methodology*. Butterworth Heinemann, Oxford, pp. 199–214.

Theologis, T. N., Jefferson, R. J., Simpson, A. H. R. W., Turner-Smith, A. R., and Fairbank, J. C. T. (1993): Quantifying the cosmetic defect of adolescent idiopathic scoliosis. *Spine* **18**, 909–12.

Theologis, T. N., Fairbank, J. C. T., Turner-Smith, A. R., and Pantazopoulos, T. (1997): Early detection of progression in adolescent idiopathic scoliosis by measurement of changes in back shape with the Integrated Shape Imaging System scanner. *Spine* **22**, 1223–7.

Thometz, J. G., Lamdan, R., Liu, X. C., and Lyon, R. (2000): Relationship between Quantec measurement and Cobb angle in patients with idiopathic scoliosis. *J Pediatr Orthop* **20**, 512–16.

Wenger, D. R., and Rang, M. (1993): *The Art and Practice of Children's Orthopaedics*. Raven Press, New York.

Womer, R. B. (1996): Problems and controversies in the management of childhood sarcomas. *Br Med Bull* **52**, 826–43.

Wood, V. E., Peppers, T. A., and Shook, J. (1997): Cleft foot closure: a simplified technique and review of the literature. *J Pediatr Orthop* **17**, 501–4.

12

Growth plate injuries
D. M. Eastwood

Fractures in childhood are common. Although the physis is the weakest link in the immature skeleton, only 18 per cent of bony injuries actually involve the growth plate (Mizuta *et al.* 1987). Physeal injuries are considered to have a favourable outcome, 'healing quickly' and 'remodelling with time'; nevertheless, any surgeon involved with such cases is fully aware that joint incongruity and premature growth arrest do occur. Some authors believe that these dreaded complications are predictable and, under certain circumstances, are preventable (Salter and Harris 1963). However, before an outcome can be so assured, a sound understanding of the pathological anatomy is required.

APPLIED ANATOMY OF THE GROWTH PLATE

The structure and strength of the physis and surrounding tissues change with growth. Similarly, the effects of trauma to this region can – and do – vary with age. The immature skeleton consists of two types of growth plate or physis:

- The *pressure physis*: this lies at right-angles to the long axis of the bone, joining epiphysis to metaphysis. It is normally subjected to compression forces and is responsible for longitudinal bone growth.

- The *traction physis*: this links the apophysis (with its major muscle attachments) to the bone shaft. It does not usually lie perpendicular to the long axis of the bone. By exerting tension on the physis, the muscles shape the apophysis and the bone itself.

Histologically, both physes consist of four main layers: the germinal layer; the proliferative zone; the hypertrophic zone; and the zone of transformation. The perichondrial ring, which is contiguous with the articular cartilage and receives the metaphyseal periosteum, surrounds the physis. The ring plays a critical role in the structural integrity of the immature bone and, by contributing cells to the germinal layer of the physis, it is partly responsible for latitudinal bone growth.

The growth plate itself is devoid of vascular channels. It receives nutrition from three sources. Epiphyseal vessels nourish the germinal cells. Damage to these vessels causes irreparable alteration to the physeal growth potential. The periosteal vasculature supplies the perichondrial ring and the peripheral physis. The nutrient artery feeds the metaphyseal side of the central 75 per cent of the physis. Vascular damage slows the transformation of cartilage to bone, leading to temporary widening of the affected physis (Ogden *et al.* 1996).

The physis interdigitates with the metaphysis, and the resistance to transverse or shear stresses is enhanced by this increased contact area. Early descriptions of growth plate injuries included a plane of cleavage through the junctional zone of the physis where there is chondrocyte hypertrophy. The germinal cells responsible for bone growth remained with the epiphysis, their fate being decided by the state of the epiphyseal vasculature. More recent pathological and radiological evidence suggests that in over 50 per cent of cases the cleavage plane may traverse any zone of the plate (Jaramillo *et al.* 2000) accounting, perhaps, for some of the seemingly unpredictable growth disturbances noted in the past. This variation in fracture line propagation occurs particularly in adolescent patients, as distinct from infants (Jaramillo *et al.* 2000), and in sites where the physis undulates (Bright *et al.* 1974).

ASSESSMENT OF PHYSEAL INJURY

Classification

Several general systems for classifying growth plate injuries have been proposed. Poland was one of the first to propose a classification by defining four broad categories of separation based on the anatomical features of injury (cited in Petersen 1996). As radiographic imaging improved, further injury patterns were identified and modifications to Poland's classification were made.

Aitken (1965) described three fracture types. He felt that deformity secondary to malunion or growth disturbance was rare, but emphasized that a compression injury could lead to major growth problems. The system described by Weber (1980) was based on fracture line propagation and helped the clinician to distinguish fractures which had a good prognosis and could be treated closed, from those with a poorer prognosis that required operative treatment.

The Salter-Harris (Salter and Harris 1963) classification has gained the most widespread acceptance (Fig. 12.1). This system is based on the mechanism of injury, the relationship of the fracture line to the germinal cells of the physis and outcome as regards growth disturbance. In general, fracture types I, II, and III had a good prognosis for growth, whilst types IV and V did not. Rang (cited in Weber 1980) extended the Salter-Harris classification by describing a type VI injury with localized damage to the perichondrial ring and a significant risk of growth disturbance (Fig. 12.1).

Most recently, Petersen *et al.* (1994) developed a classification based on an epidemiological review of almost 1000 injuries over a 10-year period

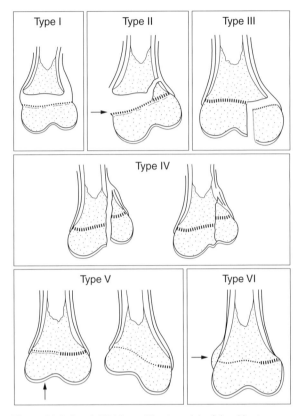

Figure 12.1 Rang's (1969) modification of the Salter-Harris (1963) classification of epiphyseal injuries. Adapted from Weber (1980).

(Fig. 12.2). Six specific fracture types are described, five of which corresponded closely to five in the extended Salter-Harris classification system (Petersen 1994a, b). The Petersen classification has an anatomical basis depicting physeal injury as a continuum from relatively minor involvement of the physis (type I) through complete transphyseal involvement (type III) to longitudinal disruption of the physis with or without loss of a fragment of physeal plate (types V or VI). This concept of progressive physeal damage led Petersen (1994a) to subdivide the type II injury depending on the size of the metaphyseal fragment. The larger the fragment, the less the physeal damage.

Both the Salter-Harris (Salter and Harris 1963) and the Petersen (1994b) systems are concise and are useful clinically. However, certain injury patterns such as the distal tibial triplane fracture are still not readily accommodated by such systems. Ogden (1981)

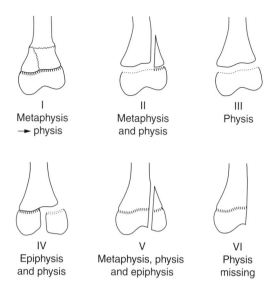

Figure 12.2 Petersen's (1994b) classification of physeal injuries.

I
Metaphysis
→ physis

II
Metaphysis
and physis

III
Physis

IV
Epiphysis
and physis

V
Metaphysis, physis
and epiphysis

VI
Physis
missing

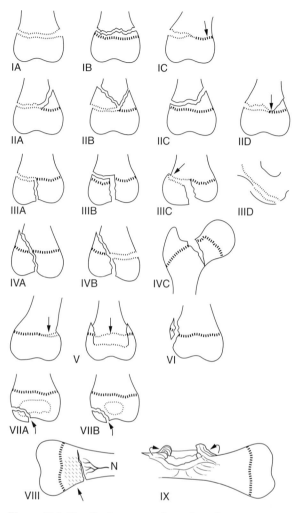

Figure 12.3 Classification system of growth mechanism injuries according to Ogden (1981).

expanded the basic Salter-Harris system to define specific subgroups that he felt explained the increasingly recognized but 'unexpected' cases of growth disturbance. His system also describes additional fracture patterns (types VII, VIII and IX) that affect areas of the growth mechanism outside the physeal plate (Fig. 12.3).

Imaging techniques

PLAIN RADIOGRAPHS

The assessment of growth plate injuries poses particular problems as the physis itself is radiolucent. Nevertheless, plain radiography remains the most important imaging tool. It is always essential that radiographs are of good quality and that two views taken at 90° to each other are obtained. Not all injuries to the developing skeleton are easily seen on standard views, and 15–20 per cent of fractures may only be evident on oblique films (Petersen 1994a; Rogers 1970). Occasionally, the actual fracture line may never be discerned. Whenever possible, radiographs should be taken perpendicular to the physis, and equivalent views of the contralateral physis may be required for comparison. Accurate interpretation of these radiographs is a prerequisite for application of all the classification systems.

When assessing an injured child, it is important to suspect physeal injury and to understand where the weak points lie in an immature skeleton. A child with a lax knee secondary to trauma is more likely to have a physeal injury than a collateral ligament rupture (Skak *et al.* 1987). The physeal injury may not be apparent on plain radiographs, but stress views or other imaging techniques (e.g. magnetic resonance imaging; MRI) will define the problem (Close and Strouse 2000). If a collateral ligament injury has occurred it is usually an avulsion fracture of the proximal insertion. This is an injury which damages the perichondrial ring and is associated with growth disturbance (Hresko and Kasser 1989). Careful analysis of plain films may show small lamellar fragments of bone within the physis, indicating that the fracture line has violated at least part of the zone of provisional calcification.

In selected cases, modalities such as hypocycloidal tomograms (rather than linear tomograms) may be helpful in defining the plane of injury and the fracture fragments.

OTHER TECHNIQUES

Arthrography (Yates and Sullivan 1987) has been of some value in young children with elbow injuries, while *ultrasonography* has the advantage of not using ionizing radiation. The important radiolucent structures of the physis and the unossified portion of the epiphysis are more readily visible – this is useful in evaluating birth injuries (Dias *et al.* 1988). Both of these techniques are currently being superseded by MRI (Anderson *et al.* 1998; Carey *et al.* 1998; Close and Strouse 2000; Lohman *et al.* 2001), which affords excellent visualization of cartilaginous structures. Imaging takes time, and sedation or a general anaesthetic may be required in the young child. When possible, the plane of imaging should correlate with the plane of the physis, and the choice of sequences depends on whether a bony or cartilaginous injury predominates. Displaced fractures are easier to visualize (Jaramillo *et al.* 2000), but the clinical value may lie in identifying non-displaced fractures (Close and Strouse 2000).

Although MRI cannot specifically identify individual physeal layers, it can demonstrate fracture lines which are juxta-epiphyseal (with fracture through the germinal or proliferative zones), central or juxta-metaphyseal (hypertrophic zone) (Smith *et al.* 1994; Jaramillo *et al.* 2000). In animal studies following controlled fractures of the distal femur, 11 of 14 fracture lines became juxta-epiphyseal compared with seven of 14 similar fractures in the proximal tibia (Jaramillo *et al.* 2000). The juxta-epiphyseal damage was central in the distal femur and smaller and more variable in site in the proximal tibia.

The value of MRI probably varies with the site of injury, and authors disagree as to whether the MRI appearances affect clinical management (Close and Strouse 2000; Carey *et al.* 1998; Lohman *et al.*

2001). The plain-film diagnosis of fracture type may change on MRI – commonly a Salter-Harris type III injury becomes a type IV.

Clinical factors

In all patients, taking a full history and conducting a complete clinical examination is essential. A detailed account of the mechanism of injury – including the force involved – will help to assess the severity of physeal damage. It must be remembered that physeal injury may be due to repetitive stress (Tolat *et al.* 1992; Caine *et al.* 1997) or to many other aetiologies (Petersen 1996).

EARLY ASSESSMENT OF OUTCOME

Once the injury has been defined, its likely outcome can be determined, and suitable parameters for measuring this can be identified. In certain respects the outcome measures for growth plate injuries should not differ greatly from those used to assess other skeletal injuries, and factors such as fracture union and malunion, range of movement and deformity should be measured (c.f. Chapter 20). However, each of these will be influenced by growth of the immature skeleton and by the child's unique capability of adapting to handicap. Functional health questionnaires and assessments are unhelpful in this group of children (Haynes and Sullivan 2001).

Fracture union

Fracture union is usually assessed both clinically and radiologically. Radiological union is difficult to define when fracture lines involve radiolucent plates, and hence its value as an outcome measure is limited. Growth plate injuries unite rapidly, but clinical assessment of fracture union is considered to be too subjective to be of scientific value (Radford 1993).

Objective techniques such as those evaluating fracture stiffness are now more available and more reliable, but may not be easily applicable to a child with a growth plate injury (c.f. Chapter 20). The non-union of a fracture following injury to a compression physis is extremely rare (Beekman and Sullivan 1941).

Malunion

There are no generally accepted criteria for measuring the cosmetic, functional or psychological effects of residual deformity. In the child, functional hindrance following malunion is rare; minor angulatory deformity should remodel with growth, provided that the growth plate has not been damaged. Angular deformity in excess of 20° will probably not correct, especially if the angulation is not in the axis of movement of the adjacent joint (Evans 1990). Similarly, rotational abnormalities do not correct spontaneously. Remodelling is not a reliable phenomenon and there must be at least two years of growth remaining (estimated by skeletal age rather than chronological age) if significant correction is to be achieved (Ogden et al. 1996). Radiographic evaluation of deformity may be useful in an individual case to assess progress with time, but as an outcome measure it is impracticable. The deformity is rarely maximal in the standard radiographic planes and is essentially unique to each case.

Joint incongruity may complicate physeal injuries that involve the articular surface. It will not remodel with time and indeed may progress if growth has been disrupted. The development of osteoarthritis, secondary to joint incongruity, may be used as an outcome measure for growth plate injuries. Very few long-term follow-up studies of growth plate injuries addressing this issue have been conducted, and most of these reports have many deficiencies (Caterini et al. 1991a, b).

Joint movement

Joint stiffness is an important outcome measure following adult trauma. In the child, post-traumatic stiffness is uncommon unless there is direct damage to a joint. Subjective complaints of stiffness are extremely unusual, and restricted movements at one joint are often compensated for by improved movement in adjacent joints.

Symptoms

Few published data exist on the subject of symptoms following skeletal injury in children, and the evidence to support any objective assessment of such symptoms is sparse. Pain assessment in children has been documented (McGrath 1989; McGrath et al. 1986), but evaluating persistent discomfort – as distinct from pain – is more difficult (c.f. Chapter 7). A review of 281 wrist injuries by Fodden (1992) showed that at three years after injury, seven patients complained of symptoms such as aching, crepitus and weakness. In this study, all three patients with premature physeal fusion were symptomatic, although only one patient had a recognized physeal injury. In contrast, in a study of distal ulnar physeal injuries the majority of patients were asymptomatic, even with significant growth arrest (Golz et al. 1991). It seems unlikely that the presence or absence of symptoms could be used as anything more than a very general measure of outcome. Complex regional pain syndromes are infrequent in childhood, and trauma is the precipitating factor in only 50 per cent of cases.

LATE ASSESSMENT OF OUTCOME

Skeletal injury in childhood, particularly when the physis is involved, may result in disturbance of the growth mechanism. In this respect, the outcome following fracture differs considerably from injuries in adults, and hence a unique form of measurement is required.

Growth disturbance

The most feared (but uncommon) outcome of physeal injury is growth retardation with formation of a bone bridge across the physis. The most likely outcome is restoration of normal anatomy with a normal growth potential. The reported risk of growth disturbance following physeal injury is from 1.4 to 33 per cent (Mizuta *et al.* 1987; Smith 1924), with significant clinical effects complicating between 0.6 and 10 per cent of cases (Mizuta *et al.* 1987; Rogers 1970). This wide variation reflects the lack of adequate studies that follow *all* physeal injuries to skeletal maturity, and the problems of identifying growth arrest and defining what is 'significant growth disturbance'. Recognition of growth arrest requires a high index of suspicion. Complete physeal closure is usually well seen on plain radiographs, but the identification of a partial growth arrest and the underlying bony bar is not always straightforward. Careful attention must be paid to the siting and orientation of the radiographs, and both the epiphysis and the metaphysis must be scrutinized for evidence of disordered bone growth.

HARRIS LINES

These metaphyseal lines (Harris 1926) often appear after trauma (Siffert and Katz 1983; Ogden 1984). A line parallel to the physeal contour indicates that bone growth has resumed and the risk of significant physeal damage is minimal. If the lines are present in both limbs, the rates of growth can be compared and matched with expected growth rates. If the metaphyseal line and the physis converge, then eccentric physeal damage has occurred and a bony bar or physeal bridge has formed. Harris lines are most obvious in regions of rapid growth such as the distal femur and the proximal tibia, but are of doubtful value as an outcome measure. In fact, they are much less visible in areas of slow growth, except for specific injuries about the knee and perhaps the ankle. The resolution and visualization of arrest lines is significantly better on MRI than on plain films (Futami *et al.* 2000).

It is important to identify growth arrest early. If plain radiographs leave any doubt as to whether or not physeal damage exists, then additional imaging techniques should be employed. In order to plan further treatment appropriately, a map of the location, size and contour of the bar must be made (Carlson and Wenger 1984). Traditionally, this has been

drawn with the help of multiplanar tomograms – the mapping process takes time and is subject to interpretation, it also has a high radiation exposure. Helical CT scans allow rapid acquisition of data, for a lower radiation exposure and the ability to reconstruct the images in any plane (Loder *et al.* 1997); moreover, they are useful for delineating mature bars. More recently, MRI has been used to delineate the bone bridge. Disturbances of growth can be identified within a few weeks of injury (Jaramillo *et al.* 1990; Ogden *et al.* 1996; Futami *et al.* 2000), although the exact mechanism by which a bony bar develops has yet to be fully understood (Lee *et al.* 2000).

Occasionally, the only method of identifying physeal closure is by assessing its overall effect on bone growth. This gives an indirect measure. The measurement of limb length discrepancy remains a problem, and clinical methods may still be as accurate as radiological methods (Eastwood and Cole 1995).

Classification of growth arrest

The following classification system relates growth arrest to outcome and treatment options.

COMPLETE GROWTH ARREST

Complete growth arrest is uncommon, but it usually leads to a progressive limb length discrepancy (Shapiro 1982). The clinical effect of this depends on the age at which the arrest occurs, the growth potential of the particular physis involved, and whether the involved bone is part of a paired unit. There are some suggestions that loss of growth from one physis will be partially compensated for by accelerated growth from the plate at the opposite end of the bone (Petersen 1996). Shapiro's study (Shapiro 1982) has clearly shown that no such tendency occurs.

PARTIAL GROWTH ARREST

Partial growth arrest with bone bridge formation is more common. The size and location of the physeal tether determine the clinical deformity, while

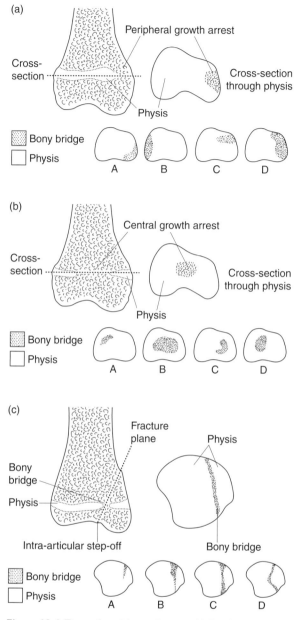

Figure 12.4 Types of partial growth arrest. (a) Peripheral; (b) central; and (c) linear. Adapted from Petersen (1996).

descriptive terms:

- *Peripheral*: this type of partial arrest may result in progressive limb-length discrepancy, but more commonly it is associated with an increasing angulatory deformity.

- *Central*: a central partial arrest is less common and, radiographically, is manifested as a tenting of the physis as the peripheral plate continues to grow. Overall, longitudinal growth may be significantly restricted but angulatory deformity is unusual. Significant incongruity may develop at the joint secondary to distortion of the physis and the epiphysis.

- *Linear*: this subgroup is secondary to a malunion of the Petersen type IV or V (Salter-Harris III or IV) fracture, and again is associated with incongruity of the articular margin.

Occasionally, small bone tethers may be overcome by the forces within the physis, but once a substantial tether has developed, then the progression of deformity has an almost linear relationship with time (Osterman 1972). If damage occurs when the ossification centre is very small, the bone bridge may not form until the ossific nucleus expands to oppose the area of physeal damage. In such instances, there will be a considerable delay before radiological or clinical deformity is apparent. However, it may then progress rapidly. Bony bars occupying more than 50 per cent of the physis are not usually amenable to surgical intervention (Petersen 1996).

Although growth retardation following physeal injury causes most concern, growth acceleration may also occur. A fracture adjacent to a physis is known to stimulate growth (Shapiro 1981; Taylor *et al.* 1987), although the effect is usually only detectable for the first year post-injury. Physeal injury itself may accelerate growth, but the hyperaemic response to injury is short – as is the subsequent growth disturbance – and the result is rarely of clinical significance. Metallic implants used in the internal fixation of some fractures act as a chronic stimulus for accelerated longitudinal growth in experimental animals (Wilson 1970; Castle 1971), but the relevance of this in man has not been addressed fully.

the age at injury and potential growth remaining define the ultimate severity. Both Bright and Ogden have classified partial growth arrests into three types. Unfortunately, they used the numbers 1 to 3 in opposite directions (Petersen 1996) (Fig. 12.4). It is preferable therefore to use the following

VARIABLES THAT MAY AFFECT OUTCOME

The measures discussed above assess early and late outcome following physeal injury. However, the outcome of any individual injury is highly dependent on a number of variables.

Severity of injury

Overall, as with all injuries, the more severe the damage the poorer the outcome. In the commonly used classification systems, injuries associated with an open wound, significant soft tissue damage or comminution are associated with ascending fracture type and are more likely to be complicated by infection or bone bridge formation. Fracture outcome is often related to initial displacement – thus, the greater the initial displacement the worse the eventual outcome, even if the reduction is satisfactory, though with respect to physeal injuries few data exist to support such beliefs. One report commenting on injuries to the proximal femur considered that the severity of the initial displacement was of more prognostic value in children and adolescents than in infants (Caterini et al. 1991a). Certainly, in injuries involving intra-articular epiphyses, severe displacement is associated with a high risk of avascular necrosis and growth plate arrest (Dale and Harris 1958).

Mechanism of injury

Whilst the Salter-Harris classification (Salter and Harris 1963) was based partially on mechanism of injury and detailed the shearing, avulsion, splitting and crushing elements which could affect the physis, an understanding of the degree of force applied and how the growing skeleton reacts to it is also required (Riseborough et al. 1983). In the adolescent age group the periosteal/perichondrial sheath, in thickness and in strength, resembles that of the adult, and the force required to disrupt the physis is relatively less than that needed to rupture the thicker sheath in the younger child (Riseborough et al. 1983). Considerable force is required to fracture physes such as those of the distal ulna and metacarpal heads, and this may account for the high incidence of growth disturbance (Golz et al. 1991; Light and Ogden 1987). On occasion, the applied force is sufficient to cause physeal damage without disrupting the periosteum. A history of a glancing blow to a subcutaneous physis such as that of the distal tibia may increase suspicion of a perichondrial injury and encourage patient follow-up. Similarly, repetitive application of subcritical forces may result in fatigue failure of the physis (Caine et al. 1997).

Age

The younger the child is when the growth plate injury occurs, the greater is the potential effect of the injury on growth. However, the peak age for physeal injury is 12 years, and by this age many physes have only a limited growth potential. The fracture types most associated with growth disturbance are more common in the adolescent patient (Petersen et al. 1994). The size of the physis, its contour and its rate of growth all change with increasing age, and each of these factors may influence outcome. The size of the growth arrest does not increase with time, but the size of the unaffected physis does; thus, a growth arrest affecting 50 per cent of the physis of a two-year-old child will represent a smaller proportion of the physis in the same child aged 10 years.

Site

Extra-articular epiphyses derive their blood supply from soft tissue attachments remote from the physis, whilst intra-articular epiphyses such as those of the proximal femur and the proximal radius are supplied by vessels arising from the periosteal vasculature which penetrate the periphery of the physis (Dale and Harris 1958). These vessels are often damaged when epiphyseal displacement occurs, and growth disturbance is more common when this type of physis is injured.

The growth potential of physes vary considerably; thus, 70 per cent of femoral length arises from the distal physis, whereas 80 per cent of humeral length derives from the proximal physis. Injuries to the proximal tibia and distal femur represent only 3 per cent of injuries (Petersen 1996; Ogden 1981), but they are among the sites most frequently complicated by physeal arrest and significant clinical problems. The distal radius is the most frequently injured physis and yet growth disturbance at this site has been regarded as extremely uncommon. Recent studies, however, suggest that if these injuries are followed closely to maturity and their outcome evaluated carefully, a higher incidence of 'problems' such as a change in ulnar variance may be identified (Golz et al. 1991; Fodden 1992). Physeal damage leading to limb-length discrepancy is more likely to be of clinical significance in the lower limb than the upper limb.

Certain physes are subjected to particular stresses and develop an undulating structure. Fracture lines through these physes are more likely to cross through various layers of the plate, increasing the risk of damage to the germinal cell layer (Jaramillo et al. 2000; Alexander 1976).

Fracture type

Many fracture classifications have attempted to link outcome with fracture type and although popular, the Salter-Harris system (Salter and Harris 1963) has been only partially successful in this respect. Petersen's classification (Petersen 1994b) is more useful, with both the need for immediate and delayed surgery increasing with increasing physeal damage and ascending fracture type:

- Petersen Type I: Essentially a metaphyseal fracture with extension towards the physis. The obvious damage to the physis is minimal. It is usually due to compression forces and premature physeal closure has been noted.

- Petersen Type II (Salter-Harris Type II): Classically, this is the most common type of physeal injury identified, and accounts for 53–75 per cent of cases (Rogers 1970; Oh et al. 1974; Petersen 1994b). It is considered a 'safe' physeal injury, and reduction is usually both easy to obtain and maintain. However, increasingly, complications have been recognized (Light and Ogden 1987; Fodden 1992), particularly in the irregular physes (Riseborough et al. 1983; Berson et al. 2000; Jaramillo et al. 2000).

- Petersen Type III (Salter-Harris Type I): This injury accounts for between 6 and 26 per cent of cases (Rogers 1970; Oh et al. 1974) and is truly a 'fracture' through cartilage alone. If the plane of cleavage is through the junctional zone of the physis, the outcome should be excellent unless the epiphysis is intra-articular. It commonly occurs as a birth injury or in the younger child, and is frequently over-diagnosed on assessment of a tender lateral malleolus (Petersen 1994b; Lohman et al. 2001).

- Petersen Type IV (Salter-Harris Type III): This fracture accounts for 6–10 per cent of cases (Rogers 1970; Mizuta et al. 1987), most commonly towards the end of growth. In order to re-establish joint congruity an operative approach is often needed. The outcome will be good, assuming that the physis is not further damaged or rendered avascular by soft tissue stripping during surgery. Growth arrest is common, but usually complete.

- Petersen Type V (Salter-Harris Type IV): Between 6 and 10 per cent of fractures fall into this category (Mizuta et al. 1987; Petersen 1994b). Fractures are frequently comminuted and often open. Premature growth arrest is common (partial, linear), even when an open approach has achieved an anatomical reduction.

- Petersen Type VI (Salter-Harris Type VI): These rare injuries are often open. If a 'part is missing', as described by Petersen (1994a), then the physeal damage is obvious and a significant growth problem can be expected. These cases may be suitable for the anticipatory Langenskiold procedure recently reported by Foster *et al.* (2000). Sometimes the diagnosis is made in retrospect after a glancing blow to a subcutaneous physis or when a small avulsion fracture involving the perichondrial ring was 'missed'. Angular deformity can develop rapidly.

- Salter-Harris Type V: Theoretically, this is a compression injury to the physis that is severe enough to damage the growth potential of the germinal cells, but not severe enough to break any bony trabeculae. Controversy therefore exists as to whether or not this injury actually exists and, if it does, what the exact aetiology is (Keret *et al.* 1990; Petersen 1994b). Several authors have commented on eccentric or unexpected growth disturbances following trauma to non-physeal areas of the bone (Pappas and Toczylowski 1984; Petersen 1994b). Perhaps if appropriate oblique radiographs had been taken at the time of injury, extensions of the fracture line towards the physis might have been identified – the Petersen type I fracture has a low but recognized complication of growth arrest secondary to compression forces. The idea that an 'element' of a type V injury accounts for unexpected poor outcomes following other injuries is outdated. A better understanding of the pathology of physeal injury both histologically and on MRI shows that the original injury can be underestimated (Smith *et al.* 1994; Jaramillo *et al.* 2000).

Treatment

It is important to differentiate between outcome of the injury alone and outcome of the injury combined with its treatment. During a forceful manipulation, bone spikes may damage the germinal layer of the physis. Similarly, overzealous clearing of the soft tissues during an operative approach should be avoided. Direct instrument pressure on the physis and penetration of the physis by wires or screws should be minimized (Petersen 1996).

Fracture outcome is related to adequacy of reduction, which in turn may be related to severity of initial displacement, although figures relevant to growth plate injuries are difficult to find (Lombardo and Harvey 1977; Caterini *et al.* 1991a, b; Petersen *et al.* 1994). Treatment timing is also an important factor. Physeal injuries heal rapidly, and delayed primary treatment or repeated attempts to improve outcome must be judged in this light.

In certain acute physeal injuries where significant growth arrest is anticipated, the damaged area of physeal plate could be excised and the defect filled with an interpositional graft (Bright *et al.* 1974; Foster *et al.* 2000).

APOPHYSEAL INJURIES

Acute injuries to the apophyseal physis are usually caused by a sudden major muscular contraction that disrupts the integrity of the bone–physis–tendon unit. Cleavage through the growth plate is more likely to occur than tendon avulsion. The physeal vascular supply, via muscular attachments to the apophysis, is usually maintained. The exact plane of cleavage through the apophyseal physis has not been documented histologically. It has been suggested that stress fractures similar to a Petersen type IV (Salter-Harris III) or an Ogden type VII may occur and lead to an apophysitis. There is increasing evidence that the development of an apophysitis predisposes the patient to an avulsion fracture (Ogden *et al.* 1980; Merloz *et al.* 1987; Kujala *et al.* 1997).

The outcome of apophyseal plate injuries is dependent on the displacement of the apophysis and its muscular attachments. If this displacement is significant (>1–2 cm), healing often occurs with abundant callus formation and there may be a measurable reduction in muscle strength. Thus, both functionally and cosmetically, the outcome may be less than satisfactory. Non-union does occur.

Formal grading of muscle strength could be used as an objective measure of outcome in both the short- and long-term follow-up of apophyseal injuries. An alternative outcome measure is physeal arrest. Closure of the physis is common whether the injury is treated operatively, or not. If the injury occurs at an early age, then considerable disturbance of bone shape may develop, although the exact significance of this is unknown. Most commonly, these injuries occur as the physis is undergoing physiological closure, and thus growth disturbance is not a significant problem (Ogden *et al.* 1980). Patients such as elite female gymnasts appear to be at particular risk for this type of injury (Rossi and Dragoni 2001).

SUMMARY

Clear definition of an injury is required before outcome can be predicted and then measured. Whilst the Salter-Harris classification is still popular, the Petersen system has much to recommend it, and its anatomic basis of a continuum of injury is attractive for prediction of outcome. Over recent years, MRI has improved our understanding of the pathoanatomy of both physeal fractures and the subsequent growth disturbances. As a *predictive* assessment of outcome, MRI evaluation should now be considered in cases where the risk of growth disturbance is high, including young children with extensive residual growth potential, those with particularly vulnerable growth plates, and those with complex injuries.

There are few reliable, objective or appropriate measures for assessing outcome of growth plate injuries, but the identification of growth disturbance is perhaps the best available. For *process* and *endpoint* outcome assessment, careful radiographic review is essential, but MRI has a role in the early assessment of high-risk injuries to delineate the nature and extent of the physeal arrest.

Ideally, a stage will be reached when the problem can be so well defined at presentation that the 'inevitable' growth arrest can be predicted accurately and appropriate anticipatory (rather than salvage) surgery performed (Lee *et al.* 1998; Foster *et al.* 2000).

REFERENCES

Aitken, A. P. (1965): Fractures of the epiphysis. *Clin Orthop* **41**, 19–23.

Alexander, C. J. (1976): Effect of growth rate on the strength of the growth plate-shaft junction. *Skeletal Radiol* **1**, 67–76.

Anderson, S. E., Otsuka, N. Y., and Steinbach, L. S. (1998): MR imaging of paediatric elbow trauma. *Musculoskeletal Radiol Semin* **2**, 185–98.

Beekman, F., and Sullivan, J. (1941): Some observations of fractures of long bones in the child. *Am J Surg* **51**, 722.

Berson, L., Davidson, R. S., Dormans, J. P., Drummond, D. S., and Gregg, J. R. (2000): Growth disturbances after distal tibial physeal fractures. *Foot Ankle Int* **21**, 54–8.

Bright, R. W., Burstein, A. H., and Elmore, S. M. (1974): Epiphyseal-plate cartilage. A biomechanical and histological analysis of failure modes. *J Bone Joint Surg* **56-A**, 688–703.

Caine, D., Howe, W., Ross, W., and Bergman, G. (1997): Does repetitive physical loading inhibit radial growth in female gymnasts? *Clin J Sports Med* **7**, 302–8.

Carey, J., Spence, L., Blickman, H., and Eustace, S. (1998): MRI of paediatric growth plate injuries – correlation with plain film radiographs and clinical outcome. *Skeletal Radiol* **27**, 250–5.

Carlson, W. O., and Wenger, D. R. (1984): A mapping method to prepare for surgical excision of a partial physeal arrest. *J Pediatr Orthop* **4**, 232–8.

Castle, M. E. (1971): Epiphyseal stimulation. *J Bone Joint Surg* **53-A**, 326–34.

Caterini, R., Farsetti, P., d'Arrigo, C., and Ippolito, E. (1991a): Unusual physeal lesions of the lower limb. A report of 16 cases with very long follow-up observation. *J Orthop Trauma* **5**, 38–46.

Caterini, R., Farsetti, P., and Ippolito, E. (1991b): Long term follow-up of physeal injury to the ankle. *Foot Ankle* **11**, 372–83.

Close, B. J., and Strouse, P. J. (2000): MR of physeal fractures of the adolescent knee. *Pediatr Radiol* **30**, 756–62.

Dale, G. G., and Harris, W. M. (1958): Prognosis of epiphyseal separation. *J Bone Joint Surg* **40-B**, 117–22.

Dias, J. J., Lamont, A. C., and Jones, J. M. (1988): Ultrasonic diagnosis of neonatal separation of the distal humeral epiphysis. *J Bone Joint Surg* **70-B**, 825–8.

Eastwood, D. M., and Cole, W. G. (1995): A graphic method for timing the correction of leg-length discrepancy. *J Bone Joint Surg* **77-B**, 743–7.

Evans, G. (1990): Management of disordered growth following physeal injury. *Injury* **21**, 329–33.

Fodden, D. I. (1992): A study of wrist injuries in children: the incidence of various injuries and of premature closure of the distal radial growth plate. *Arch Emerg Med* **9**, 9–13.

Foster, B. K., John, B., and Hasler, C. (2000): Free fat interpositional graft in acute physeal injuries: the anticipatory Langenskiold procedure. *J Pediatr Orthop* **20**, 282–5.

Futami, T., Foster, B. K., Morris, L. L., and Le Quesne, G. W. (2000): Magnetic resonance imaging of growth plate injuries: the efficacy and indications for surgical procedures. *Arch Orthop Trauma Surg* **120**, 390–6.

Golz, R. J., Grogan, D. P., Greene, T. L., Belsole, R. J., and Ogden, J. A. (1991): Distal ulnar physeal injury. *J Pediatr Orthop* **11**, 318–26.

Harris, H. A. (1926): The growth of long bones in childhood with special reference to certain bony striations of the metaphysis and to the role of vitamins. *Arch Intern Med* **38**, 785–93.

Haynes, R. J., and Sullivan, E. (2001): The Paediatric Orthopaedic Society of North America Paediatric Orthopaedic Functional Health Questionnaire: an analysis of normals. *J Pediatr Orthop* **21**, 619–21.

Hresko, M. T., and Kasser, J. R. (1989): Physeal arrest about the knee associated with non-physeal fractures in the lower extremity. *J Bone Joint Surg* **71-A**, 698–703.

Jaramillo, D., Shapiro, F., Hoffer, F. A., Winalski, C. S., Koskinen, M. F., Frasso, R., and Johnson, A. (1990): Post-traumatic growth-plate abnormalities: MR imaging of bony-bridge formation in rabbits. *Radiology* **175**, 767–73.

Jaramillo, D., Kammen, B. F., and Shapiro, F. (2000): Cartilaginous pathology of physeal fracture separations: evaluation with MR imaging – an experimental study with histological correlation in rabbits. *Radiology* **215**, 504–11.

Keret, D., Mendez, A. A., Harcke, H. T., and MacEwen, G. D. (1990): Type V physeal injury: a case report. *J Pediatr Orthop* **10**, 545–8.

Kujala, U. M., Orava, S., Karpakka, J., Leppavuori, J., and Mattila, K. (1997): Ischial tuberosity apophysitis and avulsion among athletes. *Int J Sports Med* **18**, 149–55.

Lee, E. H., Chen, F., Dhan, J., and Bose, K. (1998): Treatment of growth arrest by transfer of cultured chondrocytes into physeal defects. *J Pediatr Orthop* **18**, 155–60.

Lee, M. A., Nissen, T. P., and Otsuka, N. Y. (2000): Utilization of a murine model to investigate the molecular process of transphyseal bone formation. *J Pediatr Orthop* **20**, 802–6.

Light, T. R., and Ogden, J. A. (1987): Metacarpal epiphyseal fractures. *J Hand Surg* **12A**, 460–4.

Loder, R. T., Swinford, A. E., and Kuhns, L. R. (1997): The use of helical computed tomographic scans to assess bony physeal bars. *J Pediatr Orthop* **17**, 356–9.

Lohman, M., Kivisaari, A., Kallio, P., Puntila, J., Vehmas, T., and Kivisaari, L. (2001): Acute paediatric ankle trauma: MRI versus plain radiography. *Skeletal Radiol* **30**, 504–11.

Lombardo, S. J., and Harvey, J. J. P. (1977): Fractures of the distal femoral epiphyses. Factors influencing prognosis: a review of 34 cases. *J Bone Joint Surg* **59-A**, 742–51.

McGrath, P. A. (1989): Evaluating a child's pain. *J Pain Sympt Manag* **4**, 198–214.

McGrath, P. J., Cunningham, S. J., Goodman, J. T., and Unruh, A. (1986): The clinical measurement of pain in children. A review. *Clin J Pain* **1**, 221–7.

Merloz, P. H., de Cheveigne, C., Butel, J., and Robb, J. E. (1987): Case report: bilateral Salter-Harris type II upper tibial epiphyseal fractures. *J Pediatr Orthop* **7**, 466–7.

Mizuta, T., Benson, W. M., Foster, B. K., Paterson, D. C., and Morris, L. L. (1987): Statistical analysis of the incidence of physeal injuries. *Paediatr Orthop* **7**, 518–23.

Ogden, J. A. (1981): Injury to the growth mechanism of the immature skeleton. *Skeletal Radiol* **6**, 237–53.

Ogden, J. A. (1984): Growth slowdown and arrest lines. *J Pediatr Orthop* **4**, 409–15.

Ogden, J. A., Tross, R. B., and Murphy, M. J. (1980): Fractures of the tibial tuberosity. *J Bone Joint Surg* **62-A**, 205–15.

Ogden, J. A., Ganey, T. M., and Ogden, D. A. (1996): The biological aspects of children's fractures. In: Rockwood, C. A., Wilkins, K. E., and Beaty, J. H. (eds), *Fractures in Children*. Volume 3; 4th edition. Lippincott, Philadelphia, pp. 19–52.

Oh, W. H., Craig, C., and Banks, H. H. (1974): Epiphyseal injuries. *Paediatr Clin North Am* **21**, 407–22.

Osterman, K. (1972): Operative elimination of partial premature epiphyseal closure. An experimental study. *Acta Orthop Scand Suppl*, 3–79.

Pappas, A. M., and Toczylowski, A. M. (1984): Asymmetrical arrest of the proximal tibial physis and genu recurvatum deformity. *J Bone Joint Surg* **66-A**, 575–81.

Petersen, H. A. (1994a): Physeal fractures: Part 2. Two previously unclassified types. *J Pediatr Orthop* **14**, 431–8.

Petersen, H. A. (1994b): Physeal fractures: Part 3. Classification. *J Pediatr Orthop* **14**, 439–48.

Petersen, H. A. (1996): Physeal and apophyseal injuries In: Rockwood, C. A., Wilkins, K. E., and Beaty, J. H. (eds), *Fractures in Children*. Volume 3; 4th edition. Lippincott, Philadelphia, pp. 103–65.

Petersen, H. A., Madhok, R., Benson, B. A., Ilstrup, D. M., and Melton, L. J. (1994):

Physeal fractures: Part 1. Epidemiology in Olmsted County, Minnesota 1979–1988. *Pediatr Orthop* **14**, 423–30.

Radford, P. J. (1993): General outcome measures. In: Pynsent, P., Fairbank, J., and Carr, A. (eds), *Outcome Measures in Orthopaedics*. Butterworth-Heinemann, Oxford, pp. 58–80.

Riseborough, E., Barrett, I., and Shapiro, F. (1983): Growth disturbances following distal femoral physeal fracture-separations. *J Bone Joint Surg Am* **65**, 885–93.

Rogers, L. F. (1970): The radiography of epiphyseal injuries. *Radiology* **96**, 289–99.

Rossi, F., and Dragoni, S. (2001): Acute avulsion fractures of the pelvis in adolescent competitive athletes: prevalence, location and sports distribution of 203 cases collected. *Skeletal Radiol* **30**, 127–31.

Salter, R. B., and Harris, W. R. (1963): Injuries involving the epiphyseal plate. *Bone Joint Surg Am* **45-A**, 587–621.

Shapiro, F. (1981): Fractures of the femoral shaft in children. The overgrowth phenomenon. *Acta Orthop Scand* **52**, 649–55.

Shapiro, F. (1982): Developmental patterns in lower-extremity length discrepancies. *J Bone Joint Surg* **64-A**, 639–51.

Siffert, R. S., and Katz, J. F. (1983): Growth recovery zones. *J Pediatr Orthop* **3**, 196–201.

Skak, S. V., Jensen, T. T., Poulsen, T. D., and Sturup, J. (1987): Epidemiology of knee injuries in children. *Acta Orthop Scand* **58**, 78–81.

Smith, B. G., Rand, F., Jaramillo, D., and Shapiro, F. (1994): Early MR imaging of lower-extremity physeal fracture separations: a preliminary report. *Pediatr Orthop* **14**, 526–33.

Smith, M. K. (1924): The prognosis in epiphyseal line fractures. *Ann Surg* **79**, 273–82.

Taylor, J. F., Warrell, E., and Evans, R. A. (1987): Response of the growth plates to tibial osteotomy in rats. *J Bone Joint Surg* **69-B**, 664–9.

Tolat, A. R., Sanderson, P. L., De Smet, L., and Stanley, J. K. (1992): The gymnast's wrist: acquired positive ulnar variance following chronic epiphyseal injury. *J Hand Surg* **17**, 678–81.

Weber, B. G. (1980): Fracture healing in the growing bone and in the mature skeleton. In: Weber, B. G., Brunner, C., and Freuler, F. (eds), *Treatment of Fractures in Children and Adolescents*. Springer-Verlag, New York, pp. 20–57.

Wilson, C. L. (1970): Experimental attempts to stimulate bone growth. *J Bone Joint Surg* **52**-**A**, 1033–40.

Yates, C., and Sullivan, J. A. (1987): Arthrographic diagnosis of elbow injuries in children. *J Pediatr Orthop* **7**, 54–60.

13

Peripheral nerve injuries
David Warwick and Peter P. Belward

INTRODUCTION

Peripheral nerves can be injured in many ways, including laceration, traction, crushing, burning and radiation. The severity of injury ranges from a brief conduction block to nerve discontinuity, and the outcome ranges from complete recovery, through partial recovery to no recovery.

Pathophysiology of nerve injury

In order to understand nerve recovery, a brief description of the pathophysiology of the injured nerve is required (Table 13.1) (Grant *et al.* 1999; Robinson 2000).

Neurapraxia is a transient injury. Larger fibres (e.g. motor) are more prone than smaller fibres (e.g. sensory), so there may be a paralysis together with some preservation of sensation. A mild insult causes a conduction block, which recovers swiftly; a more severe insult causes focal demyelination which may take a few weeks to recover. If the history suggests a relatively minor insult, and clinical examination suggests progressive recovery, then surgery is not needed.

Axonotmesis represents a more severe injury, usually from crush or traction, and there is a variable degree of damage to the infrastructure of the nerve. Wallerian degeneration occurs beyond the injury. The amount and rate of recovery depends upon the proportion of axons which can regenerate along their original tubules, in good time before the end organ degenerates irreversibly. In a grade 2 axonotmesis, where there is minimal damage and therefore scarring to the internal structure, more or less full recovery occurs. However, in a grade 4 axonotmesis, there is so much scarring that the injury does not recover at all. Distinguishing between low-grade axonotmesis (for which surgery would be an unnecessary insult) and high-grade axonotmesis (which requires surgery to be carried out as soon as possible, as the results of repair or grafting are

Table 13.1: Grades of nerve injury

Seddon (1943)	Sunderland (1978)	Pathology	Recovery	Treatment
Neurapraxia	First-degree	Transient ischaemia or focal demyelination, axon loss	Good	Watch
Axonotmesis	Second-degree	Axon loss, endoneurial tubes intact	Good to fair	Watch
	Third-degree	Axon and endoneurium loss	Fair to poor	Surgery
	Fourth-degree	Axon, endoneurium and perineurium loss, epineurium intact	Poor	Surgery
Neurotmesis	Fifth-degree	Severance of nerve	None	Early surgery

inversely proportional to the delay in operation (Birch and Raji 1991) is often a dilemma for the surgeon. Careful understanding of the mechanism of injury, and careful assessment for recovery as described below, is crucial.

Neurotmesis means a complete loss of nerve continuity. This condition is caused by laceration, heavy crushing or severe traction, and early surgery is required.

ASSESSMENT

The assessment of nerve injuries has three purposes:

1. Serial monitoring for recovery.

2. The pronouncement of final outcome.

3. Comparison of outcome in groups of patients.

SERIAL MEASURES OF RECOVERY

Tinel's percussion test (Tinel 1915; Moldaver 1978)

If and when the nerve regenerates across the site of injury or repair, the leading edge of touch fibres within the nerve are hypersensitive. Percussion at the leading edge will be interpreted by the patient as an unpleasant tingling (dysaesthesia) in the cutaneous distribution of the nerve. As the nerve recovers, the site at which tingling is produced by percussion will advance distally. The rate of advance depends upon the particular nerve, but is about 1–2 mm per day. If the sign, once established at the site of injury, does not advance at all, then – in the absence of any other signs of recovery – it is assumed that the nerve will not regenerate further and surgery should be considered. If the sign advances too slowly, or advances then fades out, then it may be assumed – again in the absence of other signs of recovery – that regeneration is failing.

The following caveats should be remembered:

- The sign does not appear immediately; there is a delay of four to six weeks after injury or repair.

- The sign will be positive, even if only a small proportion of the fibres are regenerating. Thus, even if the sign advances at the expected rate, full functional recovery is by no means certain.

- The nerve can recover successfully without an advancing Tinel's sign, so it should be interpreted alongside other clinical measures.

Progressive sensory recovery

Sensation recovers before motor function (Dellon 1981). Sensory modalities tend to appear in the following order:

- Protective sensation (pain and temperature, mediated by small-calibre fibres which regenerate more rapidly).

- Low-frequency vibration sense; moving two-point discrimination.

- Touch; high-frequency vibration.

- Two-point discrimination.

Measurement of these is discussed in greater detail below.

Progressive motor recovery

Motor recovery recovers in the following order:

- *Sequential muscle recovery*. This is best demonstrated in a high radial nerve lesion, in which brachioradialis recovers first, then ECRL, ECRB and so on, as the regeneration along the main trunk passes the motor branch to each nerve. The progression may slow down or cease, suggesting an axonotmesis or muscle failure.

- *Recovery of muscle atrophy*. This cannot be measured objectively. If the regenerating nerve does not reach the motor end plate within about 12 months of the injury, then recovery of the muscle is unlikely. This is due to breakdown of the motor end plate and irreversible muscle atrophy, and means that surgical exploration – particularly of more proximal lesions – should not be delayed so long that, with an advance of 1–2 mm per day, the nerve cannot reach the muscle in time.

- *Contraction and power*. Two scales are currently in use. The British Medical Research Council (MRC) scale (Table 13.2A; Medical Research Council 1941) is more appropriate for proximal nerve lesions, and measures global recovery of a nerve injury. It is not widely used and has been supplanted by a commonly used amended version (Table 13.2B; Merle D'Aubigne *et al.* 1956). This can be applied to individual muscles more usefully as it allows monitoring of sequential recovery of muscles and distinction to be made between varying grades of recovery in the muscles served by a motor nerve. These scales are likely to suffer from some observer variability; the main drawback is the broad range of recovery encompassed by Grade 4 or M4. Motor recovery can falter at any stage;

appearance of a Grade 1 recovery does not mean that a Grade 5 recovery will be achieved.

- *Objective measurement of power*. The Jamar grip dynamometer and the pinch dynamometer are widely used as an objective measure of power. The Jamar dynamometer has five grip settings and gives a reading in pounds per inch or kg per meter. The power grip measured depends upon the grip setting, with most power on setting 3 then 2, then 4, 5 and 1. Alteration to this distribution, or abnormal variation with rapid alternation between hands, can sometimes suggest voluntary manipulation (i.e. malingering).

ASSESSMENT OF SENSIBILITY

Touch is very complex. There are many types of cutaneous receptors, some with unique functions (e.g. specific hot and cold receptors) and others with overlapping functions. External stimuli provoke the receptors to generate an action potentials, which pass to the brain. The information is integrated and consciousness then perceives the overall modality of 'touch' or 'sensibility'. Following nerve injury, the clinician must quantify this highly complex modality both objectively and accurately. This means inference from various assessment methods which are, at best, blunt and which assess only a small part of the totality of touch (Bell-Krotoski 1991).

Autonomous areas

When sensation is tested, by whichever means, it should be remembered that there is considerable overlap between the distribution of cutaneous nerves. Only small areas are 'autonomous' – that is, supplied by one nerve alone. The autonomous areas in the upper limb are:

- Radial nerve – just beyond the anatomical snuffbox.
- Median nerve – the pulp of the index finger.
- Ulnar nerve – the pulp of the little finger.

Table 13.2: MRC grading of muscle power and motor recovery

(A) *MRC grading of muscle power*	
M0	No contraction
M1	Perceptible contraction in proximal muscles
M2	Perceptible contraction in both proximal and distal muscles
M3	All important muscles able to work against resistance
M4	All synergistic and independent movements possible
M5	Complete recovery
(B) *Motor recovery*	
Grade 0	Total paralysis
Grade 1	Flicker
Grade 2	Movement with gravity eliminated
Grade 3	Movement against gravity
Grade 4	Movement against gravity and resistance
Grade 5	Full power

Sensory assessment should be confined to these areas in order to avoid error. The territory of cutaneous nerves should not be confused with the *dermatomes*, which are areas of skin innervated by a particular level in the spinal cord.

The Medical Research Council scale (Table 13.3)

This can be used to summarize recovery in an individual patient, or to compare outcome between individuals. It is rather subjective; the only objective outcome measure within the scale is two-point discrimination which itself has drawbacks (*vide infra*).

Cutaneous sensation

Cutaneous sensation is mediated by two types of receptors. The *Pacinian corpuscles* respond quickly and fade quickly, whereas the *Merkel discs* respond slowly and fade slowly. It is difficult to measure 'touch' objectively, yet without reliable and valid instruments it is impossible to assess the outcome in an individual patient or to compare outcomes between patients or surgeons (Fess 1986). Furthermore, it is not so much the quantity of *sensation* as

Table 13.3: Medical Research Council scale for sensory recovery

S0	Absence of sensibility in the autonomous area
S1	Recovery of deep cutaneous pain sensibility within an autonomous area of the nerve
S2	Some superficial pain and touch
S2+	Touch and pain sensation in autonomous areas with persistent overreaction
S3	Return of some degree of superficial cutaneous pain and tactile sensibility within the autonomous area of the nerve
S3+	Return of sensibility as S3, with some recovery of two-point discrimination
S4	Complete recovery

the quality of *function* which is the real measure of outcome (Moberg 1960).

PAIN

Pain – which is a protective sensation – is an early sign of sensory recovery and a very important clinical goal. Pain sensation recovers in a predictable order: pressure sensation; sharp sensation with poor localization; sharp sensation with more precise localization; and normal.

Blunt and sharp needles are used to assess cutaneous sensation. The patient must distinguish between sharp and blunt (to distinguish between pain rather than pressure receptors), and the amount of pressure needed can be estimated by comparison with the uninjured side. This type of test is intrinsically subjective.

SIMPLE LIGHT TOUCH

This can be measured by stroking with the pulp of the examiner's finger or with a wisp of cotton wool. Although of some use to briefly screen for the presence or otherwise of sensation in a particular autonomous area, the test is too subjective and too dependent upon the method and force of application.

FILAMENT TESTS

These are an objective measure of light touch. These measure the *threshold* at which sensation is perceived (whereas two-point discrimination measures the *density* of sensory fibres). Horse hairs were originally used in the late nineteenth century by Von Frey, who found that hairs of increasing width would withstand increasing axial pressure before bending. When the fibre is pressed against the skin, it will bend and then a constant force is maintained. The wider the filament, the more force is required to bend it. A more formal method was devised by Semmes and Weinstein (Semmes *et al.* 1960), who used nylon monofilaments of specific diameters each mounted onto a rod. The purpose is to test the threshold at which the touch receptors on the skin are stimulated. A kit with five filaments is used (Bell-Krotoski *et al.* 1993). The tip of the smallest filament is placed gently on the skin with the hand supported from behind in putty. The tip is pushed down perpendicularly until it buckles, and the patient – while looking away – states whether or not the tip is felt. If not, a larger filament is used. The test is repeated until the patient feels the filament. The size of filament required at specific autonomous zones is mapped (with a colour-code) onto a diagram of the hand. Thus, an objective record of touch is made which can be compared over time. Repeatability is good (Bell-Krotoski and Tomancik 1987), and the results correlate with two-point discrimination (von Prince and Butler 1967). The test is responsive to change in nerve compression syndromes (Gelberman *et al.* 1983).

STATIC TWO-POINT DISCRIMINATION

This is an objective measure of the quality of sensation. It is determined by the minimum distance between two points on the skin at which the patient can distinguish a stimulus. The test is performed as follows:

- The patient is asked to look away.
- The ends of a paper clip, a drawing compass or a dedicated wheel can be used.
- The skin is touched randomly ten times with both tips, and ten times with one tip (Moberg 1964, 1990).

To pass the test, the patient must score 5 or more, when the total of incorrect one-point applications is subtracted from the total of correct two-point applications. A simpler method is for the patient to correctly state two out of three times whether one or two points are being pressed against the skin (Omer 1962). The American Society for Surgery of the Hand recommends seven correct answers out of ten.

- Starting with a distance between the tips of 15 mm, the gap is closed incrementally until the patient fails.
- The points must be applied simultaneously. The touches should be made 4 seconds apart to allow the receptors time to recover.

- The test, when conducted correctly, is very time consuming. However, if it is not conducted correctly, then it is likely to be unreliable.
- The normal values depend on the area of skin being tested (Gellis and Pool, 1977). The pulp of the finger tip is 3–5 mm, the palm of the hand 6–9 mm, the dorsum of the hand 7–10 mm, and the forearm 20–50 mm.

The American Society for Surgery of the Hand suggests the following interpretation:

- Normal   6 mm
- Fair   6–10 mm
- Poor   11–15 mm
- Protective   One point only detected
- Anaesthetic   No point detected

The test has some advantages, mainly that it is relatively straightforward to perform and can be a useful screening measure for normal sensation at the finger tips. The test correlates moderately well with the Moberg pick-up test (Chassard *et al.* 1993). Notwithstanding imperfect repeatability, it provides an objective measure of recovery in neurapraxia and low-grade axonotmesis.

The test has significant shortcomings, however. The force used is critical – just less than that needed to cause blanching beneath the tips, though this is impossible to judge accurately. Too much force may cause the pain fibres and/or adjacent tip to be stimulated. Repeatability is therefore limited (Bell-Krotoski and Bulford 1988; Bell-Krotoski *et al.* 1993). The test is not responsive to change in nerve compression syndromes (Gelberman *et al.* 1983). After repair of a divided nerve, the test is not responsive to change and rarely provides measurable values in adults. Thus, two-point discrimination usually remains poor, even when other measures of sensibility (filament tests and tactile gnosis tests) have shown improvement (Jerosch-Herold 2000; Rosen *et al.* 2000).

MOVING TWO-POINT DISCRIMINATION

Constant touch is mediated by slowly adapting fibres. However, quickly adapting fibres (which measure movement across the skin) recover earlier after nerve injuries (Dellon 1978, 1981). The test is performed as follows: the tips are spaced 10 mm apart and then passed distally along the finger pulp. The patient must distinguish between one and two tips. If the patient responds correctly to seven out of ten passes, then the tip space is narrowed. Normal moving two-point discrimination is 2 mm in the finger pulps, which is several millimetres narrower than static discrimination.

Moving two-point discrimination of greater than about 10 mm will allow the blindfolded patient to identify an object by manipulation, yet when the same object is touched without moving, it cannot be identified (Lister 1993).

LOCALIZATION

Birch *et al.* (1998) advocated a localization chart to monitor recovery, and aid rehabilitation, after nerve repair. A diagram of the hand is divided into zones, each of which has a reference number. The blindfolded patient is touched on each zone and is asked to state which zone is actually felt. The zone on the diagram is marked with the reference number of the zone stated by the patient. As the nerve recovers, the localization improves. This technique is also used as part of the sensory re-education programme, as the patient can learn to recognize erroneous touch.

VIBRATION

Tuning forks (30 Hz and 256 Hz) can be used to test sensibility in superficial and deep dermal receptors (Dellon 1980). However, the method depends too much upon the force and method of application and is therefore not reliable. Furthermore, there is no evidence that vibration correlates with functional outcome (Bell-Krotoski and Bulford 1988).

TEMPERATURE

This is measured with test-tubes filled with hot and cold water. The patient touches the tubes and must correctly assign which tubes are hot and which are cold. Temperature measurement is not widely used because of poor reliability and because there is no correlation with function (Tubiana *et al.* 1996).

SWEATING

Skin without a blood supply will not sweat properly. Sweating recovers after the return of pain and touch. It can be measured by:

- Tactile adherence (Harrison 1974). The barrel of a smooth pen is brushed along the skin. Smoothness – the absence of a slight stickiness because of sweat – suggests loss of innervation. The test needs careful comparison with the other side. Its only use is probably in the unconscious patient.

- Stains (Aschan and Moberg 1962). Sweating can be mapped out objectively with stains such as ninhydrin, which produces a purple colour on sweating skin. The test is difficult to perform however, and the presence of sweating does not correlate with sensation or function. Therefore, the test is not particularly useful, except perhaps in the detection of malingering or in unconscious or uncooperative patients. It should be remembered that sweating is not lost in brachial plexus root avulsion (because this injury is proximal to the attachment of the cervical sympathetic chain which transmits the sweating fibres).

- Wrinkling (O'Riain 1973). If a hand is immersed in warm water for 30 minutes, skin which has lost its innervation will not wrinkle whereas normally innervated skin will. This test might be useful in infants or in unconscious patients.

FUNCTIONAL TESTS

Teleologically, it is hand function, rather than any individual measure of touch, which is the final arbiter of nerve recovery, and the standard against which these measures should be compared.

Global scores

Altered function after nerve injury can, of course, be reflected in measures of general health (e.g. the SF-36)

repair in a longitudinal cohort. *Scand J Plast Reconst Hand Surg* **34**, 71–8.

Seddon, H. J. (1943): Three types of nerve injury. *Brain* **66**, 237–88.

Semmes, J., Weinstein, S., Ghent, L., and Tueber, H. (1960): *Somatosensory Changes after Penetrating Brain Wounds in Man*. Harvard University Press, Cambridge.

Sunderland, S. (1978): *Nerve and Nerve Injuries*. Churchill-Livingstone, New York.

Tinel, J. (1915): Le signe du 'fourmillement' dans les lesions des nerfs peripheriques. *Presse Med* **47**, 388–9.

Tubiana, R., Thomine, J. M., and Mackin, E. (1996): *Examination of the Hand and Wrist*. 2nd edition. E. Martin Dunitz, London.

von Prince, K., and Butler, B. (1967): Measuring sensory function of the hand in peripheral nerve injuries. *Am J Occup Ther* **21**, 385–96.

14

Spine and spinal cord
Jeremy C. T. Fairbank and Harry Brownlow

INTRODUCTION

This chapter is concerned with the assessment of outcome in spinal deformity, low back pain, cervical spine and trauma. The requirements of these four areas differ, although there is some overlap, such that disability and generic outcome measures can be applied to all four areas, and measures of deformity can be applied to trauma cases. Psychosocial factors are especially relevant to back-pain patients, although there is accumulating evidence that psychological distress can be relieved if pain and other symptoms can be treated.

This chapter is derived and updated from the earlier editions of books in this series. Some new measures have been described since they were published, and some developments have also been made on the validation and reliability of the measures.

There is interest in patient-generated outcome measures in this area, but no data have been published with regard to the spine (Ruta *et al.* 1994a, b; Carr 1996; MacDuff and Russell 1998; Bernheim 1999).

DEFORMITY

No satisfactory condition specific assessment for scoliosis has been developed, though the Scoliosis Research Society is actively developing an outcome measure for assessing the effects of scoliosis treatment. At the time of writing, little has been published using this measure, and it is not possible for us to draw any helpful conclusions about this

instrument. It is probably better to use a generic outcome measure for scoliosis treatment at present. The Cobb angle has been extensively used both as an outcome measure and an aid to decision making. There are strong theoretical reasons for not using this measure, however (cf. Chapter 1). Most clinicians acknowledge the considerable limitations in using such an inaccurate measure that only reflects part of the deformity. Understanding of the importance of the sagittal plane and surface topography is widespread among experienced scoliosis surgeons. There are measures to describe these deformities; even so, the Cobb angle (Fig. 14.1) is

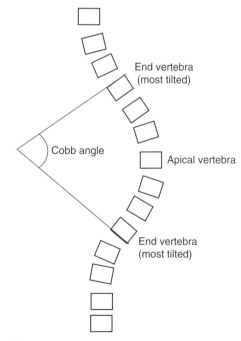

Figure 14.1 The Cobb angle.

helpful to both clinicians and their patients. No useful alternative has been found, and it is likely that this measure will remain an important outcome in the years to come.

Optimum outcome measurements

Cobb angle (in frontal and sagittal planes) (Cobb 1948).

- A measure of surface topography (to be defined).
- A measure of patient defined outcome (to be defined).

LOW BACK PAIN

There are a large number of measures available to assess low back pain. We favour the Oswestry Disability Index for more severe and chronic back pain conditions, though the Roland-Morris score is popular and probably works best in the milder varieties of back pain as are seen in general practice or in a primary physiotherapy clinic. Linear analogue scales are effective for the measurement of pain. Generic outcome measures can be used and tend to correlate with the condition-specific instruments. They are generally more complex and difficult to score than either of the suggested outcome scores.

Radiographic assessment of fusion status remains unreliable.

Optimum outcome measurements

- Oswestry Disability Index (Fairbank *et al.* 1980; Fairbank and Pynsent 2000).
- Roland-Morris Disability Questionnaire (Roland and Morris 1983; Roland and Fairbank 2000).

CERVICAL SPINE

Outcome measures for the cervical spine are generally unsatisfactory, although there is some support for the use of generic outcome measures here.

Optimum outcome measurements

- Neck Disability Index (Vernon and Mior 1991).

SPINAL CORD INJURY

Outcomes of spinal cord injury depend on clinical examination and the use of various rehabilitation outcome measures. The main problem for these patients is the neurological one. The Frankel score has been used widely and seems robust. It is also helpful in defining patient groups. In the longer term, these patients have diverse problems and outcomes require careful selection. Non-specific general outcome measures such as the Nottingham Health Profile (NHP) are the most helpful.

Optimum outcome measurements

- Frankel Score (Frankel *et al.* 1969).
- ASIA Revised Motor and Sensory Scoring System (see McGuire 1998).

INDEX OPERATIONS

A list is included of recommended index procedures for audit purposes.

Cervical spine (Table 14.1)

- Anterior cervical discectomy, decom-pression and fusion (including bone grafting/multiple levels) (cervical region)

Lumbar spine (Table 14.2)

- Posterior excision of disc prolapse including microdiscectomy (lumbar region)

- Decompression for central spinal stenosis (one or two levels)
- Primary posterior fusion ± decompression ± discectomy (lumbar region)

Spinal deformity (Tables 14.3–14.14)

- Posterior correction of scoliosis with instrumentation and fusion
- Anterior correction of scoliosis with instrumentation and fusion
- Combined anterior and posterior correction and instrumentation of scoliosis

Table 14.1: Cervical spine: range of movement

Instrument	What does it measure?	Validated?	Reliable?	Responsive?	Usage	Score
Visual inspection	Cervical range of motion	Not tested	Youdas et al. (1991)*48	Not tested	Numerous	4
Goniometer and electrogoniometer	Cervical range of motion	Alund and Larsson (1990)	Tucci et al. (1986); Youdas et al. (1991)*49	Not tested	Numerous	8
Inclinometer	Cervical range of motion	Mayer et al. (1993)	Youdas et al. (1991)	Not tested	Numerous	8
Cervical range of movement instrument (Youdas et al. 1991)	Cervical range of motion	Tousignant et al. (2000)	Ordway et al. (1997)	Not tested	Numerous	8
CMS 50 Ultrasound-based spatial kinematic analyser (Castro et al. 2000)	Cervical range of motion	Not tested	Castro et al. (2000)	Not tested	Not reported	1
CMS 70 Ultrasound-based spatial kinematic analyser (Dvir and Prushansky 2000)	Cervical range of motion	Dvir and Prushansky (2000)	Dvir and Prushansky (2000)	Not tested	Not reported	2
3-Space computerized tracking system (Tucci et al. 1986)	Cervical range of motion	Ordway et al. (1997)	Not tested	Not tested	Not reported	2
FASTRAK Computerized tracking system (Jordan et al. 2000)	Cervical range of motion	Not tested	Jordan et al. (2000)*50	Not tested	Not reported	0

Youdas et al. (1991)*48 intraclass correlation coefficient <0.8.
Youdas et al. (1991)*49 intraclass correlation coefficient <0.8.
Jordan et al. (2000)*50 variable reliability.

Table 14.2: Lumbar spine: range of movement and strength

Instrument	What does it measure?	Validated?	Reliable?	Responsive?	Usage	Score
Fingertip to floor distance	Thoracolumbar flexion	Viitanen et al. (1995)*40; Kippers and Parker (1987)*41	Viitanen et al. (1995); Pile et al. (1991); Gill et al. (1988)*42; Merritt et al. (1986)*43	Viitanen et al. (1995)	Numerous	8
Modified Schober technique (Moll and Wright 1971)	Thoracolumbar flexion	Viitanen et al. (1995)	Viitanen et al. (1995); Pile et al. (1991); Gill et al. (1988); Ensink et al. (1996)*39; Miller et al. (1992)*56	Viitanen et al. (1995)*38	Numerous	8
Moll technique (Moll and Wright 1971)	Thoracolumbar lateral flexion	Not tested	Merritt et al. (1986)	Not tested	Numerous	6
Photometric technique (Gill et al. 1988)	Thoracolumbar flexion	Not tested	Gill et al. (1988)	Not tested	Not reported	1
Double inclinometer technique (Loebl 1967)	Thoracolumbar flexion	Saur et al. (1996)	Saur et al. (1996); Chen et al. (1997)*18; Stude et al. (1994)*19; Williams et al. (1993)*20; Boline et al. (1992)*21; Mayer et al. (1997)*59; Mayer et al. (1995)*62	Not tested	Numerous	8
Flexicurve (Burton 1986)	Thoracolumbar flexion	Tillotson and Burton (1991)	Tillotson and Burton (1991); Lundon et al. (1998)	Not tested	Salisbury and Porter (1987); Stokes et al. (1987); Ettinger et al. (1994); Salminen et al. (1993); Burton et al. (1996)	8

Table 14.2: Lumbar spine: range of movement and strength – *continued*

Instrument	What does it measure?	Validated?	Reliable?	Responsive?	Usage	Score
CA-6000 Spine motion analyser (electro-goniometer)	Spine motion	Dopf *et al.* (1994); Paquet *et al.* (1991)	Dopf *et al.* (1994); Christensen and Nilsson (1998) (cervical spine); Petersen *et al.* (1994) (thoracolumbar); Paquet *et al.* (1991) (thoracolumbar)	Not tested	Numerous	8
Isostation B-200	Thoracolumbar spine motion	Not tested	Rytokoski *et al.* (1994); Dillard *et al.* (1991)*54; Hutten and Hermans (1997)*57	Not tested	Numerous	6
Cybex	Thoracolumbar spine motion	Not tested	Bo *et al.* (1997)*22	Not tested	Not reported	0
Applied Rehabilitation Concepts (ARCON) System (Hasten *et al.* 1995)	Thoracolumbar spine motion	Not tested	Not tested	Not tested	Hasten *et al.* (1996)	1
Cybex	Trunk strength	Madsen (1996)*16	Newton *et al.* (1993)	Newton *et al.* (1993)*17	Numerous	6

Viitanen *et al.* (1995)*40 Poor validity with ankylosing spondylitis.
Kippers and Parker (1987)*41 Less than half of the variations in fingertip-floor distance is explained by changes in vertebral mobility.
Gill *et al.* (1988)*42 Poor repeatability of the fingertip-floor distance.
Merritt *et al.* (1986)*43 Poor reproducibility of the fingertip-floor distance.
Ensink *et al.* (1996)*39 Schober's test result changes during the course of the day.
Miller *et al.* (1992)*56 Poor reproducibility.
Viitanen *et al.* (1995)*38 Poor responsiveness in ankylosing spondylitis patients.
Chen *et al.* (1997)*18 Poor inter- and intra-observer variability.
Stude *et al.* (1994)*19 Poor inter- and intra-observer variability.
Williams *et al.* (1993)*20 Poor inter- and intra-observer variability.
Boline *et al.* (1992)*21 Poor inter- and intra-observer variability.
Mayer *et al.* (1997)*59 Device error minimal, but unreliable as administrators not trained.
Mayer *et al.* (1995)*62 Poor inter-observer reliability.
Dillard *et al.* (1991)*54 Poor reproducibility.
Hutten and Hermans (1997)*57 Poor reproducibility.
Bo *et al.* (1997)*22 Poor inter- and intra-observer variability.
Madsen (1996)*16 Considerable individual day-to-day variability.
Newton *et al.* (1993)*17 Poor discrimination between normal people and patients.

Table 14.3: Deformity: scoliosis

Instrument	What does it measure?	Validated?	Reliable?	Responsive?	Usage	Score
Scoliometer (Bunnell 1984)	Rib hump	Pearsall et al. (1992)*7; Amendt et al. (1990)*8	Amendt et al. (1990); Pearsall et al. (1992); Cote et al. (1998); Korovessis and Stamatakis (1996); Murrell et al. (1993)	Not tested	Karachalios et al. (1999); Grossman et al. (1995); Dangerfield and Denton (1986); Samuelsson and Noren (1997)	6
Body contour formulator (Thurlbourne and Gillespie 1976)	Rib hump profile	Thurlbourne and Gillespie (1976); Pun et al. (1987)	Pun et al. (1987)	Not tested	Pun et al. (1987)	5
Moire fringe topography (Willner 1979)	Back shape	Laulund et al. (1982)*1; Adair et al. (1977)*2; Nissinen et al. (1993)*3; Pruijs et al. (1995a)*4; Sahlstrand (1986)*6	Pruijs et al. (1995a)*5	Not tested	Adair et al. (1977); Laulund et al. (1982); Nissinen et al. (1993); Pruijs et al. (1995a); Sahlstrand (1986)	0
Integrated Shape Imaging System (ISIS) (Turner-Smith et al. 1988)	Back shape	Weisz et al. (1988)	Not tested	Weisz et al. (1988); Jefferson et al. (1988)	Carr et al. (1991); Upadhyay et al. (1988); Hullin et al. (1991); Theologis et al. (1997)	8
Quantec Spinal Imaging System (Wojcik et al. 1994)	Back shape	Thometz et al. (2000); Goldberg et al. (2001)	Not tested	Not tested	Thometz et al. (2000)	2
Metrecom Skeletal Analysis System (MSAS) (Mior et al. 1996)	Back shape	Mior et al. (1996)*11	Mior et al. (1996)*12	Not tested	Not reported	0

Table 14.3: Deformity: scoliosis – *continued*

Instrument	What does it measure?	Validated?	Reliable?	Responsive?	Usage	Score
Optoelectronic evaluation of trunk shape (Dawson et al. 1993)	Trunk deformity	Dawson et al. (1993)	Dawson et al. (1993)	Not tested	Not reported	2
Cobb angle (Cobb 1948)	Coronal curvature	Pruijs et al. (1995b)	Carman et al. (1990); Morrissy et al. (1990); Goldberg et al. (1988)	Pruijs et al. (1995b)	Numerous	10
Rib-vertebra angle (Mehta 1972)	Rib inclination	Not tested	McAlindon and Kruse (1997)	Not tested	Numerous	6
End vertebra angle (Appelgren and Willner 1990)	Angle of tilt of end vertebrae	Not tested	Not tested	Not tested	Not reported	0
Angle of radiographic scoliosis (Diab et al. 1995)	Scoliosis angle	Diab et al. (1995)	Not tested	Not tested	Not reported	1
3D Reconstruction of radiological deformity (Dansereau et al. 1990)	Spine and trunk deformity	Not tested	Labelle et al. (1995)	Not tested	Aubin et al. (1997)	3

Pearsall et al. (1992)*7 Poor correlation with lumbar Cobb values, OK with thoracic.
Amendt et al. (1990)*8 Poor correlation with lumbar Cobb values, OK with thoracic.
Laulund et al. (1982)*1 High false-positive rate and poor correlation with Cobb angle.
Adair et al. (1977)*2 High false-positive rate and poor correlation with Cobb angle.
Nissinen et al. (1993)*3 High false-positive rate and poor correlation with Cobb angle.
Pruijs et al. (1995a)*4 Poor correlation with Cobb angle.
Sahlstrand (1986)*6 High false-positive rate.
Pruijs et al. (1995a)*5 Poor reproducibility.
Mior et al. (1996)*11 Poor correlation with Cobb angle.
Mior et al. (1996)*12 Large inter-observer variability.

Table 14.4: Deformity: kyphosis

Instrument	What does it measure?	Validated?	Reliable?	Responsive?	Usage	Score
Kyphometer (Debrunner, 1972)	Trunk kyphosis	Lundon et al. (1998)	Lundon et al. (1998); Ohlen et al. (1989); Mayer et al. (1995)*63		Lundon et al. (1998); Ohlen et al. (1989)	4
Arcometer (D'Osualdo et al. 1997)	Trunk kyphosis	D'Osualdo et al. (1997)	D'Osualdo et al. (1997)*58	Not tested	Not reported	2
Integrated Shape Imaging System (ISIS) (Carr et al. 1989)	Back shape	Carr et al. (1989)	Carr et al. (1989)	Carr et al. (1989)	Carr et al. (1989)	3
Kyphosis Cobb angle (Cobb 1948)	Sagittal curvature	Goh et al. (2000)	Goh et al. (2000); Carman et al. (1990)	Not tested	Numerous	8

Mayer et al. (1995)*63 Poor inter-observer reliability.
D'Osualdo et al. (1997)*58 Poor reproducibility.

Table 14.5: Deformity: rotational

Instrument	What does it measure?	Validated?	Reliable?	Responsive?	Usage	Score
Perdriolle torsion meter (Perdriolle and Vidal 1985)	Apical vertebral rotation	Richards (1992)*9; Barsanti et al. (1990); Omeroglu et al. (1996)	Richards (1992)*10; Weiss (1995)	Not tested	Lee and Nachemson (1997); Suk et al. (1995); Rajasekaran et al. (1994); Herzenberg et al. (1990); Hosman et al. (1996)	8
CT (Ho et al. 1993)	Vertebral rotation	Ho et al. (1993); Gocen et al. (1998)	Not tested	Not tested	Numerous	6
MRI (Birchall et al. 1997)	Vertebral rotation	Birchall et al. (1997)	Not tested	Not tested	Not reported	1

Richards (1992)*9 70% of measurements over-estimate rotation angle, 47% of measurements >5° wrong.
Richards (1992)*10 66% measurements differ more than 5°.

Table 14.6: Instability

Instrument	What does it measure?	Validated?	Reliable?	Responsive?	Usage	Score
Flexion/extension radiography	Cervical spine instability	Not tested	Not tested	Not tested	Numerous	4
Flexion/extension/ side-bending radiography (Dupuis et al. 1985)	Lumbar spine instability	Not tested	Dvorak et al. (1991); Pitkanen and Manninen (1994)*28	Sato and Kikuchi (1993)*51	Numerous	6
Traction/ compression radiography (Friberg 1987)	Lumbar spine instability	Pitkanen et al. (1997)*29	Not tested	Not tested	Kalebo et al. (1990)	1
Flexion/extension cineradiography (Hino et al. 1999)	Cervical instability	Not tested	Not tested	Not tested	Numerous	4
Flexion/ extension MRI	Cervical instability	Bell and Stearns (1991)	Not tested	Not tested	Not reported	2

Pitkanen and Manninen (1994)*28 Poor inter-observer variability.
Sato and Kikuchi (1993)*51 Changes in radiological features of instability did not correlate with clinical features in the same patients over 10 years.
Pitkanen et al. (1997)*29 Poor reliability and less able to distinguish instability than flexion/extension views.

Table 14.7: Fusion

Instrument	What does it measure?	Validated?	Reliable?	Responsive?	Usage	Score
Radiography	Spinal fusion	Siambanes and Mather (1998)*31; Larsen et al. (1996)*32; Brodsky et al. (1991)*33; Lang et al. (1990)*34; Blumenthal and Gill (1993)*52; Kant et al. (1995)*61	Hamill and Simmons (1997)	Not tested	Numerous	6
Flexion/ extension radiography	Spinal fusion	Larsen et al. (1996)*26; Brodsky et al. (1991)*27	Not tested	Not tested	Numerous	4

Table 14.7: Fusion – *continued*

Instrument	What does it measure?	Validated?	Reliable?	Responsive?	Usage	Score
Lateral bending radiography	Spinal fusion	Brodsky *et al.* (1991)*35	Hamill and Simmons (1997)	Not tested	Numerous	6
Tomography (Calder *et al.* 1984)	Spinal fusion	Not tested	Not tested	Not tested	Numerous	4
Computed tomography	Spinal fusion	Djukic *et al.* (1990); Brodsky *et al.* (1991)*23; Larsen *et al.* (1996)*24	Not tested	Not tested	Numerous	6
Ultrasound	Spinal fusion	Jacobson *et al.* (1997)*37	Not tested	Not tested	Not reported	0
Scintigraphy	Spinal fusion	(Bohnsack *et al.* 1999); Larsen *et al.* (1996)*25	Not tested	Not tested	Numerous	6
MRI	Spinal fusion	Lang *et al.* (1990)	Not tested	Albert *et al.* (1993)	Djukic *et al.* (1990)	5
Roentgen stereophoto-grammetry (Morris *et al.* 1985)	Spinal fusion	Not tested	Not tested	Not tested	Lee *et al.* (1994); Johnsson *et al.* (1992); Johnsson *et al.* (1999)	3
SPECT	Spinal fusion	Albert *et al.* (1998)*36	Not tested	Not tested	Not reported	0

Siambanes and Mather (1998)*31 Plain films are too unpredictable for assessing spinal fusion.
Larsen *et al.* (1996)*32 Plain films are too unpredictable for assessing spinal fusion.
Brodsky *et al.* (1991)*33 Plain films are too unpredictable for assessing spinal fusion.
Lang *et al.* (1990)*34 Plain films are too unpredictable for assessing spinal fusion.
Blumenthal and Gill (1993)*52 42% false-positive, 29% false-negative results of radiological diagnosis of fusion compared to surgical findings.
Kant *et al.* (1995)*61 Radiographs only 68% accurate.
Larsen *et al.* (1996)*26 Poor comparison with surgical exploration.
Brodsky *et al.* (1991)* 27 Poor comparison with surgical exploration.
Brodsky *et al.* (1991)*35 Poor correlation with surgical exploration of fusion mass.
Brodsky *et al.* (1991)*23 22% inaccuracy compared to surgical exploration.
Larsen *et al.* (1996)* 24 Poor comparison with surgical exploration.
Jacobson *et al.* (1997)*37 Sensitive but not specific for pseudo-arthrosis due to overlying hardware.
Larsen *et al.* (1996)* 25 Poor comparison with surgical exploration.
Albert *et al.* (1998)*36 Poor sensitivity and specificity for detection of pseudo-arthrosis.

Table 14.8: Spinal canal size

Instrument	What does it measure?	Validated?	Reliable?	Responsive?	Usage	Score
X-ray	Spinal canal size	Not tested	Not tested	Not tested	Numerous	4
X-ray ratio (Torg et al. 1986)	Spinal canal size	Blackley et al. (1999)*60	Not tested	Not tested	Numerous	4
CT	Spinal canal size	Not tested	Not tested	Not tested	Numerous	4
MRI	Spinal canal size	Not tested	Not tested	Not tested	Herno et al. (1999b)	1

Blackley et al. (1999)*60 Not valid compared to CT.

Table 14.9: Neurological outcome

Instrument	What does it measure?	Validated?	Reliable?	Responsive?	Usage	Score
MRC grade (MRC 1976)	Motor deficit	Inferred	Not tested	Not tested	Numerous	6
Trauma motor index (Lucas and Ducker 1979)	Motor deficit	Not tested	Not tested	Not tested	Gertzbein (1992); Bondurant et al. (1990); Cotler et al. (1990); Wells and Nicosia (1995)	4
Frankel score (Frankel et al. 1969)	Neurological deficit	Inferred	Davis et al. (1993)	Davis et al. (1993)*13; Gertzbein (1992); Blaustein et al. (1993)	Numerous	10
Sunnybrook Cord Injury Scale (Tator 1982)	Neurological deficit	Not tested	Davis et al. (1993)	Davis et al. (1993)*14; Segatore (1991)	Pitts et al. (1995)	5
ASIA Motor and Sensory Scoring System (Association 1984)	Neurological deficit	Not tested	Priebe and Waring (1991)*15	Not tested	Bracken et al. (1984)	1
Manabe scale (Manabe et al. 1989)	Change in Frankel grade, and pain	Not tested	Not tested	Not tested	Gertzbein (1992)	1

Table 14.9: Neurological outcome – *continued*

Instrument	What does it measure?	Validated?	Reliable?	Responsive?	Usage	Score
ASIA Revised Motor and Sensory Scoring System (McGuire 1998)	Neurological deficit	Inferred (El Masry et al. 1996) (motor only)	Cohen et al. (1998); Donovan et al. (1997)	Capaul et al. (1994)	Numerous	10
National Acute Spinal Cord Injury Study Score (NASCIS) (Bracken et al. 1984)	Neurological deficit	El Masry et al. (1996) (motor only)	Not tested	Not tested	Bracken et al. (1990); Bracken et al. (1998)	5
ASIA (Neurological) Impairment Scale (McGuire 1998)	Neurological impairment	Inferred	Not tested	Not tested	Numerous	6

Davis et al. (1993)*13 Relatively insensitive to important changes in motor, sensory, bladder and walking recovery.
Davis et al. (1993)*14 Insensitive to bladder and walking function.
Priebe and Waring (1991)*15 Poor inter-observer reliability, especially with respect to sensory testing.

Table 14.10: Functional outcome measures: general spine

Instrument	What does it measure?	Validated?	Reliable?	Responsive?	Usage	Score
Oswestry Disability Index (Fairbank et al. 1980)	Functional outcome measure for patients with back pain	Grevitt et al. (1997)	Fisher and Johnson (1997)	Beurskens et al. (1996)	Numerous	10
Million Visual Analogue Scale (Million et al. 1982)	Disability and pain questionnaire for patients with back pain	Beurskens et al. (1995)	Beurskens et al. (1995)	Beurskens et al. (1995)	Numerous	10
Roland-Morris Disability Questionnaire (Roland and Morris 1983)	Functional outcome measure for patients with back pain	Jensen et al. (1992)	Stratford and Binkley (1997)	Jensen et al. (1992)	Numerous	10
Iowa Low-Back Rating Scale (Lehmann et al. 1983)	Functional outcome measure	Lehmann et al. (1983)	Not tested	Not tested	Not reported	1

Table 14.10: Functional outcome measures: general spine – *continued*

Instrument	What does it measure?	Validated?	Reliable?	Responsive?	Usage	Score
Waddell Disability Index (Waddell and Main 1984)	Functional outcome measure for patients with back pain	Beurskens et al. (1995)	Beurskens et al. (1995)	Beurskens et al. (1995)	Numerous	10
Japanese Orthopedic Evaluation Criteria	Outcome of lumbar spinal surgery	Inferred	Not tested	Not tested	Numerous	6
Dallas Pain Questionnaire (Lawlis et al. 1989)	Impact of spinal pain on behaviour	Lawlis et al. (1989)	Lawlis et al. (1989)	Haas et al. (1995)	Numerous	8
Low-Back Outcome Scale (Greenough and Fraser 1992)	Functional outcome measure for patients with back pain	Greenough and Fraser (1992)	Not tested	Taylor et al. (1999)	Numerous	7
Distress and Risk Assessment Method (Main et al. 1992)	Distress and risk assessment	Main et al. (1992)	Not tested	Not tested	Tandon et al. (1999); Jamison (1999)	3
Von Korff's Pain Grade (Von Korff et al. 1992)	Chronic pain	Smith et al. (1997); Underwood et al. (1999)	Underwood et al. (1999)	Not tested	Not reported	4
Von Korff's Disability Grade (Von Korff et al. 1992)	Chronic disability	Underwood et al. (1999)	Underwood et al. (1999)	Not tested	Not reported	4
Low Back Pain Rating Scale (Manniche et al. 1994)	Assessment of low back pain	Manniche et al. (1994)	Manniche et al. (1994)	Not tested	Jensen et al. (1996); Manniche (1995); Laursen and Fugl (1995)	5
Clinical Low Back Pain (Aberdeen) Questionnaire (Ruta et al. 1994b)	Functional outcome measure for patients with back pain	Ruta et al. (1994b)	Ruta et al. (1994b)	Ruta et al. (1994b)	Moffett et al. (1999); Leung et al. (1999)	5
Quebec Back Pain Disability Scale (Kopec et al. 1995)	Functional outcome measure	Schoppink et al. (1996)	Schoppink et al. (1996)	Kopec et al. (1995)	Rossignol et al. (2000); Danaberg and Guiliano (1999); Vendrig et al. (2000)	8

Table 14.10: Functional outcome measures: general spine – *continued*

Instrument	What does it measure?	Validated?	Reliable?	Responsive?	Usage	Score
North American Spine Society Lumbar Spine Outcome Assessment Instrument (Daltroy et al. 1996)	Functional outcome measure	Daltroy et al. (1996)	Daltroy et al. (1996)	Not tested	Not reported	2
Core Outcome Measure (Deyo et al. 1998)	Proposed core questions of outcome of low back pain treatment	Not tested	Not tested	Not tested	Not reported	0
Back Pain Functional Scale (Stratford et al. 2000)	Functional outcome measure	Stratford et al. (2000)	Stratford et al. (2000)	Not tested	Not reported	2

Table 14.11: Functional outcome measures: cervical spine

Instrument	What does it measure?	Validated?	Reliable?	Responsive?	Usage	Score
Modified Oswestry Disability Index	Neck pain functional outcome	Not tested	Not tested	Not tested	Blunt et al. (1997); Zoega et al. (2000); Palit et al. (1999)	3
Neck Disability Index (Vernon and Mior 1991)	Neck pain functional outcome	Riddle and Stratford (1998)	Vernon and Mior (1991)	Riddle and Stratford (1998)	Numerous	9
Copenhagen Neck Functional Disability Scale (Jordan et al. 1998)	Neck pain functional outcome	Jordan et al. (1998)	Jordan et al. (1998)	Jordan et al. (1998)	Not reported	3
Neck Pain and Disability Scale (Wheeler et al. 1999)	Neck pain and disability	Wheeler et al. (1999)	Not tested	Not tested	Not reported	1

Table 14.11: Functional outcome measures: cervical spine – *continued*

Instrument	What does it measure?	Validated?	Reliable?	Responsive?	Usage	Score
Ranawat Score (Ranawat et al. 1979)	Functional outcome for cervical myelopathy	Inferred	Not tested	Not tested	Numerous	6
Japanese Orthopedic Evaluation Criteria (Association 1986)	Functional outcome for cervical myelopathy	Inferred	Not tested	Not tested	Numerous	6
Walking test (Singh and Crockard 1999)	Severity of cervical spondylotic myelopathy	Singh and Crockard (1999)	Singh and Crockard (1999)	Singh and Crockard (1999)	Not reported	3
Norris and Watt Classification (Norris and Watt 1983)	Signs and symptoms of whiplash	Not tested	Not tested	Not tested	Not reported	0
Gargan and Bannister Classification (Gargan and Bannister 1990)	Severity of symptoms after whiplash	Not tested	Not tested	Not tested	Not reported	0
Smiley Webster Functional Outcome Scale (Webster and Smiley 1957)	Functional outcome after Dens fracture	Not tested	Not tested	Not tested	Numerous	4

Table 14.12: Functional outcome measures: condition-specific; lumbar spine

Instrument	What does it measure?	Validated?	Reliable?	Responsive?	Usage	Score
Symptom Severity, Physical Function, and Satisfaction Scale (Stucki et al. 1996)	Functional outcome for spinal stenosis	Stucki et al. (1996)	Stucki et al. (1996)	Stucki et al. (1996)	Pratt et al. (2002)	4
Shuttle Walking Test (Singh et al. 1992)	Walking distance limited by pain related to spinal stenosis	Not tested	Pratt et al. (2002)	Pratt et al. (2002)	Not reported	4
Exercise Treadmill with Visual Analogue Scale Pain Test (Herno et al. 1994)	Severity of leg and back pain after exercise related to spinal stenosis	Not tested	Not tested	Not tested	Herno et al. (1999b); Herno et al. (1999c); Herno et al. (1999a)	3
Exercise Treadmill Test (Deen et al. 1998)	Walking distance limited by pain related to spinal stenosis	Not tested	Not tested	Deen et al. (1998)	Not reported	1
Exercise Treadmill Test Pre and Post Body Casting (Tokuhashi et al. 1993)	Exercise-induced leg and back pain related to lumbar instability	Not tested	Not tested	Tokuhashi et al. (1993)	Not reported	1
Macnab Classification (Macnab, 1971)	Outcome of nerve root decompression surgery	Not tested	Not tested	Not tested	Numerous	4
Staffer-Coventry Evaluation Criteria (Staffer and Coventry 1972)	Pain and functional outcome after lumbar fusion	Not tested	Not tested	Not tested	Loupasis et al. (1999)	1
Outcome Tool for Surgery for Neuromuscular Scoliosis (Samuelsson et al. 1996)	Functional outcome for neuromuscular scoliosis	Samuelsson et al. (1996)	Not tested	Not tested	Not reported	1
SRS Instrument (Haher et al. 1999)	Functional outcome for adolescent idiopathic scoliosis	Haher et al. (1999)	Haher et al. (1999)	Not tested	Bernstein and Hall (1998); White et al. (1999)	4

Table 14.13: Outcome measures of general health, mental health, and quality of life

Instrument	What does it measure?	Validated?	Reliable?	Responsive?	Usage	Score
Sickness Impact Profile (Bergner et al. 1981)	Generic measure of health	McHorney and Tarlov (1995); Deyo and Diehl (1983)	Beaton et al. (1997); Deyo and Diehl (1983)	Beaton et al. (1997); Deyo and Diehl (1983)	Numerous	10
Nottingham Health Profile (Hunt et al. 1985)	Generic measure of health	McHorney and Tarlov (1995)	McHorney and Tarlov (1995)	Beaton et al. (1997)	Numerous	10
EuroQoL (EuroQol Group 1990)	General health status	Hurst et al. (1997); Fransen and Edmonds (1999)	Hurst et al. (1997); Fransen and Edmonds (1999)	Hurst et al. (1997)	Numerous	10
Duke Health Profile (Parkerson et al. 1990)	Generic measure of health	McHorney and Tarlov (1995)	McHorney and Tarlov (1995)*46	Beaton et al. (1997)	Numerous	8
SF-36 (Ware and Sherbourne 1992)	Generic measure of health	McHorney and Tarlov (1995)	McHorney and Tarlov (1995)	Beaton et al. (1997)	Numerous	10
Quality of Life Profile (Climent et al. 1995)	Quality of life assessment for adolescents with spinal deformity	Climent et al. (1995)	Climent et al. (1995)	Not tested	Climent and Sanchez (1999)	3
COOP/WONCA Charts	Generic measure of health	McHorney and Tarlov (1995)	McHorney andTarlov (1995)*47	Kinnersley et al. (1994)	Numerous	8
Symptom Checklist-90 Revised (SCL-90R) (Derogatis et al. 1976)	Psychological screening in chronic pain patients	Kinney et al. (1991)	Not tested	Kinney et al. (1991)*55	Numerous	6
General Health Questionnaire (Goldberg and Hillier 1979)	Mental health screening questionnaire	Goldberg and Williams (1988)	Goldberg and Williams (1988)	Naughton and Wiklund (1993)*64	Numerous	7
Hospital Anxiety and Depression Scale (Zigmond and Snaith 1983)	Anxiety and depression screening questionnaire	Herrmann (1997)	Herrmann (1997)	Herrmann (1997)	Numerous	10
Modified Somatic Perception Questionnaire (Main 1983)	Anxiety screening in chronic back pain patients	Inferred	Mannion et al. (1996)*53	Greenough and Fraser (1991)	Numerous	8

Table 14.13: Outcome measures of general health, mental health, and quality of life – *continued*

Instrument	What does it measure?	Validated?	Reliable?	Responsive?	Usage	Score
Zung Depression Scale (Zung 1965)	Assessment of depression	Naughton and Wiklund (1993)	Knight et al. (1983)	Triano et al. (1993); Greenough and Fraser (1991)	Numerous	10
Beck Depression Inventory (Beck et al. 1961)	Detects levels of depression over last week	Levin et al. (1988)	Levin et al. (1988)	Naughton and Wiklund (1993)	Numerous	10
Eysenck Personality Inventory (Eysenck and Eysenck 1964)	Personality traits	Inferred	Katz and Dalby (1981)	Not tested	Numerous	8
Minnesota Multiphasic Personality Index (Graham 1977)	Personality traits	Inferred	Putnam et al. (1996)	Watkins et al. (1986)	Numerous	10

McHorney and Tarlov (1995)*46 Poor test-retest reliability.
McHorney and Tarlov (1995)*47 Poor test-retest reliability.
Kinney et al. (1991)*55 Poor responsiveness.
Naughton and Wiklund (1993)*64 GHQ was not designed to study changes with respect to treatment, but only to assess the acute mental health condition.
Mannion et al. (1996)*53 ICC = 0.67 at 6-month interval.

Table 14.14: Rehabilitation

Instrument	What does it measure?	Validated?	Reliable?	Responsive?	Usage	Score
Walking Index (Ditunno et al. 2000)	Walking scale for spinal cord injury patients	Ditunno et al. (2000)	Ditunno et al. (2000)	Not tested	Not reported	2
Energy expenditure	Energy expenditure during walking	Inferred	Sykes et al. (1996)	Waters et al. (1993)	Numerous	10
EPIC Lift Capacity Test (Matheson et al. 1995)	Lifting capacity of physically impaired adults	Not tested	Matheson et al. (1995)	Not tested	Jay et al. (2000)	2

Table 14.14: Rehabilitation – *continued*

Instrument	What does it measure?	Validated?	Reliable?	Responsive?	Usage	Score
Modified Ashworth scale (Bohannon and Smith 1987)	Muscle spasticity	Pandyan *et al.* (1999)*44	Pandyan *et al.* (1999); Gregson *et al.* (1999); Haas *et al.* (1996)*45	Numerous	Numerous	10
Katz Index (Katz and Lyerly 1963)	Independence in activities of daily living	Brorsson and Asberg (1984)	Brorsson and Asberg (1984)	Sonn (1996)	Numerous	10
Barthel Index (Mahoney and Barthel 1965)	Index of improvement of rehabilitation of the chronically ill	Inferred	Hachisuka *et al.* (1997)	Wells and Nicosia (1995)	Numerous	10
Resumption of Activities of Daily Living Scale (Williams and Myers 1998)	Independence in activities of daily living	Williams and Myers (1998)	Williams and Myers (1998)	Not tested	Not reported	2
Self-Reported Functional Measure (Hoenig *et al.* 1999)	Self-care function questionnaire for use in spinal cord dysfunction patients	Hoenig *et al.* (1999)	Not tested	Not tested	Not reported	1
Functional Independence Measure	Functional independence	Kidd *et al.* (1995); Dodds *et al.* (1993)	Kidd *et al.* (1995); Dodds *et al.* (1993)	Motor items good, but cognition items less good in spinal cord injury patients (Hall *et al.* 1999)	Numerous	10

Pandyan *et al.* (1999)*44 Measure of resistance to passive movement, which is a complex measure that can be influenced by many factors one of which may be spasticity.

Haas *et al.* (1996)*45 Varying levels of reliability, upper limbs more reliable than lower limbs; Ashworth more reliable than modified Ashworth.

OSWESTRY DISABILITY INDEX (V. 2.1)

Could you please complete this questionnaire. It is designed to give us information as to how your back (or leg) trouble has affected your ability to manage in everyday life.

Please answer **every section**. Mark **one box only** in each section that most closely describes you **today**.

Section 1: Pain intensity

☐ I have no pain at the moment.

☐ The pain is very mild at the moment.

☐ The pain is moderate at the moment.

☐ The pain is fairly severe at the moment.

☐ The pain is very severe at the moment.

☐ The pain is the worst imaginable at the moment.

Section 2: Personal care (washing, dressing, etc.)

☐ I can look after myself normally without causing extra pain.

☐ I can look after myself normally, but it is very painful.

☐ It is painful to look after myself and I am slow and careful.

☐ I need some help but manage most of my personal care.

☐ I need help every day in most aspects of self care.

☐ I do not get dressed, wash with difficulty and stay in bed.

Section 3: Lifting

☐ I can lift heavy weights without extra pain.

☐ I can lift heavy weights but it gives extra pain.

☐ Pain prevents me from lifting heavy weights off the floor but I can manage if they are conveniently positioned, e.g. on a table.

☐ Pain prevents me from lifting heavy weights, but I can manage light to medium weights if they are conveniently positioned.

☐ I can lift only very light weights.

☐ I cannot lift or carry anything at all.

Section 4: Walking

☐ Pain does not prevent me walking any distance.

☐ Pain prevents me walking more than 1 mile.

☐ Pain prevents me walking more than 1/4 of a mile.

☐ Pain prevents me walking more than 100 yards.

☐ I can only walk using a stick or crutches.

☐ I am in bed most of the time and have to crawl to the toilet.

Section 5: Sitting

☐ I can sit in any chair as long as I like.

☐ I can sit in my favourite chair as long as I like.

☐ Pain prevents me from sitting for more than 1 hour.

☐ Pain prevents me from sitting for more than 1/2 an hour.

☐ Pain prevents me from sitting for more than 10 minutes.

☐ Pain prevents me from sitting at all.

Section 6: Standing

☐ I can stand as long as I want without extra pain.

☐ I can stand as long as I want, but it gives me extra pain.

☐ Pain prevents me from standing for more than 1 hour.

☐ Pain prevents me from standing for more than 1/2 an hour.

☐ Pain prevents me from standing for more than 10 minutes.

☐ Pain prevents me from standing at all.

Section 7: Sleeping

- ☐ My sleep is never disturbed by pain.
- ☐ My sleep is occasionally disturbed by pain.
- ☐ Because of pain I have less than 6 hours sleep.
- ☐ Because of pain I have less than 4 hours sleep.
- ☐ Because of pain I have less than 2 hours sleep.
- ☐ Pain prevents me from sleeping at all.

Section 8: Sex life (if applicable)

- ☐ My sex life is normal and causes no extra pain.
- ☐ My sex life is normal, but causes some extra pain.
- ☐ My sex life is nearly normal, but is very painful.
- ☐ My sex life is severely restricted by pain.
- ☐ My sex life is nearly absent because of pain.
- ☐ Pain prevents any sex life at all.

Section 9: Social life

- ☐ My social life is normal and causes me no extra pain.
- ☐ My social life is normal, but increases the degree of pain.
- ☐ Pain has no significant effect on my social life apart from limiting my more energetic interests, e.g. sport.
- ☐ Pain has restricted my social life and I do not go out as often.
- ☐ Pain has restricted social life to my home.
- ☐ I have no social life because of pain.

Section 10: Travelling

- ☐ I can travel anywhere without pain.
- ☐ I can travel anywhere, but it gives extra pain.
- ☐ Pain is bad but I manage journeys over 2 hours.
- ☐ Pain restricts me to journeys of less than 1 hour.
- ☐ Pain restricts me to short necessary journeys under 30 minutes.
- ☐ Pain prevents me from travelling, except to receive treatment.

Scoring

For each section, the total score is 5; if the first statement is marked the score = 0; if the last statement is marked, the score = 5. Intervening statements are scored according to rank.

If more than one box is marked in each section, take the highest score.

If all 10 sections are completed, the score is calculated as follows:

Example: 16 (total scored)/50(total possible score) × 100 = 32%

If one section is missed (or not applicable) the score is calculated:

Example: 16 (total scored)/45 (total possible score) × 100 = 35.5%

And so on, such that if two or more sections are omitted, the percentage score is obtained by the same method.

THE ROLAND-MORRIS DISABILITY QUESTIONNAIRE (RDQ; WITH INSTRUCTIONS)

When your back hurts, you may find it difficult to do some things you normally do.

This list contains sentences that people have used to describe themselves when they have back pain. When you read them, you may find that some stand out because that describes you *today*. As you read the list, think of yourself *today*. When you read a sentence that describes you today, put a tick against it. If the sentence does not describe you, then leave the space blank and go on to the next one. Remember, only tick the sentence if you are sure it describes you today.

1. I stay at home most of the time because of my back.

2. I change position frequently to try and get my back comfortable.

3. I walk more slowly than usual because of my back.

4. Because of my back, I am not doing any of the jobs that I usually do around the house.

5. Because of my back, I use a handrail to get upstairs.

6. Because of my back, I lie down to rest more often.

7. Because of my back, I have to hold on to something to get out of an easy chair.

8. Because of my back, I try to get other people to do things for me.

9. I get dressed more slowly than usual because of my back.

10. I only stand for short periods of time because of my back.

11. Because of my back, I try not to bend or kneel down.

12. I find it difficult to get out of a chair because of my back.

13. My back is painful almost all the time.

14. I find it difficult to turn over in bed because of my back.

15. My appetite is not very good because of my back pain.

16. I have trouble putting on my socks (or stockings) because of the pain in my back.

17. I only walk short distances because of my back.

18. I sleep less well on my back.

19. Because of my back pain, I get dressed with help from someone else.

20. I sit down for most of the day because of my back.

21. I avoid heavy jobs around the house because of my back.

22. Because of my back pain, I am more irritable and bad-tempered with people than usual.

23. Because of my back, I go upstairs more slowly than usual.

24. I stay in bed most of the time because of my back.

Scoring the RDQ

The score is the total number of items checked – that is, from a minimum of 0 to a maximum of 24.

NECK DISABILITY INDEX (NDI) (VERNON AND MIOR 1991)

Section 1: Pain intensity

☐ I have no pain at the moment.

☐ The pain is very mild at the moment.

☐ The pain is moderate at the moment.

☐ The pain is fairly severe at the moment.

☐ The pain is very severe at the moment.

☐ The pain is the worst imaginable at the moment.

Section 2: Personal care (washing, dressing, etc.)

☐ I can look after myself normally, without causing extra pain.

☐ I can look after myself normally, but it causes extra pain.

☐ It is painful to look after myself and I am slow and careful.

☐ I need some help, but manage most of my personal care.

☐ I need help every day in most aspects of self care.

☐ I do not get dressed, I wash with difficulty and stay in bed.

Section 3: Lifting

☐ I can lift heavy weights without extra pain.

☐ I can lift heavy weights, but it gives extra pain.

☐ Pain prevents me from lifting heavy weights off the floor, but I can manage if they are conveniently positioned, for example on a table.

☐ Pain prevents me from lifting heavy weights off the floor, but I can manage light to medium weights if they are conveniently positioned.

☐ I can lift very light weights.

☐ I cannot lift or carry anything at all.

Section 4: Reading

☐ I can read as much as I want to with no pain in my neck.

☐ I can read as much as I want to with slight pain in my neck.

☐ I can read as much as I want to with moderate pain in my neck.

☐ I can't read as much as I want because of moderate pain in my neck.

☐ I can hardly read at all because of severe pain in my neck.

☐ I cannot read at all.

Section 5: Headaches

☐ I have no headaches at all.

☐ I have slight headaches which come infrequently.

☐ I have moderate headaches which come infrequently.

☐ I have moderate headaches which come frequently.

☐ I have severe headaches which come frequently.

☐ I have headaches almost all the time.

Section 6: Concentration

☐ I can concentrate fully when I want to, with no difficulty.

☐ I can concentrate fully when I want to, with slight difficulty.

☐ I have a fair degree of difficulty in concentration when I want to.

☐ I have a lot of difficulty in concentrating when I want to.

☐ I have a great deal of difficulty in concentrating when I want to.

☐ I cannot concentrate at all.

Section 7: Work

☐ I can do as much work as I want to.

☐ I can only do my usual work, but no more.

☐ I can do most of my usual work, but no more.

☐ I cannot do my usual work.

☐ I can hardly do any work at all.

☐ I can't do any work at all.

Section 8: Driving

☐ I can drive my car without any neck pain.

☐ I can drive my car as long as I want, but with slight neck pain.

☐ I can drive my car as long as I want, but with moderate neck pain.

☐ I can't drive my car as long as I want because of moderate pain in my neck.

☐ I can hardly drive at all because of severe pain in my neck.

☐ I can't drive my car at all.

Section 9: Sleeping

☐ I have no trouble sleeping.

☐ My sleep is slightly disturbed (less than 1 hour sleepless).

☐ My sleep is mildly disturbed (1–2 hours sleepless).

☐ My sleep is moderately disturbed (2–3 hours sleepless).

☐ My sleep is greatly disturbed (3–5 hours sleepless).

☐ My sleep is completely disturbed (5–7 hours sleepless).

Section 10: Recreation

☐ I am able to engage in all my recreation activities, with no neck pain at all.

☐ I am able to engage in all my recreation activities, with some pain in my neck.

☐ I am able to engage in most, but not all, of my usual recreation activities because of pain in my neck.

☐ I am able to engage in only a few of my usual recreation activities because of pain in my neck.

☐ I can hardly do any recreation activities because of pain in my neck.

☐ I can't do any recreation activities at all.

This index is scored in the same way as the Oswestry Disability Index, on which it is based.

FRANKEL SCALE (FRANKEL *ET AL.* 1969)

This version is a modification by the American Spinal Injury Association (ASIA).

- A = **Complete**. No sensory or motor function is preserved in the sacral segments S4–S5.

- B = **Incomplete**. Sensory but not motor function is preserved below the neurological level and includes the sacral segments S4–S5.

- C = **Incomplete**. Motor function is preserved below the neurological level and more than half of the key muscles below the neurological level have a muscle grade <3.

- D = **Incomplete**. Motor function is preserved below the neurological level and at least half of the key muscles below the neurological level have a muscle grade ⩾3.

- E = **Normal**. Sensory and motor function are normal.

REFERENCES

Adair, I., van Wijk, M., and Armstrong, G. (1977): Moire topography in scoliosis screening. *Clin Orthop* **129**, 165–71.

Albert, T., Lamb, D., Piazza, M., Flanders, A., Balderston, R., and Cotler, J. (1993): MRI evaluation of fusion mass incorporation after anterior cervical bony fusions: preliminary findings. *Paraplegia* **31**, 667–74.

Albert, T., Pinto, M., Smith, M., Balderston, R., Cotler, J., and Park, C. (1998): Accuracy of SPECT scanning in diagnosing pseudoarthrosis: a prospective study. *J Spinal Disord* **11**, 197–9.

Alund, M., and Larsson, S.-E. (1990): Three-dimensional analysis of neck motion. *Spine* **15**, 87–91.

Amendt, L., Ause-Ellias, K., Lundahl Eybers, J., Wadsworth, C., Nielsen, D., and Weinstein, S. (1990): Validity and reliability testing of the scoliometer. *Phys Ther* **70**, 108–16.

Appelgren, G., and Willner, S. (1990): End vertebra angle – a roentgenographic method to describe a scoliosis. *Spine* **15**, 71–4.

Association, A. S. I. (1984): *American Spinal Injury Association*. Chicago.

Association, J. O. (1986): Assessment of treatment of low back pain. *J Jap Orthop Assn* **60**, 909–11.

Aubin, C., Dansereau, J., de Guise, J., and Labelle, H. (1997): Rib cage-spine coupling patterns involved in brace treatment of adolescent idiopathic scoliosis. *Spine* **22**, 629–35.

Barsanti, C., deBari, A., and Covino, B. (1990): The torsion meter: a critical review. *J Paediatr Orthop* **10**, 527–31.

Beaton, D., Hogg-Johnson, S., and Bombardier, C. (1997): Evaluating changes in health status: reliability and responsiveness of five generic health status measures in workers with musculoskeletal disorders. *J Clin Epidemiol* **50**, 79–93.

Beck, A., Ward, C., and Mendelson, M. (1961): An inventory for measuring depression. *Arch Gen Psychiatry* **4**, 561–7.

Bell, G., and Stearns, K. (1991): Flexion-extension MRI of the upper rheumatoid cervical spine. *Orthopaedics* **14**, 969–73.

Bergner, M., Bobbitt, R., and Carter, W. (1981): The Sickness Impact Profile: development and final revision of a health status measure. *Med Care* **19**, 787–805.

Bernheim, J. (1999): How to get serious answers to serious questions: 'How have you been?' Subjective quality of life (QOL) as an individual experiential emergent construct. *Bioethics* **13**, 272–87.

Bernstein, R., and Hall, J. (1998): Solid rod short segment anterior fusion in thoracolumbar scoliosis. *J Paediatr Orthop B* **7**, 124–31.

Beurskens, A., de Vet, H., and Koke, A. (1996): Responsiveness of functional status in low back pain: a comparison of different instruments. *Pain* **65**, 71–6.

Beurskens, A., de Vet, H., Koke, A., van der Heijden, G., and Knipschild, P. (1995): Measuring the functional status of patients with low back pain. *Spine* **20**, 1017–28.

Birchall, D., Hughes, D., Hindle, J., Robinson, L., and Williamson, J. (1997): Measurement of vertebral rotation in adolescent idiopathic scoliosis using three-dimensional magnetic resonance imaging. *Spine* **22**, 2403–7.

Blackley, H., Plank, L., and Robertson, P. (1999): Determining the sagittal dimensions of the canal of the cervical spine. *J Bone Joint Surg* **81-B**, 110–12.

Blaustein, D., Zafonte, R., Thomas, D., Herbison, G., and Ditunno, J. (1993): Predicting recovery of complete motor quadriplegic patients: 24 hour v 72 hour motor index scores. *Am J Phys Med Rehabil* **72**, 306–11.

Blumenthal, S., and Gill, K. (1993): Can lumbar spine radiographs accurately determine fusion in postoperative patients? *Spine* **18**, 1186–9.

Blunt, K., Rajwani, M., and Guerriero, R. (1997): The effectiveness of chiropractic management of fibromyalgia patients: a pilot study. *J Manipulative Physiol Ther* **20**, 389–99.

Bo, K., Hilde, G., and Storheim, K. (1997): Intra- and interobserver reproducibility of Cybex EDI 320 measuring spinal mobility. *Scand J Med Sci Sports* **7**, 140–3.

Bohannon, R., and Smith, M. (1987): Interrater reliability of a modified Ashworth scale of muscle spasticity. *Phys Ther* **67**, 206–7.

Bohnsack, M., Gosse, F., Ruhmann, O., and Wenger, K. (1999): The value of scintigraphy in the diagnosis of pseudoarthrosis after spinal fusion surgery. *J Spinal Disord* **12**, 482–4.

Boline, P., Keating, J., Haas, M., and Anderson, A. (1992): Interexaminer reliability and discriminant validity of inclinometric measurement of lumbar rotation in chronic low-back pain patients and subjects without low-back pain. *Spine* **17**, 335–8.

Bondurant, F., Cotler, H., and Kulkarni, M. (1990): Acute spinal injury – a study using physical examination and magnetic resonance imaging. *Spine* **15**, 161–8.

Bracken, M., Collins, W., and Freeman, D. J. (1984): Efficacy of methylprednisolone in acute spinal cord injury. *JAMA* **251**, 45–52.

Bracken, M., Shepard, M., Collins, W., *et al.* (1990): A randomized, controlled trial of methylprednisolone or naloxone in the treatment of acute spinal-cord injury. *N Engl J Med* **322**, 1405–11.

Bracken, M., Shepard, M., Holford, T., *et al.* (1998): Methylprednisolone or tirilazad mesylate administration after acute spinal cord injury: 1-year follow up. Results of the Third National Acute Spinal Cord Injury randomized controlled trial. *J Neurosurg* **89**, 699–706.

Brodsky, A., Kovalsky, E., and Khalil, M. (1991): Correlation of radiologic assessment of lumbar spine fusions with surgical exploration. *Spine* **16**, S261–5.

Brorsson, B., and Asberg, K. (1984): Katz Index of Independence in ADL. Reliability and validity in short-term care. *Scand J Rehabil Med* **16**, 125–32.

Bunnell, W. (1984): An objective criterion for scoliosis screening. *J Bone Joint Surg* **66-A**, 1381–7.

Burton, A. (1986): Regional lumbar sagittal mobility. *Clin Biomech* **1**, 20–6.

Burton, A., Clarke, R., McClune, T., and Tillotson, K. (1996): The natural history of low back pain in adolescents. *Spine* **21**, 2323–8.

Calder, T., Dawson, E., and Bassett, L. (1984): The role of tomography in the evaluation of the postoperative spinal fusion. *Spine* **9**, 686–9.

Capaul, M., Zollinger, H., Satz, N., Dietz, V., Lehmann, D., and Schurch, B. (1994): Analyses of 94 consecutive spinal cord injury patients using ASIA definition and modified Frankel score classification. *Paraplegia* **32**, 583–7.

Carman, D., Browne, R., and Birch, J. (1990): Measurement of scoliosis and kyphosis radiographs. *J Bone Joint Surg* **72-A**, 328–33.

Carr, A. (1996): A patient-centred approach to evaluation and treatment in rheumatoid arthritis: the development of a clinical tool to measure patient-perceived handicap. *Br J Rheumatol* **35**, 921–32.

Carr, A., Jefferson, R., and Turner-Smith, A. (1991): Familial back shape in adolescent scoliosis. *Acta Orthop Scand* **62**, 131–5.

Carr, A., Jefferson, R., Turner-Smith, A., Weisz, I., Thomas, D., Stavrakis, T., and Houghton, G. (1989): Surface stereophotogrammetry of thoracic kyphosis. *Acta Orthop Scand* **60**, 177–80.

Castro, W., Sautmann, A., Schilgen, M., and Sautmann, M. (2000): Noninvasive three-dimensional analysis of cervical range of motion in normal subjects in relation to age and sex. *Spine* **25**, 443–9.

Chen, S., Samo, D., Chen, E., Crampton, A., Conrad, K., Egan, L., and Mitton, J. (1997): Reliability of three lumbar sagittal motion measurement methods: surface inclinometers. *J Occup Environ Med* **39**, 217–23.

Christensen, H., and Nilsson, N. (1998): The reliability of measuring active and passive cervical range of motion: an observer-blinded and randomized repeated-measures design. *J Manipulative Physiol Ther* **21**, 341–7.

Climent, J., Reig, A., Sanchez, J., and Roda, C. (1995): Construction and validation of a specific quality of life instrument for adolescents with spinal deformities. *Spine* **20**, 2006–11.

Climent, J., and Sanchez, J. (1999): Impact of the type of brace on the quality of life of adolescents with spinal deformities. *Spine* **24**, 1903–8.

Cobb, J. (1948): An outline for the study of scoliosis. In: *American Academy of Orthopaedic Surgeons Instructional Course Lectures*, Vol. V. J. W. Edwards, Ann Arbor.

Cohen, M., Ditunno, J. J., Donovan, W., and Maynard, F. J. (1998): A test of the 1992 International Standards for Neurological and Functional Classification of Spinal Cord Injury. *Spinal Cord* **36**, 554–60.

Cote, P., Kreitz, B., Cassidy, J., Dzus, A., and Martel, J. (1998): A study of the diagnostic accuracy and reliability of the scoliometer and Adam's forward bend test. *Spine* **23**, 796–803.

Cotler, H., Cotler, J., and Alder, M. (1990): The medical and economic impact of closed cervical spine dislocation. *Spine* **15**, 448–52.

D'Osualdo, F., Schierano, S., and Iannis, M. (1997): Validation of clinical measurement of kyphosis with a simple instrument: the arcometer. *Spine* **22**, 408–13.

Daltroy, L., Cats-Baril, W., and Katz, J. (1996): The North American Spine Society lumbar spine outcome assessment instrument: reliability and validity tests. *Spine* **21**, 741–9.

Danaberg, H., and Guiliano, M. (1999): Chronic low-back pain and its response to custom-made foot orthoses. *J Am Podiatr Med Assoc* **89**, 109–17.

Dangerfield, P., and Denton, J. (1986): The rib hump in infantile scoliosis and its relationship to vertebral rotation and the Cobb angle. *J Bone Joint Surg* **68-B**, 679.

Dansereau, J., Beauchamp, A., de Guise, J., and Labelle, H. (1990): 3-D reconstruction of the spine and the ribcage from stereoradiographic and imaging techniques. In: Proceedings of the CSME Mechanical Engineering Forum 1990 Volume 11: *Bioengineering Mechanics of Solids; Ice Mechanics Micromechanics* pp. 61–4.

Davis, L., Warren, S., Reid, D., Oberle, K., Saboe, L., and Grace, M. (1993): Incomplete neural deficits in thoracolumbar and lumbar spine fractures. *Spine* **18**, 257–63.

Dawson, E., Kropf, M., Purcell, G., Kabo, J., Kanim, L., and Burt, C. (1993): Optoelectronic evaluation of trunk deformity in scoliosis. *Spine* **18**, 326–31.

Debrunner, H. (1972): Das Kyphometer. *Z Orthop* **110**, 389–92.

Deen, H., Zimmerman, R., Lyons, M., McPhee, M., Verheijde, J., and Lemens, S. (1998): Use of the exercise treadmill to measure baseline functional status and surgical outcome in patients with severe lumbar spinal stenosis. *Spine* **23**, 244–8.

Derogatis, L., Rickels, K., and Rock, A. (1976): The SCL-90R and the MMPI: a step in the validation of a new self-report scale. *Br J Psychiatr* **128**, 280–9.

Deyo, R., Battie, M., Beurskens, A., Bombardier, C., Croft, P., Koes, B., Malmivaara, A., Roland, M., von Korff, M., and Waddell, G. (1998): Outcome measures for low back pain research. *Spine* **23**, 2003–13.

Deyo, R., and Diehl, A. (1983) Measuring physical and psychological function in patients with low-back pain. *Spine* **8**, 635–42.

Diab, K., Sevastik, J., Hedlund, R., and Sulivan, I. (1995): Accuracy and applicability of measurement of the scoliotic angle at the frontal plane by Cobb's method, by Fergusson's method and by a new method. *Eur Spine J* **4**, 291–5.

Dillard, J., Trafimow, J., and Andersson, G. (1991): Motion of the lumbar spine – reliability of two measurement techniques. *Spine* **16**, 321–4.

Ditunno, J., Ditunno, P., Graziani, V., *et al.* (2000): Walking Index for Spinal Cord Injury (WISCI): an international multicenter validity and reliability study. *Spinal Cord* **38**, 234–43.

Djukic, S., Lang, P., Morris, J., Hoaglund, F., and Genant, H. (1990): The postoperative spine. Magnetic resonance imaging. *Orthop Clin North Am* **21**, 603–24.

Dodds, T., Martin, D., Stolov, W., and Deyo, R. (1993): A validation of the functional independence measurement and its performance among rehabilitation inpatients. *Arch Phys Med Rehabil* **74**, 531–6.

Donovan, W., Brown, D., Ditunno, J. J., Dollfus, P., and Frankel, H. (1997): Neurological issues. *Spinal Cord* **35**, 275–81.

Dopf, C., Mandel, S., Geiger, D., and Mayer, P. (1994): Analysis of spine motion variability using a computerized goniometer compared to physical examination. *Spine* **19**, 586–95.

Dupuis, P., Yong-Hing, K., Cassidy, J., and Kirkaldy-Willis, W. (1985) Radiologic diagnosis of degenerative lumbar spinal instability. *Spine* **10**, 262–76.

Dvir, Z., and Prushansky, T. (2000): Reproducibility and instrument validity of a new ultrasonography-based system for measuring cervical spine kinematics. *Clin Biomech* **15**, 658–64.

Dvorak, J., Panjabi, M., Chang, D., Theiler, R., and Grob, D. (1991): Functional radiographic diagnosis of the lumbar spine. *Spine* **16**, 562–71.

El Masry, W., Tsubo, M., Katoh, S., Miligui, Y., and Khan, A. (1996): Validation of the American Spinal Injury Association (ASIA) motor score and the National Acute Spinal Cord Injury Study (NASCIS) motor score. *Spine* **21**, 614–19.

Ensink, F., Saur, P., Frese, K., Seeger, D., and Hilderbrandt, J. (1996): Lumbar range of motion: influence of time of day and individual factors on measurements. *Spine* **21**, 1339–43.

Ettinger, B., Black, D., Palermo, L., Nevitt, M., Melnikoff, S., and Cummings, S. (1994): Kyphosis in older women and its relation to back pain, disability and osteopenia: the study of osteoporotic fractures. *Osteoporos Int* **4**, 55–60.

Eysenck, H., and Eysenck, S. (1964): *Manual of the Eysenck Personality Inventory*. University of London Press, London.

EuroQoL Group (1990): EuroQoL – A new facility for the measurement for health-related quality of life. *Health Policy* **16**, 199–208.

Fairbank, J., and Pynsent, P. (2000): The Oswestry Disability Index. *Spine* **25**, 2940–53.

Fairbank, J., Couper, J., Davies, J., and O'Brien, J. (1980): The Oswestry low back pain questionnaire. *Physiotherapy* **66**, 271–3.

Fisher, K., and Johnson, M. (1997): Validation of the Oswestry Low Back Pain Disability Questionnaire, its sensitivity as a measure of change following treatment and its relationship with other aspects of the chronic pain experience. *Physiother Theory Pract* **13**, 67–80.

Frankel, H., Hancock, D., Hyslop, G., Melzak, J., Michaelis, L., Ungar, G., Vernon, J., and Walsh, J. (1969): The value of postural reduction in the initial management of closed injuries of the spine with paraplegia and tetraplegia. *Paraplegia* **7**, 179–92.

Fransen, M., and Edmonds, J. (1999): Reliability and validity of the EuroQoL in patients with osteoarthritis of the knee. *Rheumatology* **38**, 807–13.

Friberg, O. (1987): Lumbar instability: a dynamic approach by traction-compression radiography. *Spine* **12**, 119–29.

Gargan, M., and Bannister, G. (1990): Long-term prognosis of the soft-tissue injuries of the neck. *J Bone Joint Surg* **72-B**, 901–3.

Gertzbein, S. (1992): Scoliosis Research Society multicentre spine fracture study. *Spine* **17**, 528–40.

Gill, K., Krag, M., Johnson, G., Haugh, L., and Pope, M. (1988): Repeatability of four clinical methods for assessment of lumbar spinal motion. *Spine* **13**, 50–3.

Gocen, S., Aksu, M., Baktirogly, L., and Ozcan, O. (1998): Evaluation of computed tomographic methods to measure vertebral rotation in adolescent idiopathic scoliosis: an intraobserver and interobserver analysis. *J Spinal Disord* **11**, 210–14.

Goh, S., Price, R., Leedman, P., and Singer, K. (2000): A comparison of three methods for measuring thoracic kyphosis: implications for clinical studies. *Rheumatology* **39**, 310–15.

Goldberg, C., Kaliszar, M., Moore, D., Fogarty, E., and Dowling, F. (2001): Surface topography, Cobb angles, and cosmetic change in scoliosis. *Spine* **26**, E55.

Goldberg, D., and Hillier, W. (1979): A scaled version of the General Health Questionnaire. *Psych Med* **9**, 139–45.

Goldberg, D., and Williams, P. (1988): *A User's Guide to the General Health Questionnaire*. NFER-Nelson, Windsor.

Goldberg, M., Poitras, B., Mayo, N., Labelle, H., Bourassa, R., and Cloutier, R. (1988): Observer variation in assessing spinal curvature and skeletal development in adolescent idiopathic scoliosis. *Spine* **13**, 1371–7.

Graham, J. (1977): *The MMPI: A Practical Guide*. Oxford University Press, New York.

Greenough, C., and Fraser, R. (1991): Comparison of eight psychometric instruments in unselected patients with back pain. *Spine* **16**, 1068–74.

Greenough, C., and Fraser, R. (1992): Assessment of outcome in patients with low-back pain. *Spine* **17**, 36–41.

Gregson, J., Leathley, M., Moore, A., Sharma, A., Smith, T., and Watkins, C. (1999): Reliability of the Tone Assessment Scale and the Modified Ashworth Scale as clinical tools for assessing poststroke spasticity. *Arch Phys Med Rehabil* **80**, 1013–16.

Grevitt, M., Khazim, R., and Webb, J. (1997): The Short Form 36 Health Survey Questionnaire in spine surgery. *J Bone Joint Surg* **79-B**, 48–52.

Grossman, T., Mazur, J., and Cummings, R. (1995): An evaluation of the Adams Forward Bend Test and the scoliometer in a scoliosis school screening setting. *J Pediatr Orthop* **15**, 535–8.

Haas, B., Bergstrom, E., Jamous, A., and Bennie, A. (1996): The inter-rater reliability of the original and of the modified Ashworth scale for the assessment of spasticity in patients with spinal cord injury. *Spinal Cord* **34**, 560–4.

Haas, M., Jacobs, G., Raphael, R., and Petzing, K. (1995): Low back pain outcome measurement assessment in chiropractic teaching clinics: responsiveness and applicability of two functional disability questionnaires. *J Manipulative Physiol Ther* **18**, 79–87.

Hachisuka, K., Ogata, H., Ohkuma, H., Tanaka, S., and Dozono, K. (1997): Test-retest and inter-method reliability of the self-rating Barthel Index. *Clin Rehabil* **11**, 28–35.

Haher, T., Gorup, J., Shin, T., Howel, P., Merola, A., Grogan, D., Pugh, L., Lowe, T., and Murray, M. (1999): Scoliosis Research Society Instrument: results of the Scoliosis Research Society instrument for evaluation of surgical outcome in adolescent idiopathic scoliosis. *Spine* **24**, 1435–40.

Hall, K., Cohen, M., Wright, J., Call, M., and Werner, P. (1999): Characteristics of the functional independence measure in traumatic spinal cord injury. *Arch Phys Med Rehabil* **80**, 1471–6.

Hamill, C., and Simmons, E. (1997): Interobserver variability in grading lumbar fusions. *J Spinal Disord* **10**, 387–90.

Hasten, D., Johnston, F., and Lea, R. (1995): Validity of the Applied Rehabilitation Concepts (ARCON) system for lumbar range of motion. *Spine* **20**, 1279–83.

Hasten, D., Lea, R., and Johnston, F. (1996): Lumbar range of motion in male heavy laborers on the Applied Rehabilitation Concepts (ARCON) system. *Spine* **21**, 2230–4.

Herno, A., Airaksinen, O., and Saari, T. (1994): Computed tomography after laminectomy for lumbar spinal stenosis. Patient's pain patterns, walking capacity, and subjective disability had no correlation with computed tomography findings. *Spine* **19**, 1975–8.

Herno, A., Airaksinen, O., Saari, T., Pitkanen, M., Manninen, H., and Suomalainen, O. (1999a): Computed tomography findings 4 years after surgical management of lumbar spinal stenosis. *Spine* **24**, 2234–9.

Herno, A., Partanen, K., Talaslahti, T., Kaukanen, E., Turunen, V., Suomalainen, O., and Airaksinen, O. (1999b): Long-term clinical and magnetic resonance imaging follow-up assessment of patients with lumbar spinal stenosis after laminectomy. *Spine* **24**, 1533–7.

Herno, A., Saari, T., Suomalainen, O., and Airaksinen, O. (1999c): The degree of decompressive relief and its relation to clinical outcome in patients undergoing surgery for lumbar spinal stenosis. *Spine* **24**, 1010–14.

Herrmann, C. (1997): International experiences with the hospital anxiety and depression scale – a review of validation data and clinical results. *J Psychosom Res* 42, 17–41.

Herzenberg, J., Waanders, N., Closkey, R., Shultz, M., and Hesinger, R. (1990): Cobb angle versus spinous process angle in adolescent idiopathic scoliosis. *Spine* 15, 874–9.

Hino, H., Abumi, K., Kanayama, M., and Kaneda, K. (1999): Dynamic motion analysis of normal and unstable cervical spines using cineradiography. *Spine* 24, 163–8.

Ho, E., Upadhyay, S., Chan, F., Hsu, L., and Leong, J. (1993): New methods of measuring vertebral rotation from computed tomographic scans. *Spine* 18, 1173–7.

Hoenig, H., Branch, L., McIntyre, L., Hoff, J., and Horner, R. (1999): The validity in persons with spinal cord injury of a self-reported functional measure derived from the functional independence measure. *Spine* 24, 539–44.

Hosman, A., Slot, G., van Limbeek, J., and Beijneveld, W. (1996): Rib hump correction and rotation of the lumbar spine after selective thoracic rotation fusion. *Eur Spine J* 5, 394–9.

Hullin, M., McMaster, M., Draper, E., and Duff, E. (1991): The effect of Luque segmental sublaminar instrumentation on the rib hump in idiopathic scoliosis. *Spine* 16, 402–8.

Hunt, S., McEwen, J., and McKenna, S. (1985): Measuring health status: a new tool for clinicians and epidemiologists. *J R Coll Gen Pract* 35, 185–8.

Hurst, N., Kind, P., Ruta, D., Hunter, M., and Stubbings, A. (1997): Measuring health related quality of life in rheumatoid arthritis. *Br J Rheumatol* 36, 551–9.

Hutten, M., and Hermans, H. (1997): Reliability of lumbar dynamometry measurements in patients with chronic low back pain with test-retest measurements on different days. *Eur Spine J* 6, 54–62.

Jacobson, J., Starok, M., Pathria, M., and Garfin, S. (1997): Pseudarthrosis: US evaluation after posterolateral spinal fusion: work in progress. *Radiology* 204, 853–8.

Jamison, J. (1999): A psychological profile of fibromyalgia patients. *J Manipulative Physiol Ther* 22, 454–7.

Jay, M., Lamb, J., Watson, R., Young, I., Fearour, F., Alday, J., and Tindall, A. (2000): Sensitivity and specificity of the indicators of sincere effort of the EPIC lift capacity test on a previously injured population. *Spine* 25, 1405–12.

Jefferson, R., Weisz, I., Turner-Smith, A., Harris, J., and Houghton, G. (1988): Scoliosis surgery and its effect on back shape. *J Bone Joint Surg* 70-B, 261–6.

Jensen, M., Strom, S., and Turner, J. (1992): Validity of the Sickness Impact Profile Roland Scale as a measure of dysfunction in chronic pain patients. *Pain* 50, 157–62.

Jensen, T., Asmussen, K., Berg-Hansen, E., Lauritsen, B., Manniche, C., Vinterberg, H., Jensen, L., and Kramhoft, J. (1996): First time operation for lumbar disc herniation with or without free fat transplantation. *Spine* 21, 1072–6.

Johnsson, R., Axelsson, P., Gunnersson, G., and Stromqvist, B. (1999): Stability of lumbar fusion with transpedicular fixation determined by roentgen stereophotogrammetric analysis. *Spine* 27, 687–90.

Johnsson, R., Stromqvist, B., Axelsson, P., and Selvik, G. (1992): Influence of spinal immobilisation on consolidation of posterolateral lumbosacral fusion. *Spine* 17, 16–21.

Jordan, A., Manniche, C., Mosdal, C., and Hindsberger, C. (1998): The Copenhagen Neck Functional Disability Scale: a study of reliability and validity. *J Manipulative Physiol Ther* 21, 520–7.

Jordan, K., Dziedzic, K., Jones, P., Ong, B., and Dawes, P. (2000): The reliability of the three-dimensional FASTRAK measurement system in measuring cervical spine and shoulder range of motion in healthy subjects. *Rheumatology* 39, 382–8.

Kalebo, P., Kadziolka, R., and Sward, L. (1990): Compression-traction radiography of lumbar segment instability. *Spine* 15, 351–5.

Kant, A., Daum, W., Dean, S., and Uchida, T. (1995): Evaluation of lumbar spine fusion: plain radiographs versus direct surgical exploration and observation. *Spine* 20, 2313–17.

Karachalios, T., Sofianos, J., Roidis, N., Sapkas, G., Korres, D., and Nikolopoulos, K. (1999): Ten-year follow-up evaluation of a school screening program for scoliosis. *Spine* **24**, 2318–24.

Katz, L., and Dalby, J. (1981): Computer and manual administration of the Eysenck Personality Inventory. *J Clin Psychol* **37**, 586–8.

Katz, M., and Lyerly, S. (1963): Methods for measuring adjustment and social behaviour in the community. *Psych Rep* **13**, 503–35.

Kidd, D., Stewart, G., Baldry, J., Johnson, J., Rossiter, D., Petruckevitch, A., and Thompson, A. (1995): The Functional Independence Measure: a comparative validity and reliability study. *Disabil Rehabil* **17**, 10–14.

Kinnersley, P., Peters, T., and Stott, N. (1994): Measuring functional health status in primary care using the COOP-WONCA charts: acceptability, range of scores, construct validity, reliability and sensitivity to change. *Br J Gen Pract* **44**, 545–9.

Kinney, R., Gatchell, R., and Mayer, T. (1991): The SCL-90R evaluated as an alternative to the MMPI for psychological screening of chronic low-back pain patients. *Spine* **16**, 940–2.

Kippers, V., and Parker, A. (1987): Toe-touch test. A measure of its validity. *Phys Ther* **67**, 1680–4.

Knight, R., Waal-Manning, H., and Spears, G. (1983): Some norms and reliability data for the State-Trait Anxiety Inventory and the Zung Self-Rating Depression Scale. *Br J Clin Psychol* **22**, 245–9.

Kopec, J., Esdaile, J., and Abrahamowicz, M. (1995): The Quebec Back Pain Disability Scale: measurement properties. *Spine* **20**, 341–52.

Korovessis, P., and Stamatakis, M. (1996): Prediction of scoliotic Cobb angle with the use of the scoliometer. *Spine* **21**, 1661–6.

Labelle, H., Danreseau, J., Bellefleur, C., and Jequier, J. (1995): Variability of geometric measurements from three-dimensional reconstructions of scoliotic spines and rib cages. *Eur Spine J* **4**, 88–94.

Lang, P., Chafetz, N., Genant, H., and Morris, J. (1990): Lumbar spinal fusion. Assessment of functional stability with magnetic resonance imaging. *Spine* **15**, 581–8.

Larsen, J., Rimoldi, R., Capen, D., Nelson, R., Nagelberg, S., and Thomas, J. (1996): Assessment of pseudoarthrosis in pedicle screw fusion: a prospective study comparing plain radiographs, flexion/ extension radiographs, CT scanning, and bone scintigraphy. *J Spinal Disord* **9**, 117–20.

Laulund, T., Sojbjerg, J., and Horlyck, E. (1982): Moire topography in school screening for structural scoliosis. *Acta Orthop Scand* **53**, 765–8.

Laursen, S., and Fugl, I. (1995): Outcome of treatment of chronic low back pain in inpatients. *Dan Med Bull* **42**, 290–3.

Lawlis, G., Cuencas, R., Selby, D., and McCoy, C. (1989): The development of the Dallas Pain Questionnaire. *Spine* **14**, 511–16.

Lee, C., and Nachemson, A. (1997): The Crankshaft Phenomenon after posterior Harrington fusion in skeletally immature patients with thoracic or thoracolumbar idiopathic scoliosis followed to maturity. *Spine* **22**, 58–67.

Lee, S., Harris, K., Goel, V., and Clark, C. (1994): Spinal motion after cervical fusion. *Spine* **19**, 2336–42.

Lehmann, T., Brand, R., and Gorman, T. (1983): A low back rating scale. *Spine* **8**, 308–15.

Leung, A., Lam, T., Hedley, A., and Twomey, L. (1999): Use of a subjective health measure on Chinese low back pain patients in Hong Kong. *Spine* **24**, 961–6.

Levin, B., Llabre, M., and Weiner, W. (1988): Parkinson's disease and depression: psychometric properties of the Beck Depression Inventory. *J Neurol Neurosurg Psychiatr* **51**, 1401–4.

Loebl, W. (1967): Measurements of spinal posture and range in spinal movements. *Ann Phys Med* **9**, 103–10.

Loupasis, G., Stamos, K., Katonis, P., Sapkas, G., Korres, D., and Hartofilakidis, G. (1999): Seven- to 20- year outcome of lumbar discectomy. *Spine* **24**, 2313–17.

Lucas, J., and Ducker, T. (1979): Motor classification of spinal cord injuries with mobility, morbidity and recovery indices. *Am Surg* **45**, 151–8.

Lundon, K., Li, A., and Bibershtein, S. (1998): Interrater and intrarater reliability in the measurement of kyphosis in postmenopausal women with osteoporosis. *Spine* **23**, 1978–85.

MacDuff, C., and Russell, E. (1998): The problem of measuring change in individual health-related quality of life by postal questionnaire: use of the patient-generated index in a disabled population. *Qual Life Res* 7, 761–9.

Macnab, I. (1971): Negative disc exploration. *J Bone Joint Surg* 53-A, 891–903.

Madsen, O. (1996): Trunk extensor and flexor strength measured by the Cybex 6000 dynamometer. *Spine* 21, 2770–6.

Mahoney, F., and Barthel, D. (1965): Functional evaluation: the Barthel Index. *Maryland State Med J* 14, 61–5.

Main, C. (1983): The Modified Somatic Perception Questionnaire (MSPQ). *J Psychosom Res* 27, 503–14.

Main, C., Wood, P., Hollis, S., Spanswick, C., and Waddell, G. (1992): Distress and risk assessment method: a simple patient classification to identify distress and evaluate the risk of poor outcome. *Spine* 17, 42–52.

Manabe, S., Tateishi, A., Abe, M., and Ohno, T. (1989): Surgical treatment of metastatic tumors of the spine. *Spine* 14, 41–7.

Manniche, C. (1995): Assessment and exercise in low back pain. *Dan Med Bull* 42, 301–13.

Manniche, C., Asmussen, K., and Lauritsen, B. (1994): Low back pain rating scale: validation of a tool for assessment of low back pain. *Pain* 57, 317–26.

Mannion, A., Dolan, P., and Adams, M. (1996): Do 'abnormal' scores precede or follow first-time low back pain? *Spine* 21, 2603–11.

Matheson, L., Mooney, V., Grant, J., Affleck, M., Hall, H., Melles, T., Lichter, R., and McIntosh, G. (1995): A test to measure lift capacity of physically impaired adults. *Spine* 20, 2119–29.

Mayer, R., Chen, I.-H., Lavender, S., Trafimow, J., and Andersson, G. (1995): Variance in the measurement of sagittal lumbar spine range of motion among examiners, subjects, and instruments. *Spine* 20, 1489–93.

Mayer, T., Brady, S., Bovasso, E., Pope, P., and Gatchell, R. (1993): Non invasive measurement of cervical tri-planar motion in normal subjects. *Spine* 18, 2191–5.

Mayer, T., Kondraske, G., Beals, S., and Gatchell, R. (1997): Spine range of motion: accuracy and sources of error with inclinometric measurement. *Spine* 22, 1976–84.

McAlindon, R., and Kruse, R. (1997): Measurement of rib vertebral angle difference. *Spine* 22, 198–9.

McGuire, R. J. (1998): In: Levine, A. M., Eismont, F. J., Garfin, S. R., and Zigler, J. E. (eds), *Spine Trauma*. W. B. Saunders Co., Philadelphia.

McHorney, C., and Tarlov, A. (1995): Individual-patient monitoring in clinical practice: are available health status surveys adequate? *Qual Life Res* 4, 293–307.

Medical Research Council (1976): *Aids to the Examination of the Peripheral Nervous System*. Her Majesty's Stationery Office, London.

Mehta, M. (1972): The rib-vertebra angle in the early diagnosis of resolving and progressive infantile scoliosis. *J Bone Joint Surg* 54-A, 230–43.

Merritt, J., McLean, T., Erickson, R., and Offord, K. (1986): Measurement of trunk flexibility in normal subjects: reproducibility of three clinical methods. *Mayo Clin Proc* 61, 192–7.

Miller, S., Mayer, T., Cox, R., and Gatchell, R. (1992): Reliability problems associated with the modified Schober technique for true lumbar flexion measurement. *Spine* 17, 345–8.

Million, R., Hall, W., and Nilsen, K. (1982): Assessment of the progress of the back pain patient. *Spine* 7, 204–12.

Mior, S., Kopansky-Giles, D., Crowther, E., and Wright, J. (1996): A comparison of radiographic and electrogoniometric angles in adolescent idiopathic scoliosis. *Spine* 21, 1549–55.

Moffett, J., Torgerson, D., Bell-Syer, S., Jackson, D., Llewlyn-Phillips, H., Farrin, A., and Barber, J. (1999): Randomised controlled trial of exercise for low back pain: clinical outcomes, costs, and preferences. *Br Med J* 319, 279–83.

Moll, J., and Wright, V. (1971): Normal range of spinal mobility. *Ann Rheum Dis* 30, 381–6.

Morris, J., Baumrind, S., Genant, H., and Korn, E. (1985): Stereophotogrammetry of the lumbar spine. *Spine* 10, 368–75.

Morrissy, R., Goldsmith, G., Hall, E., Kehl, D., and Cowie, G. (1990): Measurement of the Cobb angle on radiographs of patients who have scoliosis. *J Bone Joint Surg* 72-A, 320–7.

Murrell, G., Coonrad, R., Moorman, C. I., and Fitch, R. (1993): An assessment of the reliability of the scoliometer. *Spine* **18**, 709–12.

Naughton, M., and Wiklund, I. (1993): A critical review of dimension-specific measures of health-related quality of life in cross-cultural research. *Qual Life Res* **2**, 397–432.

Newton, M., Thow, M., Somerville, D., Henderson, I., and Waddell, G. (1993): Trunk strength testing with iso-machines. Part 2: Experimental evaluation of the Cybex II back testing system in normal subjects and patients with chronic low back pain. *Spine* **18**, 812–24.

Nissinen, M., Heliovaara, M., Ylikoski, M., and Poussa, M. (1993): Trunk asymmetry and screening for scoliosis: a longitudinal cohort study of pubertal school children. *Acta Paediatr* **82**, 77–82.

Norris, S., and Watt, I. (1983): The prognosis of neck injuries resulting from rear end vehicle collisions. *J Bone Joint Surg* **65-B**, 608–11.

Ohlen, G., Spangfort, E., and Tingvall, C. (1989): Measurement of spinal sagittal configuration and mobility with Debrunner's kyphometer. *Spine* **14**, 580–3.

Omeroglu, H., Ozekin, O., and Bicinoglu, A. (1996): Measurement of vertebral rotation in idiopathic scoliosis using the Pedriolle torsionmeter: a clinical study on intraobserver and interobserver error. *Eur Spine J* **5**, 167–71.

Ordway, N., Seymour, R., Donelson, R., Hojnowski, L., Lee, E., and Edwards, W. (1997): Cervical sagittal range-of-motion analysis using three methods. *Spine* **22**, 501–8.

Palit, M., Schofferman, J., Goldthwaite, N., Reynolds, J., Kerner, M., Keaney, D., and Lawrence-Miyasaki, L. (1999): Anterior discectomy and fusion for the management of neck pain. *Spine* **24**, 2224–8.

Pandyan, A., Johnson, G., Price, C., Curless, R., Barnes, M., and Rodgers, H. (1999): A review of the properties and limitations of the Ashworth and Modified Ashworth Scales as measures of spasticity. *Clin Rehabil* **13**, 373–83.

Paquet, N., Maroccin, F., Richards, C., Dionne, J., and Comeau, F. (1991): Validity and reliability of a new electrogoniometer for the measurements of sagittal dorsolumbar movements. *Spine* **16**, 516–19.

Parkerson, G., Broadhead, W., and Tse, C. (1990): The Duke Health Profile: a 17-Item measure of health and dysfunction. *Med Care* **28**, 1056–72.

Pearsall, D., Reid, J., and Hedden, D. (1992): Comparison of three noninvasive methods for measuring scoliosis. *Phys Ther* **72**, 648–56.

Perdriolle, R., and Vidal, J. (1985): Thoracic idiopathic scoliosis curve evolution and prognosis. *Spine* **10**, 785–91.

Petersen, C., Johnson, R., Schuit, D., and Hayes, K. (1994): Intraobserver and interobserver reliability of asymptomatic subject's thoracolumbar range of motion using the OSI CA 6000 spine motion analyzer. *J Orthop Sports Phys Ther* **20**, 207–12.

Pile, K., Laurent, M., Salmond, C., Best, M., Pyle, E., and Moloney, R. (1991): Clinical assessment of ankylosing spondylitis: a study of observer variation in spinal measurements. *Br J Rheumatol* **30**, 29–34.

Pitkanen, M., and Manninen, H. (1994): Sidebending versus flexion-extension radiographs in lumbar spinal instability. *Clin Radiol* **49**, 109–14.

Pitkanen, M., Manninen, H., Lindgrer, K., Turunen, M., and Airaksinen, O. (1997): Limited usefulness of traction-compression films in the radiographic diagnosis of lumbar spinal instability. *Spine* **22**, 193–7.

Pitts, L., Ross, A., Chase, G., and Faden, A. (1995): Treatment with thyrotropin-releasing hormone (TRH) in patients with traumatic spinal cord injuries. *J Neurotrauma* **12**, 235–43.

Pratt, R., Fairbank, J., and Virr, A. (2002): The reliability of the Shuttle Walking Test, the Swiss Spinal Stenosis Questionnaire, the Oxford Spinal Stenosis Score, and the Oswestry Disability Index in the assessment of patients with lumbar spinal stenosis. *Spine* **27**, 84–91.

Priebe, M., and Waring, W. (1991): The interobserver reliability of the Revised American Spinal Injury Association Standards for Neurological Classification of Spinal Injury Patients. *Am J Phys Med Rehabil* **70**, 268–70.

Pruijs, J., Keessen, W., van der Meer, R., and van Wieringen, J. (1995a): School screening for scoliosis: the value of quantitative measurement. *Eur Spine J* 4, 226–30.

Pruijs, J., Stengs, C., and Keessen, W. (1995b): Parameter variation in stable scoliosis. *Eur Spine J* 4, 176–9.

Pun, W., Luk, K., Lee, W., and Leong, J. (1987): A simple method to estimate the rib hump in scoliosis. *Spine* 12, 342–5.

Putnam, S., Kurtz, J., and Houts, D. (1996): Four-month test–retest reliability of the MMPI-2 with normal male clergy. *J Pers Assess* 67,341–53.

Rajasekaran, S., Dorgan, J., Taylor, J., and Dangerfield, P. (1994): Eighteen-level analysis of vertebral rotation following Harrington-Luque instrumentation in idiopathic scoliosis. *J Bone Joint Surg* 76-A, 104–9.

Ranawat, C., O'Leary, P., Pelicci, P., Tsairis, P., Marchisello, P., and Dorr, L. (1979): Cervical fusion in rheumatoid arthritis. *J Bone Joint Surg Am* 63-A, 1003–10.

Richards, B. (1992): Measurement error in assessment of vertebral rotation using the Perdriolle torsionmeter. *Spine* 17, 513–17.

Riddle, D., and Stratford, P. (1998): Use of generic versus region-specific functional status measures on patients with cervical spine disorders. *Phys Ther* 78, 951–63.

Roland, M., and Fairbank, J. (2000): The Roland-Morris Disability Questionnaire and the Oswestry Disability Questionnaire. *Spine* 25, 3115–24.

Roland, M., and Morris, R. (1983): A study of the natural history of low back pain: Part 1. Development of a reliable and sensitive measure of disability in low-back pain. *Spine* 8, 141–4.

Rossignol, M., Abnehaim, L., Seguin, P., Neveu, A., Collet, J., Ducruet, T., and Shapiro, S. (2000): Coordination of primary health care for back pain. *Spine* 25, 251–8.

Ruta, D., Garratt, A., Leng, M., Russell, I., and MacDonald, L. (1994a): A new approach to the measurement of quality of life: the patient-generated index. *Med Care* 32, 1109–26.

Ruta, D., Garratt, A., Wardlaw, D., and Russell, I. (1994b): Developing a valid and reliable measure of health outcome for patients with low back pain. *Spine* 19, 1887–96.

Rytokoski, U., Karppi, S., Pukka, P., Soini, J., and Ronnemaa, T. (1994): Measurement of low back mobility, isometric strength and isoinertial performance with Isostation B-200 triaxial dynamometer: reproducibility of measurement and development of functional indices. *J Spinal Disord* 7, 54–61.

Sahlstrand, T. (1986): The clinical value of Moire topography in the management of scoliosis. *Spine* 11, 409–17.

Salisbury, P., and Porter, R. (1987): Measurement of lumbar sagittal mobility: a comparison of methods. *Spine* 12, 190–3.

Salminen, J., Oksanen, A., Maki, P., Pentii, J., and Kujala, U. (1993): Leisure time physical activity in the young. *Int J Sports Med* 14, 406–10.

Samuelsson, K., Larsson, E., Normelli, H., Oberg, B., Aaro, S., and Tropp, H. (1996): Development of an instrument for clinical evaluation after surgery for neuromuscular scoliosis. *Eur Spine J* 5, 400–6.

Samuelsson, L., and Noren, L. (1997): Trunk rotation in scoliosis: the influence of curve type and direction in 150 children. *Acta Orthop Scand* 68, 273–6.

Sato, H., and Kikuchi, S. (1993): The natural history of radiographic instability of the lumbar spine. *Spine* 18, 2075–9.

Saur, P., Ensink, F., Frese, K., Seeger, D., and Hildebrandt, J. (1996): Lumbar range of motion: reliability and validity of the inclinometer technique in the clinical measurement of trunk flexibility. *Spine* 21, 1332–8.

Schoppink, L., van-Tulder, M., Koes, B., Beurskens, S., and de-Bie, R. (1996): Reliability and validity of the Dutch Adaptation of the Quebec Back Pain Disability Scale. *Phys Ther* 76, 268–75.

Segatore, M. (1991): Determining the interrater reliability of motor power assessments using a spinal cord testing record. *J Neurosci Nurs* 23, 220–3.

Siambanes, D., and Mather, S. (1998): Comparison of plain radiographs and CT scans in instrumented posterior lumbar interbody fusion. *Orthopedics* 21, 165–7.

Singh, A., and Crockard, H. (1999): Quantitative assessment of cervical spondylotic myelopathy by a simple walking test. *Lancet* 354, 370–3.

Singh, S., Morgan, M., Scott, S., Walters, K., and Hardman, A. (1992): Development of a shuttle walking test of disability in patients with chronic airways obstruction. *Thorax* **47**, 1019–24.

Smith, B., Penny, K., and Purves, A. (1997): The Chronic Pain Grade Questionnaire: validity and reliability in postal research. *Pain* **71**, 141–7.

Sonn, U. (1996): Longitudinal studies of dependence in daily life activities among elderly persons. *Scand J Rehabil Med Suppl* **34**, 1–35.

Staffer, R., and Coventry, M. (1972): Anterior interbody lumbar fusion: analysis of Mayo Clinic series. *J Bone Joint Surg* **54-A**, 757–68.

Stokes, I., Bevins, T., and Lunn, R. (1987): Back surface curvature and measurement of lumbar spinal motion. *Spine* **12**, 355–61.

Stratford, P., and Binkley, J. (1997): Measurement properties of the RM-18: a modified version of the Roland-Morris Disability Scale. *Spine* **22**, 2416–21.

Stratford, P., Binkley, J., and Riddle, D. (2000): Development and initial validation of the back pain functional scale. *Spine* **25**, 2095–103.

Stucki, G., Daltroy, L., Liang, M., Lipson, S., Fossel, A., and Katz, J. (1996): Measurement properties of a self-administered outcome measure in lumbar spinal stenosis. *Spine* **21**, 796–803.

Stude, D., Goertz, C., and Gallinger, M. (1994): Inter- and intraexaminer reliability of a single, digital inclinometric range of motion measurement technique in the assessment of lumbar range of motion. *J Manipulative Physiol Ther* **17**, 83–7.

Suk, S., Lee, C., Kim, W., Chung, Y., and Park, Y. (1995): Segmental pedicle screw fixation in the treatment of thoracic idiopathic scoliosis. *Spine* **20**, 1399–405.

Sykes, L., Campbell, I., Powell, E., Ross, E., and Edwards, J. (1996): Energy expenditure of walking for adult patients with spinal cord lesions using the reciprocating gait orthosis and functional electrical stimulation. *Spinal Cord* **34**, 659–65.

Tandon, V., Campbell, F., and Ross, E. (1999): Posterior lumbar interbody fusion. Association between disability and psychological disturbance in non-compensation patients. *Spine* **24**, 1833–8.

Tator, C. (ed.) (1982): *Early Management of Acute Spinal Cord Injury*. Raven Press, New York.

Taylor, S., Taylor, A., Foy, M., and Fogg, A. (1999): Responsiveness of common outcome measures for patients with low back pain. *Spine* **24**, 1805–12.

Theologis, T., Fairbank, J., Turner-Smith, A., and Patazopoulos, T. (1997): Early detection of progression in adolescent idiopathic scoliosis by measurement of change in back shape with the integrated shape imaging system scanner. *Spine* **22**, 1223–8.

Thometz, J., Lamdan, M., Liu, X., and Lyon, R. (2000): Relationship between quantec measurement and Cobb angle in patients with idiopathic scoliosis. *J Paediatr Orthop* **20**, 512–16.

Thurlbourne, T., and Gillespie, R. (1976): The rib hump in idiopathic scoliosis. Measurement, analysis and response to treatment. *J Bone Joint Surg* **58-B**, 64–71.

Tillotson, K., and Burton, A. (1991): Noninvasive measurement of lumbar sagittal mobility. *Spine* **16**, 29–33.

Tokuhashi, Y., Matsuzaki, H., and Sano, S. (1993): Evaluation of clinical lumbar instability using the treadmill. *Spine* **18**, 2321–4.

Torg, J., Pavlov, H., Genuario, S., Sennet, B., Wisneski, R., Robie, B., and Jahre, C. (1986): Neuropraxia of the cervical spinal cord with transient quadriplegia. *J Bone Joint Surg* **68-A**, 1345–70.

Tousignant, M., de Bellefeuille, L., O'Donoghue, S., and Grahovac, S. (2000): Criterion validity of the Cervical Range of Motion (CROM) goniometer for cervical flexion and extension. *Spine* **25**, 324–30.

Triano, J., McGregor, M., Cramer, G., and Emde, D. (1993): A comparison of outcome measures for use with back pain patients: results of a feasibility study. *J Manipulative Physiol Ther* **16**, 67–73.

Tucci, S., Hicks, J., Gross, E., Campbell, W., and Danoff, J. (1986): Cervical motion assessment: a new, simple, and accurate method. *Arch Phys Med Rehabil* **67**, 225–30.

Turner-Smith, A., Harris, J., Houghton, G., and Jefferson, R. (1988): A method for analysis of back shape in scoliosis. *J Biomechanics* **21**, 497–509.

Underwood, M., Barnett, A., and Vickers, M. (1999): Evaluation of two time-specific backpain outcome measures. *Spine* **24**, 1104–12.

Upadhyay, S., Burwell, R., and Webb, J. (1988): Hump changes on forward flexion of the lumbar spine in patients with adolescent idiopathic scoliosis. *Spine* **13**, 146–51.

Vendrig, A., van-Akkerveeken, P., and McWhorter, K. (2000): Results of multimodal treatment program for patients with chronic symptoms after a whiplash injury of the neck. *Spine* **25**, 238–44.

Vernon, H., and Mior, S. (1991): The Neck Disability Index: a study of the reliability and validity. *J Manipulative Physiol Ther* **14**, 409–15.

Viitanen, J., Kautiainen, H., Suni, J., Kokko, M., and Lehtinen, K. (1995): The relative value of spinal and thoracic mobility measurements in ankylosing spondylitis. *Scand J Rheumatol* **24**, 94–7.

Von Korff, M., Ormeh, J., Keefe, F., and Dworkin, S. (1992): Grading the severity of chronic pain. *Pain* **50**, 133–49.

Waddell, G., and Main, C. (1984): Assessment of severity in low back disorders. *Spine* **9**, 204–8.

Ware, J., and Sherbourne, C. (1992): The MOS 36-Item Short-Form Health Survey (SF-36). I. Conceptual framework and item selection. *Med Care* **30**, 473–83.

Waters, R., Yakura, J., and Adkins, R. (1993): Gait performance after spinal cord injury. *Clin Orthop* **288**, 87–96.

Watkins, R., O'Brien, J., Draugelis, R., and Jones, D. (1986): Comparisons of preoperative and postoperative MMPI data in chronic back patients. *Spine* **11**, 385–90.

Webster, F., and Smiley, D. (1957): Evaluation of an operative series of lumbar disc herniations. *J Bone Joint Surg* **39**-A, 688.

Weiss, H. (1995): Measurement of vertebral rotation: Perdriolle versus Raimondi. *Eur Spine J* **4**, 34–8.

Weisz, I., Jefferson, R., Turner-Smith, A., Houghton, G., and Harris, J. (1988): ISIS scanning: a useful assessment technique in the management of scoliosis. *Spine* **13**, 405–8.

Wells, J., and Nicosia, S. (1995): Scoring acute spinal cord injury: a study of the utility and limitations of five different grading systems. *J Spinal Cord Med* **18**, 33–41.

Wheeler, A., Goolkasian, P., Baird, A., and Darden, B. (1999): Development of the Neck Pain and Disability Scale. *Spine* **24**, 1290–4.

White, S., Asher, M., Lai, S., and Burton, D. (1999): Patients perceptions of overall function, pain, and appearance after primary posterior instrumentation and fusion for idiopathic scoliosis. *Spine* **24**, 1693–9.

Williams, R., Binkley, J., Block, R., Goldsmith, C., and Minuk, T. (1993): Reliability of the modified-modified Schober and double inclinometer methods for measuring lumbar flexion and extension. *Phys Ther* **73**, 33–44.

Williams, R., and Myers, A. (1998): A new approach to measuring recovery in injured workers with acute low back pain: resumption of activities of daily living scale. *Phys Ther* **78**, 613–23.

Willner, S. (1979): Moire topography for the diagnosis and documentation of scoliosis. *Acta Orthop Scand* **50**, 295–302.

Wojcik, A., Phillips, G., and Mehta, M. (1994): Recording of the back surface and spinal shape by the Quantec Imaging System. A new technique in the scoliosis clinic. *J Bone Joint Surg* **76**-B, 10–11.

Youdas, J., Carey, J., and Garrett, T. (1991): Reliability of measurements of cervical spine range of motion – comparison of three methods. *Phys Ther* **71**, 98–104; discussion 105–6.

Zigmond, A., and Snaith, R. (1983): The Hospital Anxiety and Depression Scale. *Acta Psychiatr Scand* **67**, 478–83.

Zoega, B., Karrholm, J., and Lind, B. (2000): Outcome scores in degenerative cervical disc surgery. *Eur Spine J* **9**, 137–43.

Zung, W. (1965): A self-rated depression scale. *Arch Gen Psychiatr* **32**, 63–70.

15

Shoulder and elbow
Paul Harvie and Andrew J. Carr

INTRODUCTION

A review of the literature relating to shoulder and elbow surgery will testify to the bewildering number of outcome measures and scoring systems that are available to the orthopaedic surgeon undertaking research. Unfortunately, it is within the boundaries of clinical research where the use of outcome measures invariably stops, with few surgeons being sufficiently pro-active as to use them in their day-to-day clinical practice.

Increasingly however, orthopaedic surgeons are being asked to evaluate the outcome of their practice. Historically, this has been met with significant inertia, with surgeons being suspicious as to the potential consequences of acquiring such data. Wider issues such as increasing patient awareness and expectations, the rise in evidence-based healthcare, the possibility of league tables for surgeons and economic planning are likely to make the use of such measures mandatory in the future. Despite this, little guidance is available as to how outcomes should be assessed.

The proliferation of outcome measures in orthopaedics has paralleled the development of joint replacement surgery. This being so, outcome measures in shoulder and elbow surgery remain in their infancy compared with the hip and knee, the deficiency being particularly evident in the elbow. Both shoulder and elbow complexes involve more than one articulation and have significant pathology prone soft tissue components. Differing pathologies and patterns of trauma affect differing populations with diverse age ranges, and as a consequence it is virtually impossible to design a single outcome measure that will adequately address all populations. For example, can an elderly woman undergoing shoulder replacement for cuff tear arthropathy and a young man undergoing anterior stabilization for recurrent glenohumeral dislocation be assessed using the same outcome measure? Similarly, the child with an intercondylar fracture and elderly woman with a fractured olecranon?

With this in mind it is not surprising that, since the 1980s, there has been a proliferation of outcome measures. Both shoulder- and elbow-specific, general or condition-specific, patient-based or clinician-based outcome measures all exist, as well as those that assess the upper limb as a whole. Some 'outcome scores' merely represent the documentation of assessment 'criteria' used by individuals, often in the publication of landmark series', but lack any rigorous statistical validation. Many were never published as or intended to be used as true outcome measures, but have been perpetuated as such by their ongoing (yet still unvalidated) use in further series. More recently, outcome measures are being designed and statistically validated specifically for their use as a true outcome measure. Unfortunately, within this group it is evident that there is much duplication of effort. Whether this is due to the ambitions of individual researchers or to a lack of understanding of the methodology behind the development of similar scores, often only subtle differences exist in these newly developed outcome assessment scores. This, in addition to 'geographical' preferences in outcome measure selection, inhibits attempts at determining 'gold standard' outcome measures which would otherwise facilitate true research comparisons and systematic reviews.

This chapter includes an historical perspective covering the origin of outcome assessment. A brief synopsis on what constitutes a good outcome is also included. In addition, notable outcome measures relating to the shoulder and elbow – both in orthopaedics and trauma – are discussed in more detail. Detailed discussion of all outcome measures relating to shoulder and elbow surgery is not included, although a summary of those outcome measures found during a literature review is included, together with original references.

HISTORY OF OUTCOME ASSESSMENT

The End Result Idea

'The common sense notion that every hospital should follow every patient it treats, long enough to determine whether or not the treatment has been successful, and then to inquire, 'If not, why not?'' (Codman 1934)

'We believe it is the duty of every hospital to establish a follow-up system, so that as far as possible the result of every case will be available at all times for investigation by members of staff, the trustees or administration, or by other authorised investigators or statisticians. We believe that the publication of such material in abstract by case numbers is practical and does not entail a disproportionate expense' (Codman et al. 1913)

Ernest Amory Codman

The view expressed above may easily be interpreted as current affairs 'sound-bites' or abstracts from any recent surgical or, indeed, hospital board meeting. They were in fact made by Ernest Amory Codman nearly 90 years ago. Ernest Amory Codman (1869–1940) was an eminent pioneering surgeon at the Massachusetts General Hospital in Boston. A Harvard Medical School graduate, like many

surgeons of his era he was a generalist in that he was both a distinguished orthopaedic and general surgeon. Unlike many surgeons however he was capable of original forward thinking and made significant landmark contributions to surgery which today would be highly recognized. In orthopaedic surgery, Codman performed the first rotator cuff repair (1909) (Codman 1911), and summarized his lifetime's work in *The Shoulder* in 1934 (Codman 1934) – a work still considered by many to be one of the best pieces of work written in its field. Codman also pioneered the use of X-rays in orthopaedics, and established the Registry of Bone Sarcoma in 1921 (Codman 1922). In addition he developed the 'ether chart' with Harvey Cushing, which was the precursor of today's anaesthetic charts, and he was widely published on the topic of surgery for duodenal ulcer.

Despite this, Codman will be remembered most for his almost single-minded obsession with his End Result Idea. He firmly believed in the principle of patient follow-up and determination of the 'End Result', emphasizing the importance of recording adverse results in order to improve future treatment and establish 'gold standards' of care. He was the first surgeon to publish a clinical series' recording all data on End Result Cards. Unfortunately, Codman's peers did not share his enthusiasm with the End Result Idea. Codman's frustrations culminated at a meeting on January 6th 1915 in which he ridiculed his colleagues and hospital board members, portraying them in a large cartoon as an ostrich burying its head in the sand and choosing to ignore what is happening around it. Codman's career subsequently declined thereafter and he died in relative poverty.

Codman's original ideas form the basis of what has now developed into 'outcome measures research'.

WHAT CONSTITUTES A GOOD OUTCOME MEASURE?

The two essential requirements of an outcome measure are that it is valid – that is, it assesses what it is supposed to – and it is reliable, showing a minimal error. Equally important, the surgeon and researcher must understand and be able to interpret these factors so that an informed and rational selection of outcome measure can be made.

A detailed discussion relating to the measurement of validity and reliability is given by Pynsent (2001). At the extremes, shoulder-specific patient-based scores such as the Oxford Shoulder Score (OSS) (Dawson *et al.* 1996), Shoulder Pain and Disability Index (SPADI) (Roach *et al.* 1991) and the Simple Shoulder Test (SST) (Lippitt *et al.* 1993) have all been rigorously tested and found to be valid and reliable, but despite this they are not widely used. (Until recently, no elbow-specific, patient-based outcome measures existed that had been suitably tested. The Patient Rated Elbow Evaluation (PREE) (MacDermid 2001) and the combined clinician/patient-based American Shoulder and Elbow Surgeons Elbow Form (ASES-e) (King *et al.* 1999) have been available since 2001 and 1999, respectively.) In comparison, condition-specific, clinician-based scores relating to elbow trauma such as the Flynn Criteria (for paediatric supracondylar fracture assessment) (Flynn *et al.* 1974), Jupiter Criteria (for intercondylar fractures) (Jupiter *et al.* 1985), Khalfayan Score (for Mason II radial head fractures) (Khalfayan *et al.* 1992) and the Boenisch Score [for acromioclavicular joint (ACJ) dislocation] (Boenisch *et al.* 1991) have undergone no statistical assessment of validity or reliability, but are still used. In addition, these more accurately termed assessment 'criteria' have been found to be applied outside their initial condition specific application (Yokoyama *et al.* 1998; Kruger-Franke *et al.* 2000). Highlighting this point, the above-named Boenisch Score is a clinician-based score used in patients undergoing surgery for ACJ dislocation. It is dependent on clinical examination, isokinetic strength tests, subjective patient feelings and radiographic findings. In personal correspondence with Dr. Uli Boenisch, he is realistic and sufficiently honest to regard this score as 'worth nothing' (P. Harvie, 27 May 2002), and was therefore surprised when informed of the use of this score as an outcome measure nine years after its initial publication in a paper relating to clavicular fracture! (Kruger-Franke *et al.* 2000).

In addition to the statistical determinants of validity and reliability, an outcome measure must be easy and cheap to administer. It must be user-friendly and in a format that is easily understood by the clinician and/or patient, and ideally not be time-consuming. The SPADI uses 13 Visual Analogue Scales (VAS), the SST 12 Yes/No questions and the OSS 12 questions with five graded responses. Elbow scores such as the ASES-e and PREE use numerical scales. All are simple and rapidly completed, but even this small sample highlights variations in format, let alone content. In comparison, the American Shoulder and Elbow Surgeons (ASES) Shoulder Score (Barrett *et al.* 1987) uses a combination of VASs, numerical scales and Yes/No answers in its questionnaire and necessitates the use of a formula to convert questionnaire data into a final score [(10 − Visual Analogue Scale Pain Score) + ((5/3) × Cumulative Activities of Daily Living Score)]. Ideally, scores should be determined directly without need for further calculation. Further, any outcome measure must only be applied to a specific population consistent with that on which the outcome measure was initially based. The outcome measure must not be modified unless the user is prepared to go through the validation and reliability testing again.

PATIENT-BASED OR CLINICIAN-BASED OUTCOME MEASURES?

Patient-based outcome measures are rating scales and questionnaires that rely on responses from the patient. Historically, early outcome measures relating to shoulder and elbow surgery were almost entirely clinician-based, being used principally as research tools. These most frequently involved assessment of pain, range of movement, strength testing and function and occasionally – particularly in relation to trauma – radiographic evaluation and assessment of deformity. Problems arise however with different authors placing varying emphasis on different components, thereby rendering comparison between different outcome measures impossible.

In addition, such methods of scoring are especially liable to bias – particularly experimenter bias, whether deliberate or not – as well as inter- and intra-observer error. As a result, strict guidelines on the performance and interpretation of any clinical examination or strength test must be included in such outcome measures and strictly adhered to. Pain is subjective and difficult to assess quantitatively. The use of numerical scores, VASs and even analgesic requirements (e.g. University of California Los Angeles Shoulder Scoring System, UCLA; Amstutz *et al.* 1981 and the Hospital for Special Surgery Shoulder Rating Score, HSS; Altchek *et al.* 1990) are all used. There is no consensus on a uniform method of assessing range of movement, and the absolute measurement of strength is of questionable significance. The Constant-Murley Shoulder Score (Constant and Murley 1987) assigns 25 per cent of its score to shoulder strength. To score 100 per cent necessitates an individual being able to abduct their arm to 90° holding 25 lb (10 kg). Constant claims in his original paper that 'a normal shoulder in a 25-year-old man resists 25 lb without difficulty.' This is contentious, as in practice a significant number of young individuals with 'normal' shoulders are unable to do this. Such observations are widely reported, particularly in older groups. For example, normal subjects aged 61–70 years have a normalized score of 83/100 for males and 70/100 for females (Lippitt *et al.* 1993). Further contention exists as to the practical contribution to activities of daily living of actually being able to perform this test. Constant also places significant emphasis on range of movement (40% of the total score), with only 35 per cent being allocated to pain and function. Despite these factors, the European Shoulder and Elbow Society advocates use of the Constant score in papers presented at its meetings.

Instability is rarely addressed, the assumption being that adequate assessment of those factors formerly mentioned would adequately reflect any detrimental effects due to instability.

The notable exception is the highly specific Rowe Rating for Bankart Repairs (Rowe *et al.* 1978) and more recently the Western Ontario Shoulder Instability Index (WOSI) (Kirkley *et al.* 1998). Assessment of elbow instability is incorporated in the Broberg and Morrey Functional Rating Index (Broberg and Morrey 1986) for outcome assessment after radial head excision. This is given as a subjective statement by the patient however more recently the Leipzig Elbow Score (devised for outcome scoring after fracture dislocation of the elbow) (Korner *et al.* 1998) utilizes clinical examination for instability evaluation.

Radiographic assessment of surgical procedures may be useful in research projects, but should not be used in outcome evaluation as radiographic appearance does not correlate with functional result.

As with many complex issues where little effective progress is being made, it often pays dividends to take a step back and reappraise the problem from a different, often more simplistic perspective. In terms of outcome measures in shoulder and elbow surgery, the question must be asked, 'Whose interests are being met in terms of outcome assessment?' Formerly, it was the surgeon. Data obtained could either be applied to research publication or merely stored as a means of reaffirming (or not!) ones surgical skills. Today, it is the patient that should benefit. In general terms, patient-perceived health status and health-related quality of life are now generally accepted as the most important outcomes – barring mortality – from surgical intervention. Transposed to shoulder and elbow surgery, the main importance of the upper limb lies in its functional capacity; thus, recent trends have been towards developing patient-based outcome measures emphasizing pain relief and post-operative function in terms of activities of daily living. For example, the young man with recurrent shoulder dislocation who undergoes stabilization surgery may never re-dislocate and achieve a Good/Excellent result with Rowe's Rating. This outcome may be satisfactory in the eyes of the surgeon, but closer questioning using the patient-based Oxford Instability Score may reveal an underlying lack of confidence in returning to normal activity levels, indicating the need for further specialist input such as physiotherapy in order to achieve an outcome that is acceptable to both surgeon and patient.

It is evident that patient-based outcome measures represent the route forward in terms of outcome measure research. Indeed, this has been recognized by the Royal College of Surgeons of England who are formulating a database of outcome measures currently in use across all surgical specialities. Interestingly, such is the perceived importance of patient-based outcome measures that only such measures are to be included (The Royal College of Surgeons of England 2002).

Outcome measures of note: Orthopaedics

THE SHOULDER

Shoulder Pain And Disability Index (SPADI)

The SPADI is a shoulder-specific, patient-based index consisting of 13 items divided into two sub-scales for pain and disability. Each item utilizes VASs with pain and disability each carrying a 50 per cent weighting in terms of the overall score. Each VAS is scored from 0 to 11, with each subscale score representing the arithmetic sum of each item VAS expressed as a percentage of its maximum score; the total SPADI score is then calculated using the average of pain and disability scores. This index was developed using 37 male patients (age range 23 to 76 years) (Beaton and Richards 1998) with musculoskeletal shoulder pain; the remainder had a diagnosis of shoulder pain of neurogenic or unknown origin. Patients with fracture were excluded.

Test–retest reliability showed an Interclass Correlation Coefficient (ICC) of 0.66 for total score and Internal Consistency determined by Cronbach's alpha coefficient (Alpha) of 0.95 and validated using criterion, content, construct and discriminate validity.

The Simple Shoulder Test (SST)

The SST is a shoulder-specific, patient-based outcome score developed by Matsen and colleagues (Lippitt *et al.* 1993) and derived from the Neer and ASES scoring systems. It singularly assesses post-operative function by means of 12 questions with Yes/No answers. It was developed using a cohort of 250 patients with a broad spectrum of shoulder pathology inclusive of cases of instability but excluding patients with fracture. No formal statistical validation was performed by Matsen, but Beaton and Richards (1998) found ICC: 0.99, Alpha (not calculated) and validated using content and construct validity.

The Subjective Shoulder Rating Scale (SSRS)

Developed by Kohn *et al.* (1993), the SSRS is a four-point patient-based, shoulder-specific outcome measure that uses multiple choice questions to assess pain, motion, stability and activity. The former three are each given a 20 per cent weighting and the latter a 40 per cent weighting in the overall score. Statistical analysis based on a cohort of patients undergoing total shoulder arthroplasty and rotator cuff repair (age range 18–77 years) has been performed (ICC: 0.7, Alpha (not calculated) and validated using content and construct validity) (Beaton and Richards 1998).

The Subjective Shoulder Rating System

Developed by Kohn and Geyer (1997), the Subjective Shoulder Rating System is a shoulder-specific, patient-based outcome assessment system that assesses pain, range of motion, instability, activity and overhead work with weightings of 35 per cent, 35 per cent, 15 per cent and 15 per cent, respectively (5% of which is apportioned to overhead activity). The system was developed using a cohort of 200 patients (age range 18–71 years) with instability, sub-acromial impingement and frozen shoulder. No rigorous statistical validation was undertaken, and reliability was tested by direct correlation with scores obtained using the Constant-Murley score.

The Oxford Shoulder Score (OSS)

The OSS is a patient-based, shoulder-specific scoring system consisting of 12 questions each with 5-graded options, the score being given as the sum of the 12-graded responses. No further calculation is required, and the system assesses pain and activities of daily living (with weightings of 33.3% and 66.6%, respectively). It was initially based on a sample of 111 patients undergoing shoulder surgery, but excluded patients with instability. Reproducibility is assessed using the Coefficient of Reliability: 6.8, with Alpha: 0.92 and validated using construct validity.

It is easily understood by patients and quickly completed in the out-patient setting.

The Disabilities of the Arm, Shoulder and Hand Questionnaire (DASH)

The DASH questionnaire (Hudak *et al.* 1996) is a 30-point patient-based, non-joint-specific outcome measure. Its basis is that perfect upper-limb function necessitates perfect functioning of all upper-limb joints. It represents a distillation of 821 items from 13 different outcome scales, and utilizes 5-point scales for assessment of symptoms and disability (with weightings of 16.7% and 83.3%, respectively). Analysis [based on a cohort mean age of 45 years, with both surgical and non-surgical pathology (including instability)] found ICC: 0.92, Alpha 0.96 and validated using content, construct and discriminate validity (McConnell *et al.* 1999).

The Upper Extremity Functional Scale (UEFS)

The UEFS (Pransky *et al.* 1997) is an 8-point patient-based outcome measure used solely for individuals with chronic, non-traumatic, work-related upper-limb disorders. It is non-joint-specific and is designed to assess the outcome of treatment for any upper-extremity disorder meeting the above criteria. It assesses upper-limb function alone, utilizing numerical scales to assess each aspect. It was validated in two cohorts: 108 patients with upper-extremity disorders (including wrist and elbow tendinitis, nerve entrapment and chronic pain) all of whom were receiving workers' compensation; and 165 patients with carpal tunnel syndrome (overall age range 19–65 years). The UEFS has been validated using content, construct and discriminate validity, although retest data are not available.

Both the DASH and UEFS were developed for use with patients with any diagnosis involving the upper extremity. It can easily be assumed that these scales would not be as responsive as the shoulder-specific scales in patients with shoulder dysfunction. Beaton *et al.* (2001) have, however, shown that the DASH is more responsive than the SPADI in patients with shoulder dysfunction, thereby suggesting that a scale which assesses the entire upper extremity might be adequate for the evaluation of patients with any upper-extremity diagnosis.

The Oxford Instability Score

The Oxford Instability Score (Dawson *et al.* 1999) is a shoulder-specific, condition-specific, patient-based outcome measure that uses a 12-item questionnaire in which each question has 5-graded responses. It addresses symptoms of instability, pain and activities of daily living, with the overall score being obtained as the arithmetic sum of each graded response without any need for further calculation. It is based on a prospective study of 92 patients with shoulder instability with both the Oxford Instability and Rowe Scores showing excellent responsiveness in this cohort. [In comparison, the Constant-Murley Shoulder Score (Constant and Murley 1987) performed poorly, representing additional evidence for the suggestion that this score is not appropriate of outcome assessment in shoulder instability.] Reproducibility is assessed using the Coefficient of Reliability: 5.7, with alpha: 0.92 and validated using construct validity. This system is easily understood by patients and quickly completed in the out-patient setting.

The Constant-Murley Shoulder Score

The Constant-Murley Shoulder Score (Constant and Murley 1987) is a shoulder-specific, clinician-based outcome scoring system that assesses pain, activities of daily living, range of motion and power with weightings of 15 per cent, 20 per cent, 40 per cent and 25 per cent, respectively. The score is derived directly without any further calculation, and is the outcome measure of choice adopted by the European Shoulder and Elbow Society. The original paper included no statistical analysis of the scoring system (Constant and Murley 1987). As previously noted, Constant places heavy emphasis on range of motion and power, despite current trends towards pain and function. Furthermore, the system requires normalization for age and is not appropriate for outcome assessment in instability.

The American Shoulder and Elbow Surgeons Shoulder Score (ASES)

The ASES (Michener *et al.* 2000) is a shoulder-specific combined clinician/patient-based outcome score. The patient-based component assesses pain, instability and activities of daily living. Pain is assessed using VASs as well as Yes/No answers relating to analgesia requirements. Instability and activities of daily living are assessed using VASs and numerical scales, respectively. The clinician-based component assesses range of motion, 12 specific clinical signs, strength and instability. The final score necessitates complex calculation from data derived from each section, and no statistical analysis was performed at the time of original publication. Subsequent analysis based on populations with wide-ranging shoulder pathology including instability has been performed (ICC: 0.84, Alpha: 0.86 and validated using content, construct and discriminate validity) (Michener *et al.* 2000). The system is time-consuming and difficult to perform in the out-patient setting.

THE ELBOW

The Patient-Rated Elbow Evaluation (PREE)

The PREE is an elbow-specific, patient-based outcome measure that utilizes 20 numerical scales to assess pain and function (with weightings of 25% and 75%, respectively). The pain scale is transposed directly from the Patient Rated Wrist Evaluation (MacDermid 1996) with the disability scale being derived from biomechanical and clinical literature. It was based on a cohort of 70 patients (age range 16–81 years) with a wide spectrum of elbow pathology including fracture (ICC: 0.90, Alpha (not calculated) and validated using content and construct validity).

The American Shoulder and Elbow Surgeons Elbow Score (ASES-e)

The ASES-e (King *et al.* 1999) is an elbow-specific, combined clinician/patient-based outcome score. It includes a patient questionnaire and a clinician assessment form for recording elbow impairment. The patient questionnaire has three subscales for pain, function and patient satisfaction. Pain is a 5-item assessment scored on a scale of 1 to 10. Function is assessed by 12 items each scored on a 0 to 3 numerical scale, and patient satisfaction assessed by a single question rated on a 0 to 10 numerical scale. Statistical analysis performed on the same cohort as

the PREE has found ICC: 0.79–0.89, Alpha (not calculated) and validated using content and construct validity (MacDermid 2001). The ASES-e includes a companion impairment form for assessment of the unaffected limb, but this has not been tested for reliability and validity. In addition, the final outcome score needs formal calculation, and the overall assessment is time-consuming and difficult to use in the out-patient setting.

The Mayo Elbow Performance Score (MEPS)

The MEPS (Morrey and An 1993) is the most commonly applied elbow specific outcome measure. It is a clinician based score that assesses pain, motion, stability and function with weightings of 45 per cent, 20 per cent, 10 per cent and 25 per cent respectively. It is widely applied to all elbow pathology including trauma.

Outcome measures of note: Trauma

The unexpected nature of the vast majority of trauma implies that only very rarely are pre-morbid scores of patient shoulder or elbow function available with which to compare outcomes. As previously mentioned, both shoulder and elbow complexes involve more than one articulation but function as a whole. Historically, attempts at devising outcome measures for traumatic injuries to the shoulder and elbow have been published. Imatani's Score (Imatani *et al.* 1975) for assessment of surgery for ACJ dislocation, the Neer Rating (Neer 1970) for proximal humeral fractures, the Holdsworth and Mossad Score (Holdsworth and Mossad 1984) for olecranon fractures and/or the Broberg and Morrey (1986) Functional Scale Index for radial head excision are examples of scores that have attempted to assess the outcomes of injury to discrete areas within these joint complexes. Being able to say categorically that these outcome measures are in fact assessing what they were designed to assess is questionable. In addition, different age groups have different outcome priorities. The development of a patient-based outcome measure to assess, for example, supracondylar fractures in

Table 15.1: A summary of outcome scoring methods

Name	Source reference	Shoulder-specific?	Condition-specific?	Common use?	Range (points) (Worse ↔ Best)	Comments
The Shoulder: Clinician-based scores						
Imatani Score	(Imatani et al. 1975)	Yes	No	No (Imatani et al. 1975)	0 ↔ 100	Initially applied to ACJ dislocation. Based on cohort of 23 patients with complete ACJ separation. Broadly extended to general shoulder assessment
Rowe's Rating Sheet for Bankart Repairs: Rowe Score	(Rowe et al. 1978)	Yes	Yes	Yes (Dawson et al. 1999) (Cole et al. 2000)	0 ↔ 100 Excellent 90–100 Good 75–89 Fair 50–74 Poor <50	Based on cohort of 162 Bankart repairs in 161 patients. More broadly applied to surgery for instability
University of California Los Angeles Shoulder Scoring System (UCLA)	(Amstutz et al. 1981)	Yes	No	Yes (Roddey et al. 2000)	3 ↔ 30 Composite ×3 (1–10)	Designed for assessment of total shoulder arthroplasty. Condition specific variations for: 1) Rotator cuff repair (Ellman et al. 1986) 2) Post-traumatic hemiarthroplasty (Kay and Amstutz 1988) 3) Sub-acromial decompression (Ellman and Kay 1991). Should be assessed 1–10 for each component, and not a cumulative score. Poor result in any component indicates overall failure
Constant (Constant-Murley) Score	(Constant and Murley 1987)	Yes	No	Yes (Constant and Murley 1987) (Conboy et al. 1997) (Dawson et al. 2001)	0 ↔ 100	Adopted by European Shoulder & Elbow Society. Not applicable to instability (Conboy et al. 1997). May be imprecise for long-term follow-up (Dawson et al. 2001)

Table 15.1: A summary of outcome scoring methods – *continued*

Name	Source reference	Shoulder-specific?	Condition-specific?	Common use?	Range (points) (Worse ↔ Best)	Comments
						Needs age/gender adjustment for true inter-score comparisons (Lippitt et al. 1993) (Kuhn and Blasier 1997)
Swanson Shoulder Assessment	(Swanson et al. 1989)	Yes	Yes	No	6 ↔ 30 Excellent >28 Good 23–27.9 Fair 18–22.9 Poor <18	Based on cohort of 35 Swanson Bipolar Shoulder Arthroplasties for rheumatoid, primary osteo- and post-traumatic osteoarthritis
Hospital for Special Surgery Shoulder Rating Score (HSS)	(Altchek et al. 1990)	Yes	No	No	0 ↔ 100 Excellent 90–100 Good 70–89 Fair 50–69 Poor <50	Based on cohort of 40 patients undergoing sub-acromial decompression for impingement Associated partial-/full-thickness rotator cuff tears in some cases Derived from HSS Scale (Range 0–100, 1982) (Warren et al. 1982) for shoulder arthroplasty and extended 1997 (L'Insalata et al. 1998)

The Shoulder: Combined clinician-/patient-based scores

Name	Source reference	Shoulder-specific?	Condition-specific?	Common use?	Range (points) (Worse ↔ Best)	Comments
American Shoulder & Elbow Surgeons Scoring System (ASES)	(Barrett et al. 1987)	Yes	No	Yes (Kelly et al. 1987) (Hawkins et al. 1989; Kelly 1990) (Richards et al. 1994)	0 ↔ 100	Derived from Neer System 1974 (Neer 1974) and later modified by Cofield 1983 (Neer et al. 1982) (Cofield 1983) (Cofield 1984)
Athletic Shoulder Outcome Scoring System	(Tibone and Bradley 1993)	Yes	No	No	0 ↔ 100 Excellent 90–100 Good 70–89 Fair 50–69 Poor <50	Allows for high treatment expectations in this group Includes component for instability

The Shoulder: Patient based scores

Measure	Reference				Range	Notes
Shoulder Severity Index (SSI)	(Patte 1987)	Yes	No	No (Beaton and Richards 1998) (Patte 1987) (Beaton and Richards 1996)	0↔100	
Shoulder Pain And Disability Index (SPADI)	(Pransky et al. 1997)	Yes	No	No (Roach et al. 1991) (Beaton and Richards 1996) (Williams et al. 1995) (Heald et al. 1997)	100↔0	Uses Visual Analogue Scales Comprised of Pain Scale (5 items) and Disability Scale (8 items)
Simple Shoulder Test (SST)	(Morrey and An 1993)	Yes	No	No (Lippitt et al. 1993) (Beaton and Richards 1998) (Beaton and Richards 1996) (Goldberg et al. 2001a) (Duckworth et al. 1999) (Goldberg et al. 2001b) (Matsen 1996)	0↔12	Based on cohort of 250 patients with shoulder pathology Instability but No fractures included in cohort
Subjective Shoulder Rating Scale	(Kohn et al. 1993)	Yes	No	No (Beaton and Richards 1998) (Beaton and Richards, 1996)	0↔5	4-point (pain, motion, stability, activity) MCQ Questionnaire
Shoulder Surgery Score – Oxford Shoulder Score (OSS)	(Dawson et al. 1996)	Yes	No	No (Dawson et al. 1996) (Conboy et al. 1997)	60↔12	Based on cohort of 111 patients undergoing shoulder surgery Not applicable to surgery for instability (Conboy et al. 1997) Assesses Pain and Activities of Daily Living
Disabilities of the Arm, Shoulder and Hand Questionnaire (DASH)	(Hudak et al. 1996)	No	No	Yes (McConnell et al. 1999) (Beaton et al. 2001) (Atroshi et al. 2000) (Skutek et al. 2000)	0↔100	30-point index assessing entire upper limb Optionally assesses sports/ performing arts/work Also applied to shoulder trauma (van der Windt et al. 1998)

Table 15.1: A summary of outcome scoring methods – *continued*

Name	Source reference	Shoulder-specific?	Condition-specific?	Common use?	Range (points) (Worse ↔ Best)	Comments
Subjective Shoulder Rating System (SSRS)	(Kohn and Geyer 1997)	Yes	No	No	0 ↔ 100	Initially created in 1988, published in 1996 Based on patients with anterior instability, sub-acromial impingement and frozen shoulder Not principally for arthroplasty/fracture assessment
American Academy of Orthopaedic Surgeons (Upper Extremity Scoring System) (AAOS)	(AAOS 1996)	No	No	No	190 ↔ 38	
Western Ontario Shoulder Instability Index (WOSI)	(Kirkley et al. 1998)	Yes	Yes	No (Kirkley et al. 1998) (Kirkley et al. 1999)	2100 ↔ 0	Applied to both surgically and conservatively managed patients with instability Based on initial cohort of 100 patients Uses Visual Analogue Scales 21 items covering symptoms/sports, recreation and work/lifestyle/emotions
Symptoms and Function of the Shoulder Scale	(L'Insalata et al. 1998)	Yes	No	No	17 ↔ 100	Derived from HSS Shoulder Rating Score – HSS
Penn Shoulder Score	(Leggin et al. 1997)	Yes	No	No	1 ↔ 80	
Upper-Extremity Functional Scale (UEFS)	(Pransky et al. 1997)	No	No	No	8 ↔ 80	Applied to subjects with chronic, non-traumatic work-related, upper-extremity disorders
Shoulder Disability Questionnaire	(van der Heijden et al. 2000)	Yes	No	No (van der Windt et al. 1998) (Guyatt et al. 1987)	100 ↔ 0	16 Pain-Disability-related questions Yes/No answers All questions relate to preceding 24 hours only

Measure	Reference				Score	Comments
Oxford Shoulder Instability Score	(Dawson et al. 1999)	Yes	No		60 ↔ 12	Specifically for assessment of shoulder instability. Based on cohort of 92 patients with shoulder instability treated operatively or conservatively. Assesses symptoms of Pain and Instability as well as activities of daily living
The Elbow: Clinician-based scores						
Ewald Scale	(Ewald 1975)	Yes	No	No (Ewald et al. 1993) (Schemitsch et al. 1996)	0 ↔ 100	Initially applied to total elbow arthroplasty
Hospital for Special Surgery Elbow Assessment	(Inglis and Pellicci 1980)	Yes	No	No (Turchin et al. 1998) (Figgie et al. 1989)	0 ↔ 100	Initially used for assessment of elbow arthroplasty (Pynsent et al. 1993). Also applied to elbow trauma (Eygendaal et al. 2001) (Chen et al. 2001)
Souter-Strathclyde Assessment	(Souter 1985)	Yes	No	No (Souter 1990) (Burnett and Fyfe 1991)	Not numerically scored	Involves pre-, per- and post-operative assessment of 154, 152 and 121 items respectively. Includes radiographic assessment. Developed for assessment of Souter-Strathclyde Arthroplasty (Pynsent et al. 1993). Extended for use in 'elbow prosthesis trials' and adopted by British Orthopaedic Association (Pynsent et al. 1993)
Broberg and Morrey Scale (Functional Rating Index)	(Broberg and Morrey 1986)	Yes	No	No (Turchin et al. 1998) (Figgie et al. 1989) (Packer et al. 1994)	0 ↔ 100 Excellent 95–100 Good 80–94 Fair 60–79 Poor <60	Most commonly applied to trauma (Wallenbock and Potsch 1997) (Ikeda et al. 2001) (Ring et al. 1998) (Ring et al. 1997) (Broberg and Morrey 1987)

Table 15.1: A summary of outcome scoring methods – *continued*

Name	Source reference	Shoulder-specific?	Condition-specific?	Common use?	Range (points) (Worse ↔ Best)	Comments
Mayo Elbow Performance Score (MEPS)	(Morrey and An 1993)	Yes	No	Yes (Lee and Morrey 1997) (Kudo 1998) (Connor and Morrey 1998) (Gill and Morrey, 1998) (Mansat and Morrey 1998) (Gill et al. 2000)	0 ↔ 100	Also applied to trauma (Rodgers et al. 1996) (Cobb and Morrey 1997); (Schneeberger et al. 1997)
The Elbow: Combined clinician-/patient-based scores						
American Shoulder and Elbow Surgeons Elbow Form (ASES-e)	(King et al. 1999)	Yes	No	Yes (MacDermid 2001)	0 ↔ 100	Also applied to trauma (MacDermid 2001) Patient-based component assessing pain, function and patient satisfaction Clinician-based component assessing elbow impairments
The Elbow: Patient-based scores						
Disabilities of the Arm, Shoulder and Hand Questionnaire (DASH)	(Hudak et al. 1996)	No	No	Yes (McConnell et al. 1999) (Beaton et al. 2001) (Atroshi et al. 2000) (Skutek et al. 2000)	0 ↔ 100	Also applied to trauma (Maro et al. 2001) 30-point index assessing entire upper limb Optionally assesses sports, performing arts and work
Patient-Rated Elbow Evaluation (PREE)	(MacDermid 2001)	Yes	No	No (MacDermid 2001)	0 ↔ 100	Extended from Patient Rated Wrist Evaluation (MacDermid 1996); (MacDermid et al. 1998)

Trauma Outcome Scoring Methods

The Shoulder: Clinician-based shoulder scores

Arner Assessment	(Arner et al. 1957)	Yes	Yes	No	Not numerically scored	Assessment of surgical management of ACJ dislocation Extended by Walsh in 1985 (Walsh et al. 1985) and further by MacDonald in 1988 (MacDonald et al. 1988)
Neer Rating	(Neer 1970)	Yes	Yes	Yes (Svend-Hansen, 1974) (Hagg and Lundberg 1994) Kocialkowski and Wallace 1990) (Jakob et al. 1990)	0↔100 Excellent >89 Satisfactory 80–89 Unsatisfactory 70–79 Failure <70	Based on cohort of 117 patients with 3- and 4-part proximal humeral fractures Result in any patient with significant pain is failure
Wolfgang Rating	(Wolfgang 1974)	Yes	Yes	No	0↔17 Excellent 14–17 Good 11–13 Fair 8–10 Poor <8	Based on cohort of 74 open rotator cuff repairs in 73 patients
Imatani Score	(Imatani et al. 1975)	Yes	Yes	No	0↔100	Based on cohort of 23 patients with complete ACJ separation
Rowe's Rating Sheet for Bankart Repairs: Rowe Score	(Rowe et al. 1994)	Yes	Yes	Yes (Rowe et al. 1994) (Cole et al. 2000); (Weber et al. 1984); (Tsai et al. 1991)	0↔100 Excellent 90–100 Good 75–89 Fair 50–74 Poor <50	Initially applied to Bankart repairs More broadly applied to surgery for instability
University of California Los Angeles Shoulder Scoring System (UCLA)	(Amstutz et al. 1981)	Yes	No	Yes (Roddey et al. 2000) (Hessman et al. 1998) (Bosch et al. 1998) (Hessman et al. 1999) Kim and Ha, 2000) (Skutek et al. 2001)	3↔30 Composite ×3 (1–10)	Widespread assessment of shoulder trauma Should be assessed 1–10 for each component and not a cumulative score Poor score in any component indicates overall failure

Table 15.1: A summary of outcome scoring methods – *continued*

Name	Source reference	Shoulder-specific?	Condition-specific?	Common use?	Range (points) (Worse ↔ Best)	Comments
Post and Singh Assessment	(Post and Singh 1983)	Yes	Yes	No	Post-operative pain relief 0 ↔ 75 Excellent 70–75 Good 60–69 Fair 50–59 Poor <50 outcome scores Post-operative function Excellent >160' Good 125–160' Fair 75–124' Poor <75'	Based on cohort of 59 open rotator cuff repairs in 55 patients Assesses Pain (major component) and Function (minor component) Different pre- and post-operative assessment criteria Separate Pain and Function Pain-numerical, Function-overhead range of movement
Constant (Constant-Murley) Score	(Constant and Murley 1987)	Yes	No	Yes (Constant and Murley 1987) (Conboy et al. 1997) (Dawson et al. 2001) (Hessman et al. 1998) (Bosch et al. 1998) (Hessman et al. 1999)	0 ↔ 100	Adopted by European Shoulder and Elbow Society Not applicable to instability (Conboy et al. 1997) May be imprecise for long-term follow-up (Dawson et al. 2001) Needs age/gender adjustment for true inter-score comparison (Lippitt et al. 1993) (Kuhn and Blasier 1997) 25% of score allocated to Power
Hospital for Special Surgery Shoulder Rating Score (HSS)	(Altchek et al. 1990)	Yes	No (Bosch et al. 1998)	No (Bosch et al. 1998)	0 ↔ 100 Excellent 90–100 Good 70–89 Fair 50–69 Poor <50	Fracture patients NOT included in initial cohort

The Shoulder: Patient-based shoulder scores

Walsh Questionnaire	(Walsh et al. 1985)	Yes	Yes	No (Kuhn and Blasier 1997)	5 ↔ 20	Extension of Arner assessment for ACJ dislocation
Shoulder Pain and Disability Index (SPADI)	(Roach et al. 1991)	Yes	No	Yes (Roach et al. 1991) (Roddey et al. 2000) (Beaton and Richards 1996) (Williams et al. 1995) (Heald et al. 1997)	0 ↔ 100	Broadly applied to shoulder trauma BUT patients with fractures EXCLUDED from original cohort (Roach et al. 1991)
Simple Shoulder Test (SST)	(Lippitt et al. 1993)	Yes	No	No (Roach et al. 1991) (Beaton and Richards 1996) (Williams et al. 1995) (Skutek et al. 2001)	0 ↔ 12	Broadly applied to trauma but No patients with fractures included in original cohort (Morrey and An 1993)
Disabilities of the Arm, Shoulder and Hand Questionnaire (DASH)	(Hudak et al. 1996)	Yes	No	Yes (McConnell et al. 1999) (Beaton et al. 2001) (Atroshi et al. 2000) (Skutek et al. 2000)	0 ↔ 100	Broadly applied to shoulder trauma 30-point index assessing entire upper limb Optionally assesses sports, performing arts and work
Shoulder Surgery Score – Oxford Shoulder Score (OSS)	(Dawson et al. 1996)	Yes	No	No (Dawson et al. 1996) (Conboy et al. 1997)	60 ↔ 12	Not applicable to surgery for instability (Flynn et al. 1974)
Western Ontario Shoulder Instability Index (WOSI)	(Kirkley et al. 1998)	Yes	Yes	No (Kirkley et al. 1998) (Kirkley et al. 1999)	2100 ↔ 0	Applied to both surgically and conservatively managed patients with instability Based on initial cohort of 100 patients Uses Visual Analogue Scales 21 items covering symptoms/sport, recreation and work/lifestyle/emotions

Table 15.1: A summary of outcome scoring methods – *continued*

Name	Source reference	Shoulder-specific?	Condition-specific?	Common use?	Range (points) (Worse ↔ Best)	Comments
Vienna Shoulder Score (VSS)	(Gaebler et al. 1997)	Yes	No	No	40 ↔ 0	Based on cohort of 157 patients with clavicular fractures Applied to all 'shoulder girdle' trauma
Shoulder Disability Questionnaire	(van der Heijden et al. 2000)	Yes	No	No (van der Windt et al. 1998) (Guyatt et al. 1987)	100 ↔ 0	16 Pain-Disability-related questions Yes/No answers All questions relate to preceding 24 hours only
Oxford Shoulder Instability Score	(Dawson et al. 1999)	Yes	Yes	No	60 ↔ 12	Specifically for assessment of shoulder instability Based on cohort of 92 patients with instability treated operatively or conservatively Assesses symptoms of Pain and Instability as well as Activities of Daily Living
The Elbow: Clinician-based scores						
Bruce Assessment	(Bruce et al. 1974)	Yes	Yes	No	0 ↔ 100 Excellent 96–100 Good 91–95 Fair 81–90 Poor <81	Based on cohort of 35 patients with Monteggia fractures
Hospital for Special Surgery Elbow Assessment (HSS)	(Inglis and Pellicci 1980)	Yes	No	No	0 ↔ 100	Initially developed for elbow arthroplasty assessment (Pynsent et al. 1993)
Holdsworth and Mossad	(Holdsworth and Mossad) 1984	Yes	Yes	No	1 ↔ 16 Excellent 14–16 Good 11–13 Poor <11	Based on cohort of 52 patients undergoing tension band wiring of olecranon fracture
Broberg and Morrey Scale	(Broberg and Morrey 1986)	Yes	Yes	Yes (Wallenbock and Potsch 1997)	0 ↔ 100 Excellent 95–100	Based on cohort of 21 patients undergoing delayed radial head excision

Measure			References	Score	Comments
(Functional Rating Index)			(Ikeda et al. 2001) (Ring et al. 1998) (Ring et al. 1997) (Broberg and Morrey 1987)	Good 80–94 Fair 60–79 Poor <60	after fracture
Mayo Elbow Performance Score (MEPS) (Morrey and An 1993)	Yes	No	Yes (Gill et al. 2000) (Rodgers et al. 1996) (Cobb and Morrey 1997) (Schneeberger et al. 1997)	0 ↔ 100	Most frequently applied elbow score
Leipzig Elbow Score (Korner et al. 1998)	Yes	Yes	No (MacDermid 2001)	0 ↔ 100 Excellent 90–100 Good 80–89 Moderate 65–79 Poor <65	Based on cohort of 41 patients with elbow fracture-dislocations. Includes component for radiographic assessment
The Elbow: Combined clinician-/patient-based scores					
American Shoulder and Elbow Surgeons Elbow Form (ASES-e) (Gill and Morrey 1998)	Yes	No	Yes (Gill and Morrey 1998)	0 ↔ 100	Most frequently applied elbow score. Patient-based component assessing pain, function and patient satisfaction. Clinician-based component assessing elbow impairments
The Elbow: Patient-based scores					
Disabilities of the Arm, Shoulder and Hand (DASH) (Hudak et al. 1996)	No	No	Yes (McConnell et al. 1999) (Beaton et al. 2001) (Atroshi et al. 2000) (Skutek et al. 2000)	0 ↔ 100	30-point index assessing entire upper limb. Optionally assesses sports, performing arts and work
Patient-Rated Elbow Evaluation (PREE) (MacDermid 2001)	Yes	No	No (MacDermid 2001)	0 ↔ 100	Extended from Patient Rated Wrist Evaluation (MacDermid 1996) (MacDermid et al. 1998)

children may be a worthwhile exercise. However, in older age groups – where a proximal humeral or olecranon fracture may be part of a more complex pattern of trauma (e.g. associated fractured neck of femur) – the outcome may more realistically be assessed using a generic health assessment tool such as the SF-36 (Ware and Sherbourne 1992), particularly where significant co-morbidities are present which will in turn affect overall outcome.

In practical terms, with the current drive towards patient-based outcome measures, many of the historic clinician-based trauma scores are obsolete. Despite this however no patient-based trauma scores have filled this void. The Vienna Shoulder Score (Gaebler et al. 1997) is a patient-based score applied to clavicular fractures, but unsurprisingly this has not been statistically validated. Walsh, in his assessment of shoulder strength following ACJ injury, uses a patient-based questionnaire (in addition to formal strength testing), but all scores obtained 'were not subjected to any statistical analysis' (Walsh et al. 1985).

Despite this, the use of patient-based outcome scores such as the DASH, UEFS, SPADI and SST are frequently used as outcome measures in published trauma series. It is interesting to note that in the initial validation of these scores no trauma patients were included. Consequently, further validation and reliability testing should be undertaken for their specific application to trauma case series.

CONCLUSION

A wide variety of outcome measures are currently in use. Of these, many are being used on populations of patients which are different from those for which the system was initially developed. In addition, many outcome measures in fact have no statistical validation and consequently are of little true clinical application.

The improvements being made by repeated attempts at further refining old and developing new outcome measures is diminishing. The time may have come to accept the tools we currently have (even with their inherent limitations), but most importantly to encourage learned societies both nationally and internationally to arrive at a consensus as to which outcome measures should be utilized in specific circumstances so that true comparisons and systematic reviews may be undertaken.

A summary of the outcome scoring methods described in the previous sections is listed in Table 15.1.

REFERENCES

AAOS (1996): *Academy Proceeds on Outcomes Database*, pp. 29–30, AAOS, Atlanta.

Altchek, D. W., Warren, R. F., Wickiewicz, S. M. J., Ortiz, G., and Schwartz, E. (1990): Arthroscopic acromioplasty: technique and results. *J Bone Joint Surg* **72A**, 1198–207.

Amstutz, H. C., Sew Hoy, A. L., and Clarke, I. C. (1981): UCLA anatomic total shoulder arthroplasty. *Clin Orthop* **155**, 7–20.

Arner, O., Sandahl, U., and Ohrling, H. (1957): Dislocation of the acromio-clavicular joint. *Acta Chir Scand* **113**, 140–52.

Atroshi, I., Gummesson, C., Andersson, B., Dahlgren, E., and Johansson, A. (2000): The disabilities of the arm, shoulder and hand (DASH) questionnaire: reliability and validity of the Swedish version evaluated in 176 patients. *Acta Orthop Scand* **71**, 613–18.

Barrett, W. P., Franklin, J. L., Jakins, S. E., Wyss, C. R., and Matsen, F. A. (1987): Total shoulder arthroplasty. *J Bone Joint Surg Am* **69**, 865–72.

Beaton, D. E., Katz, J. N., Fossel, A. H., Wright, J. G., Tarasuk, V., and Bombardier, C. (2001): Measuring the whole or the parts? Validity, reliability and responsiveness of the Disabilities of the Arm, Shoulder and Hand outcome measure in different regions of the upper extremity. *J Hand Ther* **14**, 128–46.

Beaton, D. E., and Richards, R. R. (1996): Measuring the function of the shoulder: a cross-sectional comparison of five questionnaires. *J Bone Joint Surg* **78A**, 882–90.

Beaton, D. E., and Richards, R. R. (1998): Assessing the reliability and responsiveness of 5 shoulder questionnaires. *J Shoulder Elbow Surg* 7, 565–72.

Boenisch, U., Huyer, C., and Wasmer, G. (1991): Standardised shoulder examination with reference to computerised isokinetic strength testing (Cybex II). *Sportverletzung Sportsschaden* 5, 5–11.

Bosch, U., Skutek, M., Fremerey, R. W., and Tscherne, H. (1998): Outcome after primary and secondary hemiarthroplasty in elderly patients with fractures of the proximal humerus. *J Shoulder Elbow Surg* 7, 479–84.

Broberg, M. A., and Morrey, B. F. (1986): Results of delayed excision of the radial head after fracture. *J Bone Joint Surg* 68, 669–74.

Broberg, M. A., and Morrey, B. F. (1987): Results of treatment of fracture-dislocations of the elbow. *Clin Orthop* 216, 109–19.

Bruce, H. E., Harvey, J. P., and Wilson, J. C. (1974): Monteggia fractures. *J Bone Joint Surg* 56A, 1563–76.

Burnett, R., and Fyfe, I. S. (1991): Souter-Strathclyde arthroplasty of the rheumatoid elbow. *Acta Orthop Scand* 62, 52–4.

Chen, R. S., Lui, C. B., Lin, X. S., Feng, X. M., Zhu, J. M., and Ye, F. Q. (2001): Supracondylar extension fracture of the humerus in children. Manipulative reduction, immobilization and fixation using U-shaped plaster slab with the elbow in full extension. *J Bone Joint Surg* 83, 883–7.

Cobb, T. K., and Morrey, B. F. (1997): Total elbow arthroplasty as primary treatment for distal humeral fractures in elderly patients. *J Bone Joint Surg* 79A, 826–32.

Codman, E. A. (1911): Complete rupture of the supraspinatus tendon. Operative treatment of two successful cases. *Boston Med Surg J* 162, 708–10.

Codman, E. A. (1922): The registry of cases of bone sarcoma. *Surg Gynecol Obstet* 34, 335–43.

Codman, E. A. (1934): *The Shoulder Rupture of the Supraspinatus Tendon and Other Lesions In or About the Subacromial Bursa* (Preface: xii). Thomas Todd Printers, Boston.

Codman, E. A., Chipman, W. W., Clark, J. G., Kanavel, A. B., and Mayo, W. J. (1913): Standardisation of Hospitals: Report of the committee appointed by the Clinical Congress of Surgeons of North America. *Trans Clin Cong Surg North Am* 4, 2–8.

Cofield, R. H. (1983): Unconstrained total shoulder prostheses. *Clin Orthop* 173, 97–108.

Cofield, R. H. (1984): Total shoulder arthroplasty with Neer prosthesis. *J Bone Joint Surg* 66A, 899–906.

Cole, B. J., L'Insalata, J., Irrang, J., and Warner, J. J. (2000): Comparison of arthroscopic and open anterior shoulder stabilization. A two to six-year follow-up study. *J Bone Joint Surg* 82A, 952–3.

Conboy, V. B., Morris, R. W., Kiss, J., and Carr, A. J. (1997): An evaluation of the Constant-Murley shoulder assessment. *J Bone Joint Surg* 79, 695–6.

Connor, P. M., and Morrey, B. F. (1998): Total elbow arthroplasty in patients who have juvenile rheumatoid arthritis. *J Bone Joint Surg* 80A, 678–88.

Constant, C. R., and Murley, A. H. G. (1987): A clinical method of functional assessment of the shoulder. *Clin Orthop* 214, 160–4.

Dawson, J., Fitzpatrick, R., and Carr, A. (1996): Questionnaire on the perception of patients about shoulder surgery. *J Bone Joint Surg* 78B, 593–600.

Dawson, J., Fitzpatrick, R., and Carr, A. (1999): The assessment of shoulder instability. The development and validation of a questionnaire. *J Bone Joint Surg* 81, 420–6.

Dawson, J., Hill, G., Fitzpatrick, R., and Carr, A. (2001): The benefits of using patient-based methods of assessment. Medium-term results of an observational study of shoulder surgery. *J Bone Joint Surg* 83B, 877–82.

Duckworth, D. G., Smith, K. L., Campbell, B., and Matsen, F. A. I. (1999): Self-assessment questionnaires document substantial variability in the clinical expression of rotator cuff tears. *J Shoulder Elbow Surg* 8, 330–3.

Ellman, H., Hanker, G., and Bayer, M. (1986): Repair of the rotator cuff: end-result study of factors influencing reconstruction. *J Bone Joint Surg* 68A, 1136–44.

Ellman, H., and Kay, S. P. (1991): Arthroscopic subacromial decompression for chronic impingement. *J Bone Joint Surg* 73B, 395–8.

Ewald, F. C. (1975): Total elbow replacement. *Orthop Clin North Am* 3, 685–96.

Ewald, F. C., Simmons, E. D. J., Sullivan, J. A., Thomas, W. H., Scott, R. D., Poss, R., Thornhill, T. S., and Sledge, C. B. (1993): Capitellocondylar total elbow replacement in rheumatoid arthritis. Long term results. *J Bone Joint Surg Am* **75**, 498–507.

Eygendaal, D., Verdegaal, S. H., Obermann, W. R., van Vugt, A. B., Poll, R. G., and Rozing, P. M. (2001): Posterolateral dislocation of the elbow joint. Relationship to medial instability. *J Bone Joint Surg Am* **83A**, 785–6.

Figgie, M. P., Inglis, A. E., Mow, C. S., and Figgie, H. E. (1989): Total elbow arthroplasty for complete ankylosis of the elbow. *J Bone Joint Surg Am* **78A**, 513–20.

Flynn, J. C., Matthews, J. G., and Benoit, R. L. (1974): Blind pinning of displaced supracondylar fractures of the humerus in children. *J Bone Joint Surg Br* **56**, 263–72.

Gaebler, C., Matis, N., Kwasny, O., and Vecsei, V. (1997): Vienna Shoulder Score (VSS) and Vienna Shoulder Formula (VSF) for follow-up and assessment of shoulder and shoulder girdle injuries. *Swiss Surg* **3**, 69–75.

Gill, D. R., Cofield, R. H., and Morrey, B. F. (2000): Ipsilateral total shoulder and elbow arthroplasties in patients who have rheumatoid arthritis. *J Bone Joint Surg* **81A**, 1128–37.

Gill, D. R., and Morrey, B. F. (1998): The Coonrad-Morrey total elbow arthroplasty in patients who have rheumatoid arthritis: a ten to fifteen year follow-up study. *J Bone Joint Surg* **80A**, 1327–35.

Goldberg, B. A., Lippitt, S. B., and Matsen, F. A. I. (2001a): Improvement in comfort and function after cuff repair without acromioplasty. *Clin Orthop* **390**, 142–50.

Goldberg, B. A., Nowinski, R. J., and Matsen, F. A. I. (2001b): Outcome of nonoperative management of full-thickness rotator cuff tears. *Clin Orthop* **382**, 99–107.

Guyatt, G. H., Walter, S., and Norman, G. (1987): Measuring change over time: assessing the usefulness of evaluation instruments. *J Chronic Dis* **40**, 171–8.

Hagg, O., and Lundberg, B. (1994): Aspects of prognostic factors in comminuted and dislocated proximal humeral fractures. In: Bateman, J. E., and Welsh, R. P. (eds), *Surgery of the Shoulder*. Marcel Decker, Philadelphia, pp. 51–9.

Harvie, P. (27 May 2002): Personal correspondence between Mr. Paul Harvie and Dr. Uli Boenisch, Oxford.

Hawkins, R. J., Bell, R. H., and Jallay, B. (1989): Total shoulder arthroplasty. *Clin Orthop* **242**, 188–94.

Heald, S. L., Riddle, D. L., and Lamb, R. L. (1997): The shoulder pain and disability index: construct validity and responsiveness of a region-specific disability measure. *J Phys Ther* **77**, 1079–89.

Hessman, M., Gotzen, L., Gehling, H., Baumgaertel, F., and Klingelhoeffer, I. (1998): Operative treatment of displaced proximal humeral fractures: two-year results in 99 cases. *Acta Chir Belg* **98**, 212–19.

Hessman, M., Baumgaertel, F., Gehling, H., Klingelhoeffer, I., and Gotzen, L. (1999): Plate fixation of proximal humeral fractures with indirect reduction: surgical technique and results utilising three shoulder scores. *Injury* **30**, 453–62.

Holdsworth, B. J., and Mossad, M. M. (1984): Elbow function following tension band fixation of displaced fractures of the olecranon. *Injury* **16**, 182–7.

Hudak, P. L., Amadio, P. C., and Bombardier, C. (1996): Development of an upper extremity outcome measure: the DASH (disabilities of the arm, shoulder and hand). The Upper Extremity Collaborative Group (UECG). *Am J Ind Med* **30**, 602–8.

Ikeda, M., Fukushima, Y., Kobayashi, Y., and Oka, Y. (2001): Comminuted fractures of the olecranon. Management by bone graft from the iliac crest and multiple tension-band wiring. *J Bone Joint Surg* **83**, 805–8.

Imatani, R. J., Hanlon, J. J., and Cady, G. W. (1975): Acute, complete acromio-clavicular separation. *J Bone Joint Surg* **57A**, 328–32.

Inglis, A. E., and Pellicci, P. M. (1980): Total elbow replacement. *J Bone Joint Surg* **62A**, 1252–8.

Jakob, R. P., Miniaci, A., Anson, P. S., Jaberg, H., Osterwalder, A., and Ganz, R. (1990): Four-part valgus impacted fractures of the proximal humerus. *J Bone Joint Surg* **73**, 295–8.

Jupiter, J. B., Neff, U., Holzach, P., and Allgower, M. (1985): Intercondylar fractures of the humerus. An operative approach. *J Bone Joint Surg* **67**, 226–39.

Kay, S. P., and Amstutz, H. C. (1988): Shoulder hemiarthroplasty at UCLA. *Clin Orthop* **228**, 42–4.

Kelly, I. G. (1990): Surgery of the rheumatoid shoulder. *Ann Rheum Dis* **49** (Suppl. 2), 824–9.

Kelly, I. G., Foster, R. S., and Fisher, W. D. (1987): Neer total shoulder replacement in rheumatoid arthritis. *J Bone Joint Surg* **69B**, 328–32.

Khalfayan, E. E., Culp, R. W., and Alexander, H. (1992): Mason Type-II radial head fractures: operative versus non-operative treatment. *J Orthop Trauma* **6**, 283–9.

Kim, S. H., and Ha, K. I. (2000): Arthroscopic treatment of symptomatic shoulders with minimally displaced greater tuberosity fracture. *Arthroscopy* **16**, 695–700.

King, G. J. W., Richards, R. R., Zuckermam, J. D., Blasier, R., Dillman, C., Friedman, R. J., Gartsman, G. M., Iannotti, J. P., Murnahan, J. P., Mow, V. C., and Woo, S. L. (1999): A standardised method for assessment of elbow function. *J Shoulder Elbow Surg* **8**, 351–4.

Kirkley, A., Griffin, S., McLintock, H., and Ng, L. (1998): The development and evaluation of a disease-specific quality of life measurement tool for shoulder instability. The Western Ontario Shoulder Instability Index (WOSI). *Am J Sports Med* **26**, 764–72.

Kirkley, A., Griffin, S., Richards, C., Miniaci, A., and Mohtadi, S. (1999): Prospective randomised clinical trial comparing the effectiveness of immediate arthroscopic stabilization versus immobilization and rehabilitation in first traumatic anterior dislocation of the shoulder. *Arthroscopy* **15**, 507–14.

Kocialkowski, A., and Wallace, W. A. (1990): Closed percutaneous K-wire stabilisation for displaced fractures of the surgical neck of the humerus. *Injury* **58**, 209–12.

Kohn, D., and Geyer, M. (1997): The subjective shoulder rating system. *Arch Orthop Trauma Surg* **116**, 324–8.

Kohn, D., Geyer, M., and Wulker, N. (1993): The subjective shoulder rating scale: an examiner-independent scoring system. International Congress of Shoulder Surgery.

Korner, J., Lill, H., Verheyden, P., and Josten, C. (1998): Die Komplexverletzung des Ellenbogengelenkes – Management und Ergebnisse. *Akt Traumatol*, pp. 205–15.

Kruger-Franke, M., Kohne, G., and Rosemeyer, B. (2000): Outcome of surgically treated lateral clavicular fractures. *Unfallchirurg* **103**, 538–44.

Kudo, H. (1998): Non-constrained elbow arthroplasty for mutilans deformity in rheumatoid arthritis; a report of 6 cases. *J Bone Joint Surg* **80B**, 234–9.

Kuhn, J. E., and Blasier, R. B. (1997): Evaluating outcomes in the treatment of shoulder disorders. In: Norris, T. R. (ed.), *Orthopaedic Knowledge and Update – Shoulder and Elbow*. ASES/AAOS, Rosemont pp. 47–55.

L'Insalata, J. C., Warren, R. F., Cohen, S. B., Altchek, D. W., and Peterson, M. G. (1998): A self-administered questionnaire for assessment of symptoms and function of the shoulder. *J Bone Joint Surg* **80**, 766–7.

Lee, B. P., and Morrey, B. (1997): Arthroscopic synovectomy of the elbow for rheumatoid arthritis: a prospective study. *J Bone Joint Surg* **79B**, 770–2.

Leggin, B. G., Shaffer, M. A., Meuman, R. M., Iannotti, J. P., Williams, G. R., and Brenneman, S. K. (1997): *Reliability, Validity and Responsiveness of a Shoulder Outcome Scoring System*. The Research Section of the Combined Sections Meeting of the American Physical Therapy Association, Dallas.

Lippitt, S. B., Harryman, D. T. I., Matsen, F. A. I., and Hawkins, R. J. E. (1993): A practical tool for evaluation of function: the simple shoulder test. In: *The Shoulder: A Balance of Mobility and Stability*. AAOS, Rosemont, IL.

MacDermid, J. C. (1996): Development of a scale for patient rating of wrist pain and disability. *J Hand Ther* **9**, 178–83.

MacDermid, J. C. (2001): Outcome evaluation in patients with elbow pathology: issues in instrumental development and evaluation. *J Hand Ther* **14**, 105–14.

MacDermid, J. C., Turgeon, T., Richards, R. S., Beadle, M., and Roth, J. H. (1998): Patient rating of wrist pain and disability: a reliable and valid measurement tool. *J Orthop Trauma* **12**, 577–86.

MacDonald, P. B., Alexander, M. J., Frejuk, J., and Johnson, G. (1988): Comprehensive functional analysis of shoulders following complete acromioclavicular separation. *Am J Sports Med* **16**, 475–80.

Mansat, P., and Morrey, B. F. (1998): The column procedure: a limited lateral approach for extrinsic contracture of the elbow. *J Bone Joint Surg* **80A**, 1603–15.

Maro, J. K., Werier, J., MacDermid, J. C., and Patterson, S. D. (2001): Arthroplasty with a metal radial head for unreconstructable fractures of the radial head. *J Bone Joint Surg Am* **83A**, 1201–11.

Matsen, F. A. I. (1996): Early effectiveness of shoulder arthroplasty for patients who have primary glenohumeral degenerative joint disease. *J Bone Joint Surg* **78A**, 260–4.

McConnell, S., Beaton, D. E., and Bombardier, C. (1999): *The DASH Outcome Measure User's Manual*. Institute for Work and Health, Toronto.

Michener, L. A., McClure, P. W., and Sennett, B. J. (2000): American Shoulder and Elbow Surgeons Standardised Shoulder Assessment Form: reliability, validity, and responsiveness. *J Orthop Sports Phys Ther* **30**, A30.

Morrey, B. F., and An, K.-N. (1993): Functional evaluation of the elbow. In: Morrey, B. F. (ed.), *The Elbow and its Disorders*. 3rd edition. W. B. Saunders, Philadelphia, pp. 74–83.

Neer, C. S. (1970): Displaced proximal humeral fractures Part I. Classification and evaluation. *J Bone Joint Surg* **52A**, 1077–89.

Neer, C. S. I. (1974): Replacement arthroplasty for glenohumeral osteoarthritis. *J Bone Joint Surg* **56A**, 1–13.

Neer, C. S. I., Watson, K. C., and Stanton, F. J. (1982): Recent experience in total shoulder replacement. *J Bone Joint Surg* **64A**, 319–37.

Packer, T. L., Wyss, U. P., and Costigan, P. (1994): Elbow kinematics during sit-to-stand-to-sit of subjects with rheumatoid arthritis. *Arch Phys Med Rehab* **75**, 900–7.

Patte, D. (1987): *Directions for the use of the Index Severity for Painful and/or Chronically Disabled Shoulders*. Abstracts of the First Open Congress of the European Society of the Shoulder and Elbow (SECEC), pp. 36–41.

Post, M., and Singh, M. (1983): Rotator cuff tears. *Clin Orthop* **173**, 78–91.

Pransky, G., Feuerstein, M., Himmelstein, J., Katz, J. N., and Vickers-Lahti, M. (1997): Measuring functional outcomes in work-related upper extremity disorders. *J Occup Environ Med* **39**, 1195–202.

Pynsent, P. B. (2001): Choosing an outcome measure. *J Bone Joint Surg* Br **83B**, 792–4.

Pynsent, P. B., Fairbank, J. C. T., and Carr, A. J. (1993): *Outcome Measures in Orthopaedics*. Butterworth Heinemann, Oxford.

Richards, R. R., An, K.-N., and Bigliani, L. U. (1994): A standardised method for assessment of shoulder function. *J Shoulder Elbow Surg* **3**, 347–52.

Ring, D., Jupiter, J. B., Sanders, R. W., Mast, J., and Simpson, N. S. (1997): Transolecranon fracture-dislocation of the elbow. *J Orthop Trauma* **11**, 545–50.

Ring, D., Jupiter, J. B., and Simpson, N. S. (1998): Monteggia fractures in adults. *J Bone Joint Surg* **80**, 1733–44.

Roach, K. E., Budiman-Mak, E., Songsiridej, N., and Lertratanakul, Y. (1991): Development of a shoulder pain and disability index. *Arthritis Care Res* **4**, 143–9.

Roddey, T. S., Olson, S. L., Cook, K. F., Gartsman, G. M., and Hanten, W. (2000): Comparison of the University of California-Los Angeles Shoulder Scale and the Simple Shoulder Test with the Shoulder Pain and Disability Index: single-administration reliability and validity. *Phys Ther* **80**, 759–68.

Rodgers, W. B., Kharrazi, F. D., Waters, P. M., Kennedy, J. G., McKee, M. D., and Lhowe, D. W. (1996): The use of osseous suture anchors in the treatment of severe, complicated elbow dislocations. *Am J Orthop* **25**, 794–8.

Rowe, C. R., Patel, D., and Southmayd, W. W. (1978): The Bankart procedure. A long-term end-result study. *J Bone Joint Surg* **60A**, 1–16.

Schemitsch, E. H., Ewald, F. C., and Thornhill, T. S. (1996): Results of total elbow arthroplasty after excision of the radial head and synovectomy in patients who had rheumatoid arthritis. *J Bone Joint Surg Am* **78A**, 1541–7.

Schneeberger, A. G., Adams, R., and Morrey, B. F. (1997): Semiconstrained total elbow replacement for the treatment of post-traumatic osteoarthrosis. *J Bone Joint Surg* **79A**, 1211–22.

Skutek, M., Fremerey, R. W., Zeichen, J., and Bosch, U. (2000): Outcome analysis following open rotator cuff repair. Early effectiveness validated using four different shoulder assessment scales. *Arch Orthop Traum Surg* **120**, 432–6.

Skutek, M., Zeichen, J., Fremerey, R. W., and Bosch, U. (2001): Outcome analysis after open reconstruction of rotator cuff ruptures. A comparative assessment of recent evaluation procedures. *Unfallchirurg* **104**, 480–7.

Souter, W. (1985): Anatomical trochlear stirrup arthroplasty of the rheumatoid elbow. *J Bone Joint Surg* **67B**, 676.

Souter, W. A. (1990): Surgery of the rheumatoid elbow. *Ann Rheum Dis* **49** (Suppl. 2), 871–82.

Svend-Hansen, H. (1974): Displaced proximal humeral fractures. A review of 49 patients. *Acta Orthop Scand* **45**, 359–64.

Swanson, A. B., de Groot Swanson, G., Sattel, A. B., Cendo, R. D., Hynes, D., and Jar-Ning, W. (1989): Bipolar implant shoulder arthroplasty. *Clin Orthop* **249**, 227–47.

The Royal College of Surgeons of England (2002): www.rcseng.ac.uk/surgical/research/ceu/projects_ongoing?proj_outcomes_html, The Royal College of Surgeons of England Website.

Tibone, J. E., and Bradley (1993): Evaluation of treatment outcomes for the athlete's shoulder. In: Matsen, F. A. I., Fu, F. H., and Hawkins, R. J. (eds), *The Shoulder: A Balance of Mobility and Stability*. AAOS, Rosemont, IL, pp. 519–29.

Tsai, T. N., Wredmark, T., Johansson, C., Gibo, K., Engstrom, B., and Tornqvist, H. (1991): Shoulder function in patients with unoperated anterior shoulder instability. *Am J Sports Med* **19**, 469–73.

Turchin, D. C., Beaton, D. E., and Richards, R. R. (1998): Validity of observer-based aggregate scoring systems as descriptors of elbow pain, function and disability. *J Bone Joint Surg Am* **80**, 154–62.

van der Heijden, G. J. M. G., Leffers, P., and Bouter, L. M. (2000): Shoulder disability questionnaire: design and responsiveness of a functional status measure. *J Clin Epidemiol* **53**, 29–38.

van der Windt, D. A., van der Heijden, G. J. M. G., de Winter, A. F., Koes, B. W., Deville, W., and Bouter, L. M. (1998): The responsiveness of the Shoulder Disability Questionnaire. *Ann Rheum Dis* **57**, 82–7.

Wallenbock, E., and Potsch, W. (1997): Resection of the radial head: an alternative to use of a prosthesis? *J Traum-Inj Inf Crit Care* **43**, 959–61.

Walsh, J. K., Peterson, D. A., Shelton, G., and Neumann, R. D. (1985): Shoulder strength following acromioclavicular injury. *Am J Sports Med* **13**, 153–8.

Ware, J. E., and Sherbourne, C. D. (1992): The MOS 36-item short-form health survey (SF36). I. Conceptual framework and item selection. *Med Care* **30**, 473–83.

Warren, R. F., Ranawat, C. S., and Inglis, A. E. (1982): *Total Shoulder Replacement Indications and Results of the Neer Nonconstrained Prosthesis*. AAOS: Symposium on Total Joint Replacement of the Upper Extremity, St. Louis, pp. 56–67.

Weber, B. G., Simpson, L. A., and Hardegger, F. (1984): Rotational humeral osteotomy for recurrent anterior dislocation of the shoulder associated with large Hill-Sachs lesion. *J Bone Joint Surg* **66**, 1443–50.

Williams, J. W., Holleman, D. R., and Simel, D. L. (1995): Measuring shoulder function with the Shoulder Pain and Disability Index. *J Rheumatol* **22**, 727–32.

Wolfgang, G. L. (1974): Surgical repair of tears of the rotator cuff of the shoulder. *J Bone Joint Surg* **56A**, 14–26.

Yokoyama, K., Itoman, M., Kobayashi, A., Shindo, M., and Futami, T. (1998): Functional outcomes of 'floating elbow' injuries in adult patients. *J Orthop Trauma* **12**, 284–90.

16

The wrist

Joseph J. Dias

INTRODUCTION

A review of the currently available literature on the wrist clearly demonstrates that outcome measures overlap those for the hand. The most common outcomes reported for different wrist disorders are range of movement and grip strength. The commonest form used is the Mayo Clinic wrist score (Cooney *et al.* 1987) with the Disabilities of the Arm, Shoulder and Hand (DASH) (Hudak *et al.* 1996) being used as a disability score more recently, and the Patient Evaluation Measure (PEM) (Dias *et al.* 2001) being used in some studies from the UK. The evolution of wrist scores lags far behind those for the knee and shoulder. This chapter provides information on some of the objective and subjective outcome measures used in reporting on disorders of the wrist.

The wrist joint is the most complex joint in the body including, as it does, ten bones, a multitude of intrinsic and extrinsic ligaments with five primary motors for the wrist joint and four for forearm rotation. Its main function is the fine positioning of the hand and provision of a stable foundation so that a specific task can be efficiently performed. The wrist and forearm work essentially as a single unit in most tasks, and it is probably artificial to separate the two. Assessment of wrist function is a composite assessment and it is often difficult to attribute impairment to a single anatomical structure. Indirect measures, such as grip strength are required to provide a 'rough' guide on outcome.

Most studies, which assess outcome of wrist injury and disease, have concentrated on movement and strength. Very few include a functional assessment or even accurately document the patient's problems.

TREATMENT AIMS

The aim of treatment of any wrist condition is to resolve the patient's problems with the least impairment, disability, handicap and especially distress.

Assessment of outcome must be: (i) appropriate to the goals established prior to intervention; and (ii) appropriately timed. An illustrative example is a patient with an acute scaphoid fracture. The patient expects to have a pain-free mobile and strong wrist. The orthopaedic goal is union of the fracture in addition to the patients' goal. Immobilization of the injured wrist in a plaster cast for eight weeks without union may, after an interval, meet the patient's expectation, but not that of the surgeon. The surgeon would expect further change for the worse with regard to the onset of degenerative arthritis. The short-term impairment of wrist motion is a direct consequence of intervention – that is, immobilization in a plaster cast.

OUTCOME ASSESSMENT

From the patient's point of view the principal positive outcome is the resolution of symptoms. It is therefore of primary importance carefully to document the patient's problem so that comparison may be made after intervention. This, together with a record of complications, provides a distilled view of the outcome.

Pain

With regard to the wrist, the most common presenting problem is pain. Injury, inflammation, abnormal movement, impingement, tension and pressure on a nerve account for most causes of wrist pain. A careful assessment of the type, site, severity, aggravating, relieving and associated factors of the pain before and after treatment is, therefore, a fundamental requirement in assessing outcome. In the case of the wrist, severe unremitting pain is uncommon, and so a careful assessment of function before treatment is required. Such an assessment must take into account the patient's level of activities and dominance, in addition to assessing the patient's own reaction to their pain.

The single most difficult aspect in assessing pain is the determination of severity, and this has been discussed in Chapter 7.

Often, the primary goal in most wrist conditions is to abolish pain. Therefore, the outcome of most wrist conditions can be assessed in terms of pain relief which may be significant if it results in better function. Intervention can make the pain worse or may leave the pain unchanged. The best outcome is complete pain relief.

Appearance of the wrist and hand

The appearance of the wrist and hand involves swelling and deformity:

- *Swelling*: Outcome following surgery for a discrete swelling around the wrist relates to its persistence or re-appearance. Recurrence can be quantified in terms of duration. In this context, 'recurrence' includes both a true recurrence and a new swelling, but at the same site. A common example is a wrist ganglion.

- *Deformity*: Assessing outcome for deformity correction is less ambiguous. The measurement

may be either clinical or radiographic. However, provided that a single observer carries out the measurement and the method is reproducible, the degree of correction may be adequately assessed.

Loss of movement

This can be the result of an abnormality of the motor (tendon division or neuromuscular abnormality) or stiffness or pain. In the former, the movement of the wrist is passively possible but actively either incomplete or impossible. Measuring movement, calculating impairment or documenting circumduction may be used to assess the range.

RANGE OF WRIST MOVEMENT

Wrist movement is complex as it allows circumduction of the hand and involves movement of the wrist and forearm.

In the clinical environment, the assessment of wrist movement is carried out by measuring the range of wrist movement using an ordinary goniometer. A single observer is more reliable than multiple observers (Horger 1990). The range of extension, flexion, radial and ulnar inclination is measured.

Wrist movement is usually measured with the forearm in full pronation and the fingers extended so that the middle finger is in line with the middle metacarpal. The neutral position is one in which the middle metacarpal is in line with the radius. Extension is measured with the goniometer on the palmar aspect and aligned with the forearm and middle metacarpal, while flexion is measured with the goniometer on the dorsum of the middle metacarpal and along the dorsal aspect of the forearm. This method has the least error and is slightly more reliable than the ulnar or radial alignment (LaStayo and Wheeler 1994). The variability may increase in the presence of disease, particularly if pain and swelling are attributes such as in complex regional pain syndromes (Geertzen *et al.* 1998). For practical purposes it is easier to measure extension and palmar flexion from the ulnar side. One limb of the goniometer is placed along the ulna and the centre of rotation over the tip of the ulnar styloid. The hand is then moved into maximum extension and the distal limb of the goniometer is brought to lie in line with the middle metacarpal. The change in angle from the neutral position is then noted as the angle of active/passive extension. Similarly, the range of flexion is assessed by moving the hand into maximum flexion (American Academy of Orthopaedic Surgeons 1965).

Radial and ulnar inclination are measured with the elbow flexed and the forearm pronated. The forearm and hand lie on the table with the palm facing downwards. In the neutral position, the middle metacarpal is in line with the radius. One limb of the goniometer is placed parallel to the axis of the radius while the centre of rotation is placed over the head of the capitate. The distal limb of the goniometer is placed along the middle metacarpal. The hand is then moved into maximum radial and ulnar inclination and the angles measured (Moore 1949; International Federation of Societies for Surgery of the Hand 2001).

Forearm rotation is measured with the elbow flexed and the forearm placed in the midprone position so that the plane of the palm lies in the parasagittal plane. The forearm is rotated into maximum supination or pronation and the angle of the plane of the palm to the neutral is measured (American Academy of Orthopaedic Surgeons 1965).

IMPAIRMENT ASSESSMENT

Based on these measurements it is possible to assess the percentage of impairment of wrist movement, which in turn can be related to the loss of the whole arm and impairment to the whole body. This method of assessment is well documented and was standardized by the International Federation of Societies for Surgery of the Hand in 1980. Each part of the upper limb is assigned a percentage value in terms of impairment to the whole limb. The wrist is assigned 60 per cent. Flexion extension arc of movement is given 70 per cent of this value, while radio-ulnar inclination represents 30 per cent. The usual range of wrist motion is 60° each of extension and flexion, and from 20° of radial inclination to 30° of ulnar inclination. The impairment is assessed by

adding that of flexion-extension and radio-ulnar inclination (Swanson *et al.* 1997).

WRIST CIRCUMDUCTION

The introduction of biaxial flexible goniometers has made it possible to assess both motions simultaneously. This is done by fixing the two end blocks of the electro-goniometer at the neck of the middle metacarpal and at the forearm, and then performing a circumduction motion of the wrist with or without constraint of forearm rotation. When connected to the appropriate software, the system can generate figures of wrist circumduction.

These describe the arc of wrist movement, and in the normal wrist are oval with the long axis inclined from dorsal and radial to palmar and ulnar. This figure gives a more functional assessment of wrist movement; these are called Lissajous's figures. Comparison of these figures assists in determining the deviation from normal and establishing any change with time especially after intervention (Ojima *et al.* 1991; Rawes *et al.* 1996).

COMPARISON

In the assessment of movement of the wrist the contralateral unaffected wrist usually serves as a frame of reference. However, the difference between the dominant and non-dominant sides must be considered. This varies for each individual and is not available when both wrists are affected. The range of movement may itself vary during the course of the day depending on the presence of stiffness or pain, and this may confound any single measurement. In assessing outcome, however, the direction and magnitude of change are of greater value.

Instability

Patients can present with abnormality of movement. This accompanies wrist pain and presents as an associated click or clunk in the distal radio-ulnar joint or the proximal carpal row or its component bones. *Instability* is defined as sudden change in alignment between the bones of the wrist on movement or load (International Federation of Societies for Surgery of the Hand 2001). Standard clinical tests are used to establish the presence or absence of instability in different locations. Quantifying the degree of instability is difficult and arbitrary. Likewise, the transition between constitutional laxity and instability is arbitrary. In broad terms, the joint in question may be considered as stable, unstable only if provoked by a test or action, and unprovoked with the patient being able to demonstrate the click or clunk at will. Most authors then categorize the provoked instability as mild, moderate or severe (Feinstein *et al.* 1999). This categorization is subjective however, and is an 'art' rather than science. Outcomes for instability surgery are usually reported as 'absence of symptoms' and objective measures of range and strength rather than the 'improvement' in instability.

Abnormal movement should be distinguished from joint laxity. A routine assessment for joint laxity should be carried out and a comparison made to the contralateral side if it is normal. This is usually not possible in the presence of disease such as rheumatoid arthritis, which can involve both wrists.

Strength

Grip strength measurement is simple and quick and can be easily performed in a busy clinic.

Almost all conditions affecting the wrist have a direct impact on grip strength, and this establishes whether any intervention has been beneficial. Assessment of strength is indirect and depends on many factors such as motivation, intact neuromuscular structure and anatomical and functional integrity of the forearm, wrist and hand.

The most commonly recommended and reliable device to assess grip strength is the Jamar hydraulic hand dynamometer with adjustable handle settings (Mathiowetz *et al.* 1984). The device should be regularly calibrated and, if used to measure change with time, the same instrument should be used at each assessment. The handles of such a device are set at the second position unless a five-position strength is being assessed. The patient is seated with the shoulder adducted and neutrally rotated, elbow flexed at 90° and the forearm and wrist in a neutral position. The two handles are squeezed together and the strength assessed using a sealed hydraulic system. In men, grip strength varies between 30.4 and 70.4 kg, while in women it ranges from 14 to 38.6 kg. There are published norms for adults and children (Mathiowetz *et al.* 1985, 1986).

Grip strength can vary with age, time of day and dominance. The grip strength can vary between the dominant and non-dominant hand by 5 to 10 per cent (Bechtol 1954). Grip strength is weaker in the non-dominant hand in 5.4 per cent of men and 8.9 per cent of women. The position of the wrist has a significant impact on grip strength (O'Driscoll *et al.* 1992), and there is a variation in strength of around 20 per cent over a two-week period (Young *et al.* 1989). These factors must be considered when using this equipment.

The assessment of fatigue and endurance is now possible by linking a dynamometer to a computer with the appropriate software installed. Such a system may assist in identifying malingerers. These techniques are time consuming, but may be of value when used to assess outcome in prospective clinical studies.

Scores

Abolishing pain and improving function are the primary aims of most interventions for the wrist. It is therefore surprising that very few assessments of outcome for wrist disorders include an assessment of function before and after intervention.

WRIST SCORES

There are a number of wrist scores (Table 16.1), which are usually generated by a combination of symptoms, impairments, disabilities and complications, and some even include radiographic evaluation. The content and quality of 32 wrist outcome measures were systematically reviewed by Bialocerkowski *et al.* (2000). These authors found that 82 per cent of the measures contained measurement of range and/or strength, and disability was assessed by 31 per cent. However, these outcome measures were considered of generally poor quality.

Table 16.1: Outcome measures assessment

Instrument	What it measures	Validation	Reliability	Responsiveness	Usage	Score
Goniometry (American Academy of Orthopaedic Surgeons 1965)	Range	1	1	2	4	8
Strength (Mathiowetz et al. 1984)	Grip	2	2	2	4	10
Laxity/instability (Feinstein et al. 1999)	Instability	0	0	0	1	1
Green and O'Brien (Green and O'Brien 1978)	Wrist outcome	0	0	0	4	4
Mayo (Cooney et al. 1987)	Wrist outcome	0	0	0	4	4
Gartland and Werley (Stewart et al. 1985)	Wrist outcome	0	0	0	4	4
PRWE (MacDermid et al. 2000)	Wrist outcome	1	1	1	0	3
PEM (Dias et al. 2001)	Disability	2	2	2	4	10
DASH (Hudak et al. 1996)	Disability	1	1	2	4	8
MHQ (Chung et al. 1998)	Disability	1	1	0	0	2
Larsen score (O'Sullivan et al. 1990)	X-ray arthritis	2	0	1	4	7
Steinbrocker staging (Kaye et al. 1990)	X-ray arthritis	2	1	0	4	7

Green and O'Brien wrist score

Most can be traced back to the score proposed by Green and O'Brien (1978) (Table 16.2). This is a demerit score looking at a symptom (pain), disability (work), impairment in the flexion extension arc and strength and one investigation: an X-radiograph. The score is obviously meant to be generated by the doctor after a detailed interview, examination and after review of an X-radiograph. Modifications of this score have been used to report outcomes in various wrist disorders. However, the score has not been validated, nor its reliability and responsiveness checked.

Mayo wrist score

Cooney et al. (1987), from the Mayo Clinic, modified the Green and O'Brien (1978) score (Table 16.3) by changing the demerit items and excluding X-radiographic findings. Furthermore, they categorized the score as excellent, good, fair and poor, and considered a score of over 65 as satisfactory. This score has been used by a number of papers reporting outcome of wrist instability, but has not been validated nor its reliability and responsiveness determined.

Gartland and Werley (Modified) score

The commonest score used to report on outcome of a fracture of the distal radius is the Gartland and Werley score and its modifications (Stewart et al. 1985) (Table 16.4). This score is a mixture of impairments, symptoms and disability, with demerit points for each and a categorization of the outcome into excellent, good, fair and poor.

Patient-rated Wrist Evaluation

A patient-rated wrist evaluation (PRWE) has been described recently by MacDermid et al. (2000) which documents pain and disability (Table 16.5) and was established by the authors to be brief, valid and reliable in distal radius and scaphoid fracture patients (MacDermid et al. 1999). It measures pain (score 50) and disability (score 50).

Table 16.2: The Green and O'Brien wrist score. Reprinted from Green and O'Brien (1978)

Pain	25	No pain
25 points	20	Cold weather symptoms
	15	Mild, no effect on activity
	5	Moderate, affects activity
	0	Severe
Occupation	25	Same as before operation
25 points	20	Same as before operation, but with limitations
	15	Able to work, but unemployed
	10	Change to lighter job
	0	Unable to work because of pain
Range of motion	20	≥140°
20 points	15	100–140°
	10	70–100°
	5	40–70°
	0	<40°
Grip strength	10	Normal
10 points	5	>50% of normal
	0	<50% of normal
X-radiographs	20	Normal
20 points	15	Slight incongruity, malunion, rotation of scaphoid or carpal instability
	10	Moderate incongruity, malunion, rotation of scaphoid or carpal instability
	5	Severe changes noted above, or non-union or avascular necrosis
	0	Arthritic changes

Table 16.3: Mayo wrist score. Reprinted from Cooney *et al.* (1987)

Pain	25	No pain
25 points	20	Mild occasional
	15	Moderate, tolerable
	0	Severe to intolerable
Functional status	25	Returned to regular employment
25 points	20	Restricted employment
	15	Able to work, unemployed
	0	Unable to work because of pain
Range of motion		% of normal
25 points	25	100
	15	75–100
	10	50–75
	5	25–50
	0	0–25
	DF-PF Arcs if only injured hand reported	
	25	≥120
	15	90–120
	10	60–90
	5	30–60
	0	≤30
Grip strength		% of normal
25 points	25	100
	15	75–100
	10	50–75
	5	25–50
	0	0–25
Rating	Excellent	90–100
	Good	80–90
	Fair	65–80 Satisfactory if ≥65
	Poor	<65

DISABILITY ASSESSMENT

The simplest form of disability assessment for the wrist is to ask the patient to enumerate those tasks that cannot be performed and those that are difficult. Assessment of outcome could then include checking whether the difficulty of these tasks has changed and whether the tasks which could not be performed can now be done. This system assesses each individual's disability, and is independent of the

Table 16.4: The modified Gartland and Werley wrist score. Reprinted from Stewart *et al.* (1985)

Subjective evaluation

Pain	None (1)	Occasional (2)	Often (3)
Limitation of movement	None (4)	Slight (5)	Present (6)
Disability	None (7)	None if careful (8)	Present (9)
Restriction of activities	None (10)	Slight (11)	Marked (12)

Demerit points

1, 4, 7, 10 = Excellent	0
2, 5, 7, 10 = Good	2
2, 5, 8, 11 = Fair	4
3, 6, 9, 12 = Poor	6

Other multiples are averaged out, with a tendency to mark towards the poor side

e.g. 1, 4, 9, 11 = Fair

2, 4, 9, 10 = Fair

Objective evaluation

Wrist extension	if less than	45 = 5
Wrist flexion	if less than	30 = 1
Wrist ulnar inclination	if less than	25 = 3
Wrist radial inclination	if less than	15 = 1
Supination	if less than	50 = 2
Pronation	if less than	50 = 2
Circumduction	if unable to do well	1

Finger flexion	if all do not flex to distal palmar crease	1
	if one or two do not flex to distal palmar crease	1
Grip strength	if decreased compared with normal side	1

Complications

Median/ulnar/radial sensory nerve compression	Mild	1
	Moderate	2
	Severe	3

End result gradings		
	Excellent	0–2
	Good	3–8
	Fair	9–14
	Poor	15+

dominance of the hand. However, it may not allow comparison between patients.

In order to assess disability, a standard assessment of daily activities can be used, and there are many such tests for the hand (Macey and Kelly 1993). These activities should ideally be independent of dominance or sex, and should also include domestic, occupational and leisure tasks. The availability of

Table 16.5: Patient-rated wrist evaluation. Reprinted from MacDermid *et al.* (2000)

Name: Date:

PATIENT-RATED WRIST EVALUATION

The questions below will help us understand how much difficulty you have had with your wrist in the past week. You will be describing your average *wrist symptoms over the past week* on a scale of 0–10. *Please provide an answer for ALL questions. If you did not perform an activity, please ESTIMATE the pain or difficulty you would expect. If you have* never *performed the activity, you may leave it blank.*

I. PAIN

Rate the average amount of pain in your wrist over the past week by circling the number that best describes your pain on a scale from 0–10. A zero (0) means that you did not have any pain and a ten (10) means that you had the worst pain you have ever experienced or that you could not do the activity because of pain.

Sample scale ☐   0   I   2   3   4   5   6   7   8   9   10
                          No Pain   Worst Ever

RATE YOUR PAIN:	
At rest	0 I 2 3 4 5 6 7 8 9 10
When doing a task with a repeated wrist movement	0 I 2 3 4 5 6 7 8 9 10
When lifting a heavy object	0 I 2 3 4 5 6 7 8 9 10
When it is at its worst	0 I 2 3 4 5 6 7 8 9 10

How often do you have pain?   0   I   2   3   4   5   6   7   8   9   10
                                        Never   Always

---

2. FUNCTION

A. SPECIFIC ACTIVITIES

Rate the amount of difficulty you experienced performing each of the items listed below, over the past week, by circling the number that describes your difficulty on a scale of 0–10. A zero (0) means you did not experience any difficulty and a ten (10) means it was so difficult you were unable to do it at all.

Sample scale ☐   0   I   2   3   4   5   6   7   8   9   10
                          No Difficulty   Unable To Do

Turn a door knob using my affected hand	0 I 2 3 4 5 6 7 8 9 10
Cut meat using a knife in my affected hand	0 I 2 3 4 5 6 7 8 9 10
Fasten buttons on my shirt	0 I 2 3 4 5 6 7 8 9 10
Use my affected hand to push up from a chair	0 I 2 3 4 5 6 7 8 9 10
Carry a 10-lb object in my affected hand	0 I 2 3 4 5 6 7 8 9 10
Use bathroom tissue with my affected hand	0 I 2 3 4 5 6 7 8 9 10

Table 16.5: Patient-rated wrist evaluation – *continued*

B. USUAL ACTIVITIES

Rate the amount of difficulty you experienced performing your usual activities in each of the areas listed below, over the past week, by circling the number that best describes your difficulty on a scale of 0–10. By 'usual activities', we mean the activities you performed before you started having a problem with your wrist. A zero (0) means that you did not experience any difficulty and a ten (10) means it was so difficult you were unable to do any of your usual activities.

Personal care activities (dressing, washing)	0 1 2 3 4 5 6 7 8 9 10
Household work (cleaning, maintenance)	0 1 2 3 4 5 6 7 8 9 10
Work (your job or usual everyday work)	0 1 2 3 4 5 6 7 8 9 10
Recreational activities	0 1 2 3 4 5 6 7 8 9 10

Comments

Comment/Interpretations:

Pain Subscale	/50
Function Subscales (total divided by 2)	= /50
Total PRWE Score (Sum)	= /100

Where items are left blank, the average score of that subscale can be substituted

Reprinted with permission of J. C. MacDermid (MacDermid *et al.* 1999).

the Baltimore Therapeutic Equipment (BTE) work simulator has helped analyse motor performance and conduct motion time measurements in order to quantify the physical attributes of disability. It allows the evaluation of manual dexterity and helps to predict skills (Curtis and Engalitcheff 1981).

Patient-completed questionnaires to assess disability have been developed for the upper limb. The Disabilities of the Arm, Shoulder and Hand (DASH) (Hudak *et al.* 1996), the Patient Evaluation Measure (PEM) (Dias *et al.* 2001) and the Michigan Hand Questionnaire (Chung *et al.* 1998) are the three currently in use. Each is valid and reliable, and responsiveness has been demonstrated for the PEM. These systems are discussed in detail in Chapter 17.

RADIOGRAPHIC ASSESSMENT

Radiographic views

Radiographs provide a picture of the anatomical abnormality within the wrist (Wilson *et al.* 1990).

Comparison of radiographs obtained before intervention and at a reasonable time after the intervention for wrist conditions provides a further objective assessment of outcome for several conditions of the wrist which involve the bones and joints.

Radiographs provide us with information regarding the integrity of the individual bones making up the wrist, the alignment of these bones, and the state of the joints. It is usual to obtain at least two views of the wrist – the postero-anterior and the lateral. It is essential to obtain standard views if radiographs are to be used for measurement.

Any radiograph of the wrist must include at least the distal third of the radius and ulna and the whole of the middle metacarpal in the image. The middle metacarpal must always (if possible) lie in line with the radius. The distance of the radiographic plate must be standard at 1 m and the thumb placed in maximum abduction.

The posterior-anterior view must be taken with the shoulder abducted at 90° and the elbow flexed to 90°. In this position, the forearm is in the anatomical mid-prone position and not in the usual full prone position.

The position of forearm rotation when obtaining wrist radiographs is important, as in full pronation the radius lies across the ulna and hence is effectively shortened. The assessment of ulnar variance (Palmer *et al.* 1982) which assesses the proximal-distal distance of the articular surface of the ulna from that of the radius depends on accurate radiographs obtained in a mid-prone anatomical position (Epner *et al.* 1982). Measurements taken in full pronation will overestimate the ulnar plus variance when the distal ulna articular surface lies distal to that of the radius.

Standardizing the position of the wrist in these radiographs contributes greatly to comparison with future radiographs, and hence assists in the accuracy of measurements.

Radiographic anatomy

The distal radius is inclined palmarwards by 11° and ulnarwards by 26°. The distal ulna is usually level with the distal radius or within 2 mm proximal to it. The gap between the distal radius and ulna is usually less than 4 mm.

Parameters

When viewing the radiographs of the wrist, four parameters are assessed.

LINES
The proximal articular surfaces of the scaphoid, lunate and triquetrum form a uniform curve, as do the distal articular surfaces of these bones and the articular surface of the capitate and hamate. Any abnormality of these lines should suggest an abnormality of the carpal bones in their alignment (Gilula 1979).

SHAPE, SIZE AND ORIENTATION OF CARPAL BONES
Deviation from normal should be noted. The scaphoid and lunate in particular deserve attention. Abnormal increase in size usually indicates a dislocation of part of the carpus, usually around the lunate.

The orientation of the carpal bones is best seen on the lateral view. The axis of the capitate, lunate and radius are in the same line. The scaphoid is tilted forward by 56°. A deviation of more than 5° from similar measurements on the opposite unaffected wrist suggests an abnormality. The method of assessment of the axis is established and found to be reliable on standard radiographs (Larsen *et al.* 1991a, b).

JOINT SPACE
A solitary joint narrowing usually suggests a dislocation. Diffuse narrowing in the presence of cysts, sclerosis and osteophytes indicates arthritis. It is important to document the precise location and severity of joint space narrowing and include information regarding cysts, sclerosis and osteophytes. The joint space may be either normal, reduced in comparison to other joints or the opposite unaffected side, or absent. Sclerosis, cyst formation and osteophytes are usually documented as present or absent. The size of the cyst need only be noted if it is large, and especially if it is solitary. The usual site for an osteophyte, apart from the radio-ulnar joint, is the radial styloid.

There are several scoring systems to document the degree of arthritis, and these are used especially in rheumatoid arthritis. The Larsen grading system is based on reference radiographs grading each joint from grade 0 (normal) to 5 (mutilating changes). The Steinbrocker staging system (4 stages for each joint) may be used to generate a comprehensive score. Some studies (Kaye *et al.* 1990; O'Sullivan *et al.* 1990) cast doubts on their value in assessing both progression of disease and outcome. Kaye (1991) has presented a good overview of the scoring systems used for rheumatoid arthritis.

It is important to compare initial radiographs with subsequent ones if any comment regarding the onset of osteoarthritis is to be made. This is of particular importance when assessing outcome, as the professed goal of several wrist procedures is to delay the onset of osteoarthritis even when there is no good information on the natural history of the condition. For example, in the treatment of scaphoid fracture non-union the goal is to prevent osteoarthritis. There is little evidence that this goal is achieved following operations to promote union.

Gaps

The possibility of ligamentous disruption should be considered if the gap between two carpal bones is greater than 4 mm, and especially when this appearance is unilateral.

Assessment of radiographs before and after intervention when bone union is intended depends on establishing that no gap exists. It must be appreciated that unless the X-ray beam is perpendicular to the gap, none will be recorded on the radiograph. A spurious impression of bone union may be formed. When doubt exists, tomograms, magnetic resonance imaging or ultrasonographic assessment for movement at that site should be carried out. Based on the gap, implant and the graft or fracture the state of bone union may be determined as satisfactory, suggest impending union or non-union or that the fracture is ununited. Time to union is a spurious outcome measure, and its use should be discouraged (Dias 2001).

CONCLUSION

Assessment of outcome for wrist conditions – like the outcome assessment for virtually every other site – is limited, even if an accurate and reproducible protocol could be defined, by the fact that each assessment is merely a snapshot of the wrist at that moment in time. If the assessment is carried out when the wrist is at its worst, then any subsequent assessment – even in the absence of intervention – would demonstrate improvement. Conversely, assessment before intervention with the wrist at its best, compared with an assessment following treatment with the wrist at its worst, may indicate little change. This is particularly true when assessing change in pain and stiffness. Some parameters can be established eventually with confidence, such as union of a fracture. Most parameters such as range of movement, strength, function and pain vary with different

factors in any one patient, thereby making the task of assessing outcome difficult.

There is no doubt that the principal aim in assessing outcome of wrist conditions is to establish whether for each individual the goals set before intervention have been met. For most wrist disorders a regional disability questionnaire such as the PEM (Dias *et al.* 2001), DASH (Hudak *et al.* 1996) or MHQ (Chung *et al.* 1998), combined with objective standardized assessment of strength and range, provides a snapshot of the wrist condition at that time. A wrist questionnaire or form such as the PRWE (MacDermid *et al.* 2000) may be added to complete the outcome assessment. The SF-36 is inadequate for upper-limb disorders and may underestimate any benefit of intervention.

REFERENCES

American Academy of Orthopaedic Surgeons (1965): *Joint Motion: Method of measuring and recording.* AAOS, Chicago.

Bechtol, C. (1954): Grip test: The use of a dynamometer with adjustable handle spacings. *J Bone Joint Surg* **36A**, 820–32.

Bialocerkowski, A. E., Grimmer, K. A., and Bain, G. I. (2000): A systematic review of the content and quality of wrist outcome instruments. *Int J Quality Health Care* **12**, 149–57.

Chung, K. C., Pillsbury, B. S., Walters, M. R., Hayward, R. A., and Arbor, A. (1998): Reliability and validity testing of the Michigan Hand Outcomes Questionnaire. *Hand Surg* **23A**, 575–87.

Cooney, W. P., Bussey, R., Dobyns, J. H., and Linscheid, R. L. (1987): Difficult wrist fractures. Perilunate fracture-dislocations of the wrist. *Clin Orthop* **214**, 136–47.

Curtis, R. M., and Engalitcheff, J. J. (1981): A work simulator for rehabilitating the upper extremity – preliminary report. *Hand Surg* **6**, 499.

Dias, J. J. (2001): Definition of union after acute fracture and surgery for fracture nonunion of the scaphoid. *Hand Surg* **26B**, 321–5.

Dias, J. J., Bhowal, B., Wildin, C. J., and Thompson, J. R. (2001): Assessing outcome of hand disorders. Is the Patient Evaluation Measure (P.E.M.) reliable, valid, responsive and without bias? *Bone Joint Surg* 83, 235–40.

Epner, R. A., Bowers, W. H., and Guilford, W. B. (1982): Ulnar variance – The effect of wrist positioning and roentgen filming technique. *Hand Surg* 7A, 298–305.

Feinstein, W. K., Lichtman, D. M., Noble, P. C., Alexander, J. W., and Hipp, J. A. (1999): Quantitative assessment of the midcarpal shift test. J *Hand Surg* 24, 977–83.

Geertzen, J. H., Dijkstra, P. U., Stewart, R. E., Groothoff, J. W., Ten Duis, H. J., and Eisma, W. H. (1998): Variation of measurements of range of motion: a study in reflex sympathetic dystrophy patients. *Clin Rehab* 12, 254–64.

Gilula, L. A. (1979): Carpal injuries: analytic approach and case exercises. *Am J Roentgenol* 133, 503.

Green, D. P., and O'Brien, T. (1978): Open reduction of carpal dislocations indications and operative techniques. J *Hand Surg* 3A, 250–65.

Horger, M. M. (1990): The reliability of goniometric measurements of active and passive wrist motions. *Am J Occup Ther* 44, 342–8.

Hudak, P. L., Amadio, P. C., and Bombadier, C. (1996): Development of an upper extremity outcome measure: The DASH (disabilities of the arm, shoulder and hand). The Upper Extremity Collaborative Group (UECG). *Am J Ind Med* 29, 602–8.

International Federation of Societies for Surgery of the Hand (2001): *Terminology for Hand Surgery*. Harcourt Health Sciences, London.

Kaye, J. J. (1991): Radiographic methods of assessment (scoring) of rheumatic disease. *Rheum Dis Clin North Am* 17, 457–70.

Kaye, J. J., Fuchs, H. A., Moseley, J. W., Nance, E. P., Callahan, L. F., and Pincus, T. (1990): Problems with the Steinbrocker staging system for radiographic assessment of the rheumatoid hand and wrist. *Invest Radiol* 25, 536–44.

Larsen, C. F., Mathiesen, F. K., and Lindquist, S. (1991a): Measurements of carpal bone angles on lateral wrist radiographs. *Hand Surg* 16A, 888–93.

Larsen, C. F., Stigsby, B., Lindquist, S., Bellstrom, T., Mathiesen, F. K., and Ipsen, T. (1991b): Observer variability in measurements of the carpal bones angles on lateral wrist radiographs. *Hand Surg* 16A, 893–8.

LaStayo, P. C., and Wheeler, D. L. (1994): Reliability of passive wrist flexion and extension goniometric measurements: a multicenter study. *Phys Ther* 74, 162–74.

MacDermid, J. C., Turgeon, T., Richards, R. S., Beadle, M., and Roth, J. H. (1999): Patient rating of wrist pain and disability: a reliable and valid measurement tool. *Orthop Trauma* 12, 577–86.

MacDermid, J. C., Richards, R. S., Donner, A., Bellamy, N., and Roth, J. H. (2000): Responsiveness of the short form-36, disability of the arm, shoulder and hand questionnaire, patient-rated wrist evaluation, and physical impairment measurements in evaluating recovery after a distal radius fracture. *J Hand Surg* 25, 330–40.

Macey, A., and Kelly, C. (1993): The hand. In: Pynsent, P., Fairbank, J., and Carr, A. (eds), *Outcome Measures in Orthopaedics*. Butterworth Heinemann, Oxford, pp. 174–93.

Mathiowetz, V., Weber, K., Volland, G., and Kasnman, N. (1984): Reliability and validity of grip and pinch strength evaluations. *Hand Surg* 9A, 222–6.

Mathiowetz, V., Kasnman, N., Volland, G., Weber, K., Dowe, M., and Rogers, S. (1985): Grip and pinch strength: normative data for adults. *Arch Phys Med Rehabil* 66, 69–74.

Mathiowetz, V., Wiemer, D. M., and Federman, S. M. (1986): Grip and pinch strengths: norms for 6 to 19 year olds. *Am J Occup Ther* 40, 705–11.

Moore, M. L. (1949): The measurement of Joint Motion. Part II. The technic of goniometry. *Phys Ther Rev* 29, 256.

O'Driscoll, S. W., Horii, E., Ness, R., Calahan, T. D., Richards, R. R., and Au, K. N. (1992): The relationship between wrist position, grasp size, and grip strength. *Hand Surg* 17, 169–77.

O'Sullivan, H. H., Lewis, P. A., Newcombe, R. G., Broderick, N. J., Robinson, D. A., Coles, E. C., and Jessop, J. D. (1990): Precision of Larsen grading of radiographs in assessing progression of rheumatoid arthritis in individual patients. *Ann Rheum Dis* **49**, 286–9.

Ojima, H., Miyake, S., Kumashiro, M., Togami, H., and Suzuki, K. (1991): Dynamic analysis of wrist circumduction: a new application of the biaxial flexible electrogoniometer. *Clin Biomech* **6**, 221–9.

Palmer, A. K., Glisson, R. R., and Werner, F. W. (1982): Ulnar variance determination. *Hand Surg* **7A**, 376–9.

Rawes, M. L., Richardson, J. B., and Dias, J. J. (1996): A new technique for the assessment of wrist movement using a biaxial flexible goniometer. *Hand Surg* **21**, 600–3.

Stewart, H. D., Innes, A. R., and Burke, F. D. (1985): Factors affecting the outcome of Colles' fracture: an anatomical and functional study. *Injury* **16**, 289–95.

Swanson, A. B., Swans, G. D., and Goran-Hagert, C. (1997): Evaluation of impairment of hand function. In: Hunter, J. M., Schneider, L. J., and Mackin, E. J. (eds), *Tendon and Nerve Surgery in the Hand. A third decade*. Mosby, St. Louis, pp. 642–4.

Wilson, A. J., Mann, F. A., and Gilula, L. A. (1990): Imaging the hand and wrist. *Hand Surg* **15B**, 153–67.

Young, V. L., Pin, P., Kraemer, B. A., Gould, R. B., Nemergut, L., and Pellowski, M. (1989): Fluctuation in grip and pinch strength among normal subjects. *Hand Surg* **14A**, 125–9.

INTRODUCTION

Many outcome measures have been described for assessing the results of treatment of hand injuries and diseases. Some of these are general, and can be applied to any condition, whereas others are specific, such as those for assessing the results of tendon surgery and nerve repair. Most of the specific outcome measures are objective, whereas most of the general outcome measures are subjective and in the form of a questionnaire. This chapter will first consider the general outcome measures, and will then consider the specific ones. A summary of the outcome measures described can be found in Table 17.6 at the end of the chapter.

GENERAL OUTCOME MEASURES

Subjective assessment

Several generic outcome measures have been described for evaluating the outcome of hand disorders, and these are provided in the appendix. The DASH (Disabilities of the Arm, Shoulder and Hand) (Hudak *et al.* 1996) and Michigan hand questionnaires (Chung *et al.* 1998) have recently been introduced in the USA. In the United Kingdom, the patient evaluation measure (PEM), the hand clinic questionnaire (HCQ) and the hand injury severity scoring system (HOSS) have been described (Sharma and Dias 2000); however, the latter two systems are hardly ever used.

THE DASH QUESTIONNAIRE (www.dash.iwh.on.ca)

Unlike other questionnaires, the DASH questionnaire is designed to assess the function of the upper limb, and it can thus be used to assess the outcome of shoulder, elbow, and wrist or hand interventions. It particularly assesses functional disability, rather than the presence and severity of persistent symptoms and has been independently assessed (Beaton *et al.* 2001). The questionnaire consists of 30 questions, of which 21 concern the patient's ability to perform general day-to-day activities: two assess the extent to which the condition of the arm interferes with work and normal social activities, two concern persistent pain. There is one each regarding paraesthesiae, weakness and stiffness in the arm. Finally, there is a question concerning sleep disturbance, and another about the patient's level of confidence with their arm. For each question the patient grades his or her level of disability or persistent symptoms on a 1 to 5 scale, on which 1 represents no difficulty with the task or no residual symptom, and 5 indicates inability to perform the function or an extreme level of the symptom. Thus, the minimum score is 30 (no residual symptoms or disability) and the maximum score is 150. This crude score is converted into a score of between 0 and 100 by subtracting 30 and then multiplying this value by 5 and dividing it by 6.

As the DASH questionnaire has been designed to assess disability of the whole arm, and only briefly assesses persistent symptoms and does not consider deformity, it is probably inadvisable to use it for the assessment of certain hand conditions. For example, in Dupuytren's disease, the problem is deformity and risk of progression of disease, rather than functional disability, in all but the most extreme cases. The use of DASH for assessing the outcome of carpal tunnel syndrome is also questionable, as there is only one question regarding sleep disturbance, two on pain and one on tingling: most carpal tunnel sufferers would not record any disability for any of the other 26 questions. The DASH questionnaire is also unlikely to detect disability following injuries such as an amputation of the distal half of the little finger, which resulted in a painless amputation stump. Normal values for the general population in the USA are to be published shortly.

THE MICHIGAN HAND OUTCOMES QUESTIONNAIRE

This questionnaire (Chung et al. 1998) assesses six domains of hand function: overall hand function; ability to perform the activities of daily living; pain; work performance; hand cosmesis; and patient satisfaction with the hand. It is completed by the patient and contains 37 questions, each consisting of a 1 to 5 scale. Unlike other questionnaires, such as the DASH, some of the questions relate exclusively to the right or the left hand (15 questions are specifically asked of each, such that the patient actually completes 52 questions, 15 repeated for each hand). The questionnaire takes a mean of 10 (range 7–20) minutes for a patient to complete, and has been rigorously assessed for reliability and validity by its designers (Chung et al. 1998).

THE PATIENT EVALUATION MEASURE (PEM)

This was designed by Eileen Bradbury, Stewart Watson and David Marsh and, like the Michigan hand questionnaire, predominantly assesses hand symptoms rather than ability to perform activities of daily living, which is the main feature of the DASH questionnaire. Like the Michigan hand questionnaire, it is specific for the hand though, as well as enquiring about persistent hand symptoms, it also assesses the quality of treatment provided to the patient and his or her overall assessment of the outcome of the intervention/injury. The PEM initially contained 10 questions regarding the state of the hand (sensation, cold intolerance, pain, dexterity, movement, strength, function for everyday activities, function for work, hand appearance and psychological feelings towards the hand), but a further question on duration of pain (ever-present to infrequent) has subsequently been added. The patient marks his/her response to all the questions on a scale, which takes an average of 4 minutes to complete.

Best buys

All of the above questionnaires are self-administered, and can be completed by the patient alone. The DASH questionnaire is gaining worldwide popularity for assessing the outcome of wrist interventions and has been translated into, and validated in, several languages. As the DASH only measures impairments, and does not assess complications, it is probably insufficient to use it in isolation. Many feel that outcome is best assessed by using two outcome questionnaires in combination. The PEM has been utilized in several studies performed within the UK. Additionally, the Nottingham Health Questionnaire has been used in hand surgery and is able to detect the improvement in well-being caused by carpal tunnel release (Rege and Sher 2001).

Sharma and Dias (2000) assessed the validity of the HOSS, HCQ and PEM questionnaires in 35 patients with hand conditions, using grip strength in the affected hand as the 'gold standard' for comparisons with the components of each outcome measure which assessed strength. They concluded that the PEM and the HCQ had comparable consistency. However, the PEM was more reproducible and they preferred its use, either as a postal questionnaire or as a questionnaire for use in outpatient clinics. Dias et al. (2001) have also reported that the PEM correlates with assessments of persistent pain, tenderness, swelling, wrist movement and grip strength following a scaphoid fracture. The HOSS was also found to be valid and suitable for the assessment of outcome in a research clinic.

Although some of these questionnaires have been extensively validated, problems can occur if they are used on their own to assess outcome. First, it has been estimated that up to 20 per cent of the population may have trouble understanding the questionnaires and may inadvertently complete them erroneously or inaccurately. Second, these questionnaires cannot detect patients who purposely complete the form so as to overstate their disability, either for personal or financial gain. It is thus generally recommended that they are used in conjunction with some objective measure(s) of outcome (for example, grip strength and range of movement), which can be used to validate the questionnaire responses and detect inconsistencies.

A further problem with all the above questionnaires is that they specifically relate to the status of the hand or, in the case of the DASH, the arm. This does not allow the comparison of disability due to arm conditions with that due to conditions of the rest of the body, which is the objective of the general health status questionnaires. However, the use of a general health status questionnaire, such as the SF-36, to assess the impact of hand diseases and injuries and the affects of interventions on hand conditions is unsatisfactory because the SF-36 contains few questions on pain, and most of its functional assessment concerns activities involving the legs rather than the arms. There is no single ideal questionnaire for assessing hand outcome, and the researcher should be aware of a number of questionnaires and should use them appropriately.

SPECIFIC OUTCOME MEASURES

Assessment of carpal tunnel syndrome outcome

There is no reason why the PEM, HSQ or another hand outcome questionnaire cannot be used to assess the severity of carpal tunnel syndrome and the outcome of its treatment. However, the DASH score – which only contains three questions on pain and tingling and one on sleep disturbance, compared with 21 questions on hand function (which is usually unaffected in carpal tunnel syndrome) – may be inappropriate for this condition. Levine *et al.* (1993)

devised a specific questionnaire for the assessment of carpal tunnel syndrome, which has a 'symptom severity scale' which assesses symptoms (pain, numbness, tingling, hand weakness and hand dexterity) and a 'functional status scale' which assesses the patient's ability to perform eight functions. The patient is able to choose between five graded responses for each of the questions in the 'symptom severity' and the 'function status' scales. A criticism of this outcome measure is that the symptom severity scale may not detect the presence of complications, such as scar tenderness. The designers of this outcome questionnaire reported that it had good reproducibility, good internal consistency and satisfactory validity when compared with hand grip, thumb pinch strength, sensory conduction velocity and 2-point discrimination and fine touch sensation. It was also sensitive to clinical change, and the symptom severity score in a cohort of carpal tunnel patients improved from a pre-operative mean of 3.4 (SD, 0.67) to a post-operative mean of 1.9 (SD, 1.0). A similar improvement in the functional score was also observed.

MEASUREMENT OF THUMB AND FINGER MOVEMENT

Finger movement

This may be assessed by measuring the ranges of flexion and extension of the metacarpophalangeal and proximal and distal interphalangeal joints either individually or, more usually, when the patient flexes or extends the finger fully. Alternatively, it may be assessed by measuring the distance between the fingertip and palm, again when making a fist. There is no direct correlation between goniometric and 'tip to palm' measurements, so these cannot be used interchangeably (MacDermid *et al.* 2001).

Measurement of the distance between the fingertip and the palm is quick and simple, and provides a rapid assessment of finger mobility, which is widely used to monitor progress with treatment and is easily understood by the patient. However, it is subject to inter-observer error because different observers use different reference points. Some measure the distance from the nail tip to the palm, whereas others use the centre of the fingertip itself as the reference point. Furthermore, although the landmark on the palm is usually the distal palmar crease, and this works well for the middle, ring and little fingers, this crease does not usually cross the base of the index finger. This led Buck-Gramcko *et al.* (1976) to use the distal composite flexion crease as the palmar landmark: this is a line drawn between the radial end of the proximal palmar crease (on radial border of palm) and the ulnar end of the distal palmar crease (on ulnar border of palm) (Tubiana *et al.* 1996). If this method of assessment is used, it is imperative that the landmarks which have been used are clearly defined.

When measuring the ranges of active extension and flexion of the individual joints of a finger when the subject makes a fist, or extends his/her fingers fully, it is usual to measure the angles with a *small* goniometer on the extensor surface of the finger. However, these angles can be equally well measured along the midlateral lines on the sides of the fingers but they must not be visually estimated ('eyeballed'), as this is very inaccurate (Rose *et al.* 2002). Finger joint goniometry has been reported to be susceptible to inter-observer variability but have good intra-observer reproducibility (Hamilton and Lachenbruch 1969), though others have observed high inter-observer reliability (Groth *et al.* 2001).

In 1976, the Clinical Assessment Committee of the American Society for Surgery of the Hand (ASSH 1976) recommended that the outcome of interventions was assessed by comparing the pre-intervention and post-intervention ranges of total active motion (TAM) and total passive motion (TPM) of the finger. These values are determined by adding together the ranges of active/passive flexion of the metacarpophalangeal and proximal and distal interphalangeal joints and then subtracting any extension deficits/fixed flexion deformities. The active range of movements of each joint must be measured while the subject is actively trying to make a fist or straighten his finger and the passive range of motion when the examiner is passively flexing or extending the *whole*

finger. They should not be measured during isolated flexion/extension of each joint individually, as this will not detect loss of motion due to tendon adhesions proximal to the proximal interphalangeal joint which restrict motion of the distal joints, as the restriction of movement in one of the joints distal to the adhesion will depend on the position of the others (tenodesis effect). If the range of total passive motion exceeds the range of total active motion, then tendon gliding is restricted. A problem with this method of assessment is that active metacarpophalangeal joint flexion is not lost following flexor tendon injuries as the intrinsic muscles of the hand perform this function: furthermore phalangeal fractures do not usually result in loss of motion at this joint and thus in many situations it provides an optimistic measurement of outcome. It is therefore wise to also document the ranges of movement of the metacarpophalangeal and interphalangeal joints separately, as well as in combination as the TAM or TPM.

Obviously the functional disability and loss of area of space in which the fingertip can be placed is less after loss of distal interphalangeal joint movement than that after the same loss of proximal interphalangeal joint, or worse still metacarpophalangeal joint, movement. However, this is not reflected by the use of TAM and TPM, or other assessments that are based entirely on goniometry. This is also a problem with the Strickland formula for assessing the outcome of flexor tendon surgery (*vide infra*). For this reason, one may consider that the measurement of fingertip-to-palm distance is a more functional measure than assessments based entirely on goniometry.

Thumb movement

ASSESSMENT OF THUMB PALMAR AND RADIAL ABDUCTION

Measurement of abduction of the trapeziometacarpal joint at the base of the thumb is inaccurate due to the absence of clearly visible landmarks. Both palmar and radial abduction are measured using the axes of the first and second metacarpals on the dorsum of the hand as markers.

ASSESSMENT OF THUMB OPPOSITION

Kapandji (1986) developed a system for assessing thumb opposition in which the tip of the thumb is moved in sequence from one position to another, until it cannot touch the next point in the sequence. It is imperative that each point is touched in sequence, and that no intervening points are missed, as it is possible for a thumb with limited opposition to move from position 1 directly to position 10, even though it has no opposition. The ten positions to which the tip of the thumb should be moved in sequence are: position 0, lateral aspect proximal phalanx of index finger; position 1, lateral aspect of middle phalanx of index finger; position 2, lateral aspect of distal phalanx of index finger; position 3, index fingertip; position 4, middle fingertip; position 5, ring fingertip; position 6, little fingertip; position 7, distal interphalangeal joint crease of little finger; position 8, proximal interphalangeal joint crease of little finger; position 9, basal crease of little finger; and position 10, distal palmar crease near the base of the little finger (Kapandji 1986; Tubiana *et al.* 1996).

MEASUREMENT OF ANGULAR JOINT DEFORMITY IN THE SAGITTAL PLANE

This is commonly done for ulnar deviation of the metacarpophalangeal joints of the fingers in rheumatoid arthritis. With the joint extended as far as possible (passively if there is an extension lag), and without passive correction of the ulnar drift, the angle between the axes of the metacarpal and proximal phalanx is measured. Some consider that these measurements are best made on posterio-anterior radiographs of the hand.

OUTCOME OF FLEXOR TENDON INJURY

A variety of techniques have been devised for assessing the outcome of flexor tendon surgery. All concentrate on assessing restoration of movement, and none assesses hand strength or dexterity. Most of the outcome measures are based on total active motion measurements, or measurement of the fingertip-to-palm distance.

Strickland's technique

Strickland and Glogovac (1980) suggested the following formula for calculating the percentage of the normal range of active finger proximal (PIP) and distal (DIP) interphalangeal joint movement:

$$\frac{PIP + DIP \text{ flexion} - \text{extensor lag}}{175°} \times 100$$
$$= \% \text{ of normal PIP and DIP motion}$$

Strickland considered that the combined arcs of movement of the DIP and PIP joints of a normal finger produced 175° of flexion, and so excluded hyperextension from these calculations.

The outcome of flexor tendon surgery was classified as excellent, good, fair or poor according to the percentage of normal finger movement attained. The original criteria for excellent, good, poor and fair outcomes have, subsequently been changed (Table 17.1) (Strickland 1985), but many surgeons consider the modified scoring system too lenient and continue to use the original system (Moiemen and Elliott 2000).

Strickland's technique is probably the most widely used method for assessing the results of flexor tendon surgery and its use has demonstrated that the outcome of isolated flexor digitorum profundus tendon repair in zone 1 is superior to the outcome of combined flexor digitorum profundus and superficialis tendon repairs in zone 2. However, although

Table 17.1: Outcome of flexor tendon surgery according to Strickland's original and modified scoring systems. Reprinted from Strickland (1985)

	Original (Strickland and Glogovac 1980)	Modified (Strickland 1985)
Excellent	85–100	75–100
Good	70–80	50–74
Fair	50–69	25–49
Poor	0–49	0–24

Values indicate the percentage of normal finger motion regained.

the total active range of movement of the finger achieved after an isolated zone 1 flexor digitorum profundus tendon is usually better than the range regained after combined profundus and superficialis tendon repairs in zone 2, this does not demonstrate that the former tendon repair is gliding and functioning any better than the latter. This is because proximal interphalangeal joint movement usually remains normal (100°) after an isolated flexor digitorum profundus tendon injury so that, even if the tendon repair fails completely, the patient retains 57 per cent of normal movement according to Strickland's criteria. This is classified as a fair result with the original scoring scheme and as a good result with the modified scoring scheme. This point has been highlighted by Moiemen and Elliot (2000), who suggested that the outcome of isolated flexor digitorum profundus tendon injuries in zone 1 should be assessed by measuring only active distal interphalangeal joint movement:

$$\frac{\text{DIP flexion} - \text{DIP lag}}{75°} \times 100\%$$

[This assumes that the normal arc of active movement at the distal interphalangeal joint is 75° (Moiemen and Elliott 2000)]. If this technique is used to assess isolated flexor digitorum profundus injuries, it quickly becomes apparent that the results of this surgery are not as good in terms of restoration of lost movement as is generally perceived.

The Buck-Gramcko method for evaluating the outcome of flexor tendon repair (Table 17.2) is also relatively widely used, particularly in Europe (Buck-Gramcko *et al.* 1976). This considers both the composite range of flexion at the metacarpophalangeal and proximal and distal interphalangeal joints, as well as the distance between the fingertip and the 'distal composite flexion crease' in the palm. Less commonly used scoring systems also utilize fingertip-to-palm distance, either in conjunction with measurement of the finger extension deficit (Kleinert *et al.* 1973) or with the composite range of finger flexion (Tsuge *et al.* 1977). Nielsen and Jensen (1985) compared the assessments of outcome of flexor

Table 17.2: Buck-Gramcko method for assessing the functional result of flexor tendon repair (Buck-Gramcko *et al.* 1976)

			Score
Distance between	0–2.5 cm	>200°	6
fingertip and distal	2.5–4.0 cm	>180°	4
palmar crease and	4.0–6.0 cm	>150°	2
composite flexion	>6.0 cm	<150°	0
Extension deficit	0–30°		3
	31–50°		2
	51–70°		1
	>70°		0
Composite flexion	>160°		6
minus composite	>160°		4
extension	>120°		2
	<120°		0
Evaluation	Evaluation		14–15
	Good		11–13
	Fair		7–10
	Poor		0–6

English translation reprinted from the *Journal of Hand Surgery*, **10B**, Nielsen and Jensen, Methods of evaluation of the functional results of flexor tendon repairs of the fingers, 60–61, ©1985, with permission of the British Society for Surgery of the Hand.

tendon repair as graded by these three systems and found that the Buck-Gramcko system gave the most favourable evaluation of outcome.

Outcome of flexor pollicis longus tendon repair

White (1956) and Buck-Gramcko *et al.* (1976) have devised techniques specifically to assess the results of flexor pollicis longus tendon repair.

Outcome of extensor tendon repair

Miller (1942) devised a method for assessing the outcome of extensor tendon repairs (Table 17.3). The total active motion (TAM) system of the American

Table 17.3: Miller's assessment of extensor tendon repair. Reprinted from Miller (1942)

Excellent	Same range of motion as opposite side
Good	Loss of 20° flexion and/or <10° extension lag
Fair	Loss of 45° flexion and/or 45–10° extension lag
Poor	>45° loss of flexion and/or >45° extension lag

Table 17.4: Total active motion (TAM) assessment of extensor tendon repairs. Reprinted from Kleinert and Verdan (1983)

Excellent	TAM* = TAM of contralateral finger
Good	TAM >75% TAM of contralateral finger
Fair	TAM 50–75% TAM of contralateral finger
Poor	TAM <50% TAM of contralateral finger

*TAM = {(MP + PIP + DIP Flexion) − (MP + PIP + DIP extension lag)}

Society for Surgery of the Hand (Kleinert and Verdan 1983) is also widely used (Table 17.4), as is Dargan's system (Dargan 1969). Khandwala *et al.* (2000) utilized all these three methods for assessing the outcome of extensor tendon repairs, and found that Dargan's system had poor intra-observer reliability. They also considered it too lenient in its assessment of outcome and concluded that the Miller system was the most stringent of these three techniques.

Best buys for assessment of tendon injuries

At present, the system described by Strickland is probably the most widely used and generally accepted technique for assessing outcome after flexor tendon surgery. However, researchers should be aware of its drawbacks and must clearly state whether they used the stringent original (Strickland and Glogovac 1980) or subsequent more lenient (Strickland 1985) assessments of excellent, good, fair and poor outcomes. For extensor tendon outcome, Miller's technique (Miller 1942) is probably the most stringent and effective.

ASSESSMENT OF SENSATION

In 1958, Moberg (1958) challenged the usefulness of assessing sensation with long-established neurological tests which are subjective and difficult to quantify. He proposed that hand surgeons should use an objective measure of sensation which correlated with, and reflected, hand function. He was not impressed by the recently developed MRC sensory scale, which was based on the work of Highet and Holmes (1943) and Zachary and Holmes (1946). This MRC scale has subsequently been modified by a variety of authors to include Seddon's grades of outcome (Seddon 1972) and incorporate both moving (Dellon *et al.* 1987; MacKinnon and Dellon 1988) and static 2-point discrimination sensation (American Society for Surgery of the Hand) (Table 17.5).

Moberg (1962) devised a 'pick-up test' to measure hand function, and used this as the gold standard with which to assess the functional value of different sensory tests. He concluded that static 2-point discrimination sensation and sensory threshold pressure (measured with von Frey hairs) correlated best with hand function, and recommended their use in clinical practice for the assessment of hand sensation. Dellon and Kallman (1983) suggested that moving 2-point discrimination provided a better measure of functional hand sensation than static 2-point discrimination. However, Marsh (1990) subsequently challenged the use of 2-point discrimination sensation as an assessment of functional hand sensation. His results showed that the recovery of this following nerve transection and repair was influenced by the age of the patient and the length of time between nerve injury and repair. Once he had taken these factors into account, the relationship between the functional 'pick up test' and 2-point discrimination was lost. Marsh considered

Table 17.5: MRC classification of sensory recovery, including Seddon's scale (Seddon 1972) and also incorporating static and moving 2-point discrimination (PD) measures (MacKinnon and Dellon 1988)

Grade	Recovery of sensibility (MRC)	Seddon's scale	Static 2-PD (mm)	Moving 2-PD (mm)
S0	No recovery in the autonomous area	Bad		
S1	Recovery of deep cutaneous pain sensibility in the autonomous area	Bad		
S1+	Recovery of superficial pain sensibility	Bad		
S2	Recovery of superficial pain and some touch sensibility	Poor		
S2+	As in S2, but with over-response	Poor		
S3	Recovery of pain and touch sensibility with disappearance of over-response	Fair	>15	>7
S3+	As in S3, but good localization of the stimulus. Imperfect recovery of 2-PD	Good	7–15	4–7
S4	Complete recovery	Excellent	2–6	2–3

that localization of sensation correlated well with the functional ability of the hand, and his reassessment of Onne's work (Onne 1962) suggested that sensory threshold pressures (measured with Semmes-Weinstein filaments) also reflected functional hand sensation. Chassard *et al.* (1993) subsequently performed a similar study to that of Marsh (Marsh 1990) and arrived at different conclusions. These authors reported that both moving and static 2-point discrimination measurements reflected hand function, even after age at injury and delay to nerve repair were taken into account.

All of the above studies compared specific tests of sensation, such as sensory threshold pressure and 2-point discrimination against functional tests which were performed without visual sensory input or the use of sensation in areas of the hand unaffected by the nerve injury. In contrast, Jerosch-Herold (1993) evaluated sensory tests against the ability and speed at performing activities of daily living with visual sensory input. She found that moving 2-point discrimination, a stringent assessment of sensory localization and object recognition all correlated with the ability to perform activities of daily living. There is thus considerable disagreement as to the best method of assessing sensation in the hand.

Functional assessment of hand sensation

Functional sensation in the hand can be assessed by relatively time-consuming functional tests which have been used as gold standards for the validation of simpler, widely used, clinical tests of sensation. These functional tests are probably the most rigorous assessments of hand sensation but time restraints usually prevent their use in clinical practice.

MOBERG 'PICK-UP' TEST

For the Moberg 'pick-up' test (Moberg 1958) as described by Marsh (1990), the patient wears two pairs of surgical gloves, which are cut away so as only to expose the skin in the territory of the damaged nerve: this prevents sensory input from areas of normal sensation. Twenty small everyday objects, such as a safety pin, paperclip, coins and a screw, are placed on a tray under a screen so that the patient cannot see them. The patient is then asked to pick up these objects, one at a time, with his or her normal hand and place them in a bowl. The time taken to perform this task is recorded, and the patient then performs the same task with the injured hand.

The number of objects which he/she is able to place in the bowl with the injured hand in the time taken to place all 20 objects in it with the normal hand is recorded and then halved in order to obtain a score between 0 and 10.

There are numerous variations to the 'pick-up' test, which Moberg never described in particular detail. Tubiana *et al.* (1996) described its use without gloves covering areas of normal sensation, and timed the patient using only his/her injured hand to pick up and place nine objects in a container, first with their eyes open and then with their eyes shut. Whilst the patient performed these tasks, an observer watched and assessed the skill of prehension and noted which fingers were, and were not, used.

Other functional tests assess recognition of shapes and textures (Marsh 1990).

SENSORY TESTS

Two-point discrimination

Moving two-point discrimination is reported to recover earlier, and is usually several millimetres less than (better than) static two-point discrimination. Although a bent ordinary paper clip is frequently used for these tests and was good enough for Moberg, an expensive discriminator (MacKinnon and Dellon 1985) or a pair of callipers may be used.

- Static two-point discrimination: This is assessed by lightly touching the tip of the finger in random sequence with either one or two points, which are aligned along the longitudinal axis of the finger (parallel to its axis). The smallest distance between the two points at which the patient correctly discerns between one or two points on seven out of 10 occasions is recorded. As the superficial branch of the radial nerve sometimes innervates the tip of the thumb, two-point discrimination and other sensory tests are usually performed on the tips of index and middle fingers after median nerve injuries. The test becomes inaccurate if too much pressure is exerted through the two points, as sensory receptors in a wide area around each point are then activated.

- Moving two-point discrimination: Here, the two points are initially set 8 mm apart. One or two points of the testing device are then moved proximally to distally along the longitudinal axis of the finger with the two points perpendicular to the line of movement. The least distance between the two points at which the patient can correctly discriminate between one and two points on seven out of 10 occasions is recorded. Normal moving two-point discrimination is 2 mm (Dellon 1978).

Sensory threshold pressure

Five Semmes-Weinstein filaments are commonly utilized which apply forces of 0.0045 to 0.068 g (green filament: normal), 0.166 to 0.408 g (blue filament: diminished light touch), 0.697 to 2.06 g (purple: diminished protective sensation), 3.63 to 4.47 g (red: loss of protective sensation) and 4.47 g (red-lined: untestable). The hand should be supported so that the filaments cannot move the finger, allowing proprioceptive input, and the patient should not be able to see the hand. The normal hand is assessed first, starting with the lightest of the five standard filaments. These should be placed perpendicularly to the skin of the fingertips, as if they are applied at an angle the force exerted is lighter. A full description of this technique is given by Tubiana *et al.* (1996).

Stimulus localization

The fingers to be assessed are each divided into three zones (proximal, middle and distal pulp spaces), and the hand is hidden from the patient's sight. A light stroking touch is then applied to each of these zones in random order and, after each, the patient is asked to point to the zone touched. Correct localization scores two points, and localization to an adjacent zone scores one point. Marsh (1990) concluded that most patients with complete ulnar or median nerve injuries found this test relatively easy and Jerosch-Herold (1993) modified it by dividing the distal pulp spaces of each finger into four zones, and asking the patient to localize between these.

Best buys for assessment of sensation

Static and mobile two-point discrimination sensation are widely accepted, possibly erroneously, as effective, reliable (Dellon *et al.* 1987) and rapid methods of assessing sensory recovery. However, there is considerable concern as to their validity, and some wonder whether patients may detect the difference between one and two points by using other sensory modalities, such as differences in pressure when one and two points are applied. Certainly, one wonders as to the functional validity of these two tests when one sees people following a median nerve repair who, according to two-point discrimination have regained very good sensation, struggle to identify and handle small objects when blinded. Sensory threshold pressure measurement with Semmes-Weinstein filaments may be of greater value but functional tests (e.g. one version of the Moberg pick-up test) are probably the best available for assessing recovery after injuries to large peripheral sensory nerves. These tests are much more time consuming than two-point discrimination, sensory threshold pressure and sensory localization tests, but probably reflect hand function more accurately. However, as they have been used as the gold standards against which other tests are assessed, their validity and reliability are not known. Whether the areas of the hand with normal sensation should be masked or not during these tests is a point of controversy.

MEASUREMENT OF STRENGTH

Grip strength

The Jamar dynamometer is the most widely used instrument for measuring grip strength. It has an adjustable handle, so that grip strength can be measured at five different grip widths. The smallest grip width is referred to as position 1, and the largest as position 5. If grip strength is measured at all five settings (five-position grip strength test), the greatest grip strength is recorded at position 2, or occasionally position 3. Grip strength is weakest when positions 1 and 5 are used. If only one grip width is used, it is usual to use position 2. In retrospective studies that assess the outcome of hand surgery or recovery after an injury (when grip strength cannot be, or was not,

measured before the injury or operation), it is usual to compare the grip strengths of the injured and uninjured hands. However, this assessment is confused by hand dominance and some recommend that the strength of the non-dominant hand is multiplied by 1.1 (increased by 10%) before comparison. The rationale for this is that in normal subjects there is usually a 5–10 per cent difference between the strengths of the dominant and non-dominant hands, though this difference can be as much as 30 per cent (Bechtol 1954). Recent studies have suggested that the difference between the dominant and non-dominant hands is not as marked, and is usually less than 5 per cent (Armstrong and Oldham 1999; Crosby and Wehbe 1999). The situation is further confused by assessments of handedness, such as the Waterloo Score, which demonstrate that many people are not entirely right- or left-handed, and perform some activities with their right hand and others with their left (Steenhuis *et al.* 1990). A recent survey found that 33 per cent of people are to some extent ambidextrous and only 3 per cent are entirely left-handed (Tan *et al.* 1993). The correlation between grip strength and hand dominance as assessed by the Waterloo score may provide a more rational and better basis for the comparison of right- and left-hand strengths.

It is usual to measure grip strength in each hand on three occasions during an assessment of hand strength. Although some authors report the best of the three grip strengths, most report the mean of the three attempts which is more reproducible (ASSH 1976).

Although grip strength assessment provides numerical data which are usually assessed with parametric statistics, its results should be considered with caution. First, it is important that grip meters are regularly calibrated as they lose their accuracy over time. Thus, comparison of the grip strengths obtained in different studies, or in the same study but with different grip meters, must be viewed with caution. Furthermore, the validity of serial measurements of grip strength taken over a period of months or years must also be viewed with caution, even if the same grip meter was used on each occasion, unless calibration was regularly performed.

The second problem with measurement of grip strength is that, although apparently objective, it is susceptible to subjective control and patients may feign weakness for financial or social gain. Several tests have been devised to detect feigned weakness, but although the five-position grip strength test may have good specificity, it only has 15 per cent sensitivity (Tredgett *et al.* 1999). The assessment of fatigue on rapid repeat testing has poor sensitivity and specificity (Tredgett and Davis 2000). The rapid exchange grip strength test however does have reasonable sensitivity and specificity, though like all tests is not entirely accurate (Joughin *et al.* 1993). The rapid exchange grip strength test is frequently performed incorrectly, and the reader is advised to carefully study its method of application, and not assume how it is performed.

It is important that grip strength is always measured in a standard fashion, with the subject in an upright chair and with the shoulder adducted and resting by the side of the torso, the elbow flexed to 90° and the forearm in neutral rotation. Another problem in the assessment of grip strength is that it may be subject to temporal variation: grip strength is said to be weakest on waking in the morning and to increase by as much as 30 per cent to reach its maximum strength in the late afternoon (Bechtol 1954), though Young *et al.* (1989) failed to observe such changes. The latter group measured hand grip strength (mean of the recordings at each of the five settings of the Jamar grip meter) on the morning and afternoons of two days of each of three consecutive weeks, and found that these 12 measures of grip strength fluctuated by a mean of approximately 20 per cent, but was not significantly stronger in the morning or afternoon. Temperature may also affect the strength of the hand, a cold hand being weaker than a warm one (Wiles and Edwards 1982).

MRC assessment of recovery of motor nerve function

Recovery of motor function in the forearm and the hand is traditionally assessed using the MRC scale of muscle strength:

MRC grade	
M0	Nil
M1	Muscle fasciculation
M2	Muscle contraction which cannot counteract gravity
M3	Muscle contraction which can counteract gravity
M4	Diminished muscle strength
M5	Normal muscle strength

This system works reasonably well for large muscles in the proximal arm and leg, though it is less satisfactory for the assessment of intrinsic hand muscle function because there is little gravity to overcome. Schreuders *et al.* (2000) assessed the measurement of the strength of abduction of the index and little fingers and palmar abduction of the thumb with a hand-held dynamometer and concluded that, with this technique, only differences of more than 35 per cent could be interpreted as real changes in the intrinsic muscle strength of an individual. However the intra-class correlation for both intra- and inter-observer reliability was greater than 0.9, indicating that the force measurements achieved with this technique are suitable for the comparison of strength between groups of patients.

Thumb pinch strength

As with the assessment of grip strength, it is important that pinch meters are regularly calibrated, and it is also advisable to use the same pinch meter throughout a study. Thumb pinch strength is measured with the subject in the same position as for the assessment of grip strength, and it is usual to assess both thumb key pinch and tip pinch strengths. Thumb key pinch strength is measured with the subject making a fist and the pinch meter lying between the radial border of the index finger (resting on the proximal interphalangeal joint) and the tip of the thumb which lies in neutral rotation. The pinch meter should be gently held by the observer as, if it is firmly held, the subject may pinch against the observer's resisting force, producing an erroneously high measurement. Thumb tip pinch strength is measured between the tips of the index finger and the opposed thumb, with the middle, ring and little fingers flexed into the palm in order to allow maximum force generation in the flexor digitorum profundus muscle (Hook and Stanley 1986).

Young *et al.* (1989) measured thumb key pinch strength in the mornings and afternoons of two days during each of three consecutive weeks. They recorded the mean of three measurements on each occasion, and found that the key pinch strengths of individual patients varied by a mean of 15 per cent, though key pinch was not significantly stronger in the afternoons than the mornings. This fluctuation in key pinch strength could not be attributed to a learning effect, as the greatest measure of grip strength often occurred at one of the earlier assessments.

Table 17.6: A summary of outcome measures

Instrument name	What it measures	Validation	Reliability	Responsiveness	Usage	Score
Outcome questionnaires						
Carpal Tunnel Questionnaire (Levine *et al.* 1993)	Carpal tunnel syndrome	1	1	1	4	7
DASH (Hudak *et al.* 1996)	Arm function	2	2	2	4	10
Hand Clinic Questionnaire (HCQ) (Sharma and Dias 2000)	General hand outcome	2	2	–	0	4
Hand Outcome Severity Score (HOSS) (Sharma and Dias 2000)	General hand outcome	2	Moderate only		1	3
Michigan Hand Questionnaire (Chung *et al.* 1998)	General hand outcome	1	1	1	3	6
Patient Evaluation Measure (PEM) (Sharma and Dias 2000)	General hand outcome	2	2	2	3	9
Sensation						
Mobile 2-point discrimination (Dellon 1978)	Sensory function	0–2	1		4	5–7
Static 2-point discrimination (Moberg 1958)	Sensory function	0–2	1		4	5–7
Sensory Threshold Pressure (Semmes-Weinstein Filaments) (Marsh 1990)	Sensory function	2			4	6
Sensory localization (Jerosch-Herold 1993; Marsh 1990)	Sensory function	2			1	3
Finger movement						
Finger joint goniometry (Groth *et al.* 2001; Hamilton and Lachenbruch 1969)	Finger joint mobility	2	2	2	4	10
Strickland (Strickland 1985; Strickland and Glogovac 1980)	Finger flexor tendon surgery outcome	–	–	–	4	4

Table 17.6: A summary of outcome measures – *continued*

Instrument name	What it measures	Validation	Reliability	Responsiveness	Usage	Score
Buck-Gramcko (Buck-Gramcko *et al.* 1976)	Thumb and finger flexor tendon surgery outcome	–	–	–	4	4
Miller (Miller 1942)	Extensor tendon surgery	–	–	–	3	3
Total active and passive motion (ASSH 1976; Kleinert and Verdan 1983)	Finger mobility and extensor tendon surgery outcome				4	3
Dargan system (Dargan 1969)	Extensor tendon surgery	–	–	–	3	3
Muscle strength						
5-position grip strength test (Tredgett *et al.* 1999)	Feigned hand weakness	–	–	–	2	2
Rapid exchange grip strength test (Joughin *et al.* 1993; Westbrook *et al.* 2002)	Feigned hand weakness	2	1	–	3	6
Intrinsic muscle dynamometer (Schreuders *et al.* 2000)	Intrinsic muscle strength	2	1	1	2	6
Other						
Percival Score (Percival *et al.* 1991)	Outcome of thumb pollicization	–	–	–	4	4

REFERENCES

Armstrong, C., and Oldham, J. (1999): A comparison of dominant and non-dominant hand strengths. *J Hand Surg* **24B**, 421–5.

ASSH (1976): Clinical Assessment Committee Report. American Society for Surgery of the Hand.

Beaton, D. E., Katz, J. N., Fossel, A. H., Wright, J. G., Tarasuk, V., and Bombardier, C. (2001): Measuring the whole or the parts? Validity, reliability, and responsiveness of the disabilities of the arm, shoulder and hand outcome measure in different regions of the upper extremity. *J Hand Ther* **14**, 128–46.

Bechtol, C. (1954): The use of a dynamometer with adjustable hand spacings. *J Bone Joint Surg* **36A**, 820–32.

Buck-Gramcko, D., Dietrich, F., and Gogge, S. (1976): Bewertungskriterein bei nachuntersuchungen von beugeshnenwiederherstellungskriterein. *Handchir Mikrochir Plast Chir* **8**, 65–9.

Chassard, M., Pham, E., and Comtet, J. J. (1993): Two-point discrimination tests versus functional sensory recovery in both median and ulnar nerve complete transections. *J Hand Surg* **18B**, 790–6.

Chung, K., Pillsbury, M., Walters, M., and Hayward, R. (1998): Reliability and validity testing of the Michigan hand outcomes questionnaire. *J Hand Surg* **23A**, 575–87.

Crosby, C., and Wehbe, M. (1999): Hand strength: normative values. *J Hand Surg* **19A**, 665–70.

Dargan, E. (1969): Management of extensor tendon injuries of the hand. *Surg Gynecol Obstet* **128**, 1269–73.

Dellon, A. (1978): The moving two-point discrimination test: clinical evaluation of the quickly-adapting fiber/receptor system. *J Hand Surg* **3**, 474–81.

Dellon, A. L., and Kallman, C. H. (1983): Evaluation of functional sensation in the hand. *J Hand Surg* **8**, 865–70.

Dellon, A., Mackinnon, S., and Crosby, P. (1987): Reliability of two-point discrimination measurements. *J Hand Surg* **12A**, 693–6.

Dias, J., Bhowal, B., Wildin, C., and Thompson, J. (2001): Assessing the outcome of disorders of the hand. *J Bone Joint Surg* **83B**, 235–40.

Groth, G. N., VanDeven, K. M., Phillips, E. C., and Ehretsman, R. L. (2001): Goniometry of the proximal and distal interphalangeal joints, Part II: placement preferences, interrater reliability, and concurrent validity. *J Hand Ther* **14**, 23–9.

Hamilton, G. F., and Lachenbruch, P. A. (1969): Reliability of goniometers in assessing finger joint angle. *Phys Ther* **49**, 465–9.

Highet, W., and Holmes, W. (1943): Traction injuries to the lateral popliteal nerve and traction injuries to peripheral nerves after suture. *Br J Surg* **30**, 212–33.

Hook, W. E., and Stanley, J. K. (1986): Assessment of thumb to index pulp to pulp pinch grip strengths. *J Hand Surg Br* **11B**, 91–2.

Hudak, P. L., Amadio, P. C., and Bombardier, C. (1996): Development of an upper extremity outcome measure: the DASH (disabilities of the arm, shoulder and hand) [corrected]. The Upper Extremity Collaborative Group (UECG) [published erratum appears in *Am J Ind Med* 1996, 30, 372]. *Am J Ind Med* **29**, 602–8.

Jerosch-Herold, C. (1993): Measuring outcome in median nerve injuries. *J Hand Surg* **18B**, 624–8.

Joughin, K., Gulati, P., Mackinnon, S., McCabe, S., Murray, J., Griffiths, S., and Richards, R. (1993): An evaluation of rapid exchange and simultaneous grip tests. *J Hand Surg* **18**, 245–52.

Kapandji, A. (1986): Cotation cliniquede l'opposition et de la contreopposition du pouce. *Ann Chir de la Main et le Membre Superiere* **5**, 67–73.

Khandwala, A., Webb, J., Harris, S., Foster, A., and Elliot, D. (2000): A comparison of dynamic extension splinting and controlled active mobilization of complete divisions of extensor tendons in zones 5 and 6. *J Hand Surg* **25B**, 140–6.

Kleinert, H., and Verdan, C. (1983): Report of the committee on tendon injuries. *J Hand Surg* **8**, 794–8.

Kleinert, H., Kutz, J., Atasoy, E., and Stormo, A. (1973): Primary repair of flexor tendons. *Orthop Clin North Am* **4**, 865–76.

Levine, D., Simmons, B., Koris, M., Daltroy, L., Hohl, G., Fossel, A., and Katz, J. (1993): A self-administered questionnaire for the assessment of severity of symptoms and functional status in carpal tunnel syndrome. *J Bone Joint Surg* **75A**, 1585–92.

MacDermid, J., Fox, E., Richards, R., and Roth, J. (2001): Validity of pulp to palm distance as a measure of finger flexion. *J Hand Surg* **26**, 432–5.

MacKinnon, S., and Dellon, A. (1985): Two-point discrimination tester. *J Hand Surg* **10A**, 906–7.

MacKinnon, S., and Dellon, A. (1988): *Surgery of the Peripheral Nerves*. Thieme, New York.

Marsh, D. (1990): The validation of measures of outcome following suture of divided peripheral nerves supplying the hand. *J Hand Surg* **15B**, 25–34.

Miller, H. (1942): Repair of severed tendons of the hand and wrist. Statistical analysis of 300 cases. *Surg Gynecol Obstet* **75**, 693–8.

Moberg, E. (1958): Objective methods for determining the functional value of sensibility in the hand. *J Bone Joint Surg* **40B**, 454–76.

Moberg, E. (1962): Criticism and study of methods for examining sensibility in the hand. *Neurology* **12**, 8–19.

Moiemen, N., and Elliott, D. (2000): Primary flexor tendon repair in zone 1. *J Hand Surg* **25B**, 78–4.

Nielsen, A., and Jensen, P. (1985): Methods of evaluation of the functional results of flexor tendon repair of the fingers. *J Hand Surg* **10B**, 60–1.

Onne, L. (1962): Recovery of sensibility and sudomotor activity in the hand after nerve suture. *Acta Chir Scand Suppl* 300.

Percival, N., Sykes, P., and Chandraprakasam, T. (1991): A method of assessment of pollicisation. *J Hand Surg Br* **16B**, 141–3.

Rege, A., and Sher, J. (2001): Can outcome of carpal tunnel release be predicted? *J Hand Surg* **26B**, 148–50.

Rose, V., Nduka, C., Pereira, J., Pickford, M., and Belcher, H. (2002): Visual estimation of finger angles: do we need goniometers? *J Hand Surg* **27**, 382–4.

Schreuders, T., Roebroeck, M., van der Kar, T., Soeters, J., Hovius, S., and Stam, H. (2000): Strength of the intrinsic muscles of the hand measured with a hand-held dynamometer: reliability in patients with ulnar and median nerve paralysis. *J Hand Surg* **25B**, 560–5.

Seddon, H. (1972): *Surgical Disorders of the Peripheral Nerves*. Churchill Livingstone, Edinburgh.

Sharma, R., and Dias, J. (2000): Validity and reliability of three generic outcome measures for hand disorders. *J Hand Surg* **25B**, 593–600.

Steenhuis, R. E., Bryden, M. P., Schwartz, M., and Lawson, S. (1990): Reliability of hand preference items and factors. *J Clin Exp Neuropsychol* **12**, 921–30.

Strickland, J. (1985): Results of tendon surgery in zone 2. *Hand Clinics* **1**, 167–79.

Strickland, J., and Glogovac, S. (1980): Digital function following flexor tendon repair in zone 2: a comparison of immobilization and controlled passive motion techniques. *J Hand Surg* **5**, 537–43.

Tan, U., Komsuoglu, S., and Akgun, A. (1993): Inverse relationship between the size of pattern reversal visual evoked potentials from the left brain and the degree of left-hand preference in left-handed normal subjects: importance of the left brain. *Int J Neurosci* **72**, 79–87.

Tredgett, M., and Davis, T. (2000): Rapid repeat testing of grip strength for detection of faked hand weakness. *J Hand Surg* **25B**, 372–5.

Tredgett, M., Pimble, L., and Davis, T. (1999): The detection of feigned hand weakness using the five position grip strength test. *J Hand Surg* **24B**, 426–8.

Tsuge, K., Ikuta, Y., and Matsuishi, Y. (1977): Repair of flexor tendons by intratendinous tendon suture. *J Hand Surg* **2**, 436–40.

Tubiana, R., Thomine, J.-E., and Mackin, E. (1996): *Examination of the Hand and Wrist*. Martin Dunitz, London.

Westbrook, A. P., Tredgett, M. W., Davis, T. R., and Oni, J. A. (2002): The rapid exchange grip strength test and the detection of submaximal grip effort. *J Hand Surg* **27**, 329–33.

White, W. (1956): Secondary restoration of finger function by digital tendon grafts. *Am J Surg* **91**, 662–8.

Wiles, C. M., and Edwards, R. H. (1982): The effect of temperature, ischaemia and contractile activity on the relaxation rate of human muscle. *Clin Physiol* **2**, 485–97.

Young, V., Pin, P., Kraemer, A., Gould, R., Mnemergut, L., and Pellowski, M. (1989): Fluctuation in grip and pinch strength among normal subjects. *J Hand Surg* **14A**, 125–9.

Zachary, R., and Holmes, W. (1946): Primary suture of nerves. *Surg Gynecol Obstet* **82**, 632–51.

CARPAL TUNNEL SYNDROME ASSESSMENT (Levine *et al.* 1993)*

a) SYMPTOM SEVERITY SCALE

The following questions refer to your symptoms for a typical 24-hour period during the past two weeks (circle one answer to each question).

How severe is the hand or wrist pain that you have at night?
1   I do not have hand or wrist pain at night
2   Mild pain
3   Moderate pain
4   Severe pain
5   Very severe pain

How often did hand or wrist pain wake you up during a typical night in the past two weeks?
1   Never
2   Once
3   Two or three times
4   Four or five times
5   More than five times

Do you typically have pain in your hand or wrist during the daytime?
1   I never have pain during the day
2   I have mild pain during the day
3   I have moderate pain during the day
4   I have severe pain during the day
5   I have very severe pain during the day

How often do you have hand or wrist pain during the daytime?
1   Never
2   Once or twice a day
3   Three to five times a day
4   More than five times a day
5   The pain is constant

How long, on average, does an episode of pain last during the daytime?
1   I never get pain during the day
2   Less than 10 minutes
3   10 to 60 minutes
4   Greater than 60 minutes
5   The pain is constant throughout the day

Do you have numbness (loss of sensation) in your hand?
1   No
2   I have mild numbness
3   I have moderate numbness
4   I have severe numbness
5   I have very severe numbness

Do you have weakness in your hand or wrist?
1   No weakness
2   Mild weakness
3   Moderate weakness
4   Severe weakness
5   Very severe weakness

* Reprinted from *The Journal of Bone and Joint Surgery*, **75A**, Levine *et al.*, A self-administered questionnaire for the assessment of severity of symptoms and functional status in carpal tunnel syndrome, 1585–92, 1993.

CARPAL TUNNEL SYNDROME ASSESSMENT (Levine et al., 1993) – *continued*

Do you have tingling sensations in your hand?
1 No tingling
2 Mild tingling
3 Moderate tingling
4 Severe tingling
5 Very severe tingling

How severe is numbness (loss of sensation) or tingling at night?
1 I have no numbness or tingling at night
2 Mild
3 Moderate
4 Severe
5 Very severe

How often did hand numbness or tingling wake you up during a typical night during the past two weeks?
1 Never
2 Once

3 Two or three times
4 Four or five times
5 More than five times

Do you have difficulty with the grasping and use of small objects such as keys or pens?
1 No difficulty
2 Mild difficulty
3 Moderate difficulty
4 Severe difficulty
5 Very severe difficulty

Analysis of data
The overall symptom severity score is calculated as the mean of the scores for each of the eleven individual questions.

b) FUNCTIONAL STATUS SCALE

On a typical day during the past two weeks, have hand and wrist symptoms caused you to have any difficulty doing the activities listed below?

Please circle one number that best describes your ability to do the activity.

Activity	No difficulty	Mild difficulty	Moderate difficulty	Severe difficulty	Cannot do due to hand or wrist symptoms
Writing	1	2	3	4	5
Buttoning of clothes	1	2	3	4	5
Holding a book while reading	1	2	3	4	5
Gripping of a telephone handle	1	2	3	4	5
Opening of jars	1	2	3	4	5
Household chores	1	2	3	4	5
Carrying of grocery bags	1	2	3	4	5
Bathing and dressing	1	2	3	4	5

The overall score for functional status was calculated as the mean of the eight items. Items that were left unanswered or that were not applicable were not included in the calculation of the overall score.

DASH – (DISABILITIES OF THE ARM, SHOULDER AND HAND) QUESTIONNAIRE (Hudak *et al.* 1996)*

INSTRUCTIONS: This questionnaire asks about your symptoms as well as your ability to perform certain activities.

Please answer every question, based on your condition in the **last week**, by circling the appropriate number.

If you did not have the opportunity to perform an activity in the past week, please make your best guess as to which response would have been most accurate.

It doesn't matter which hand or arm you use to perform the activity; please answer based on your ability, regardless of how you perform the task.

Please rate your ability to do the following activities in the *last week* by circling the number in the box below the appropriate response

	No difficulty	Mild difficulty	Moderate difficulty	Severe difficulty	Unable
Open a tight or new jar	1	2	3	4	5
Write	1	2	3	4	5
Turn a key	1	2	3	4	5
Prepare a meal	1	2	3	4	5
Push open a heavy door	1	2	3	4	5
Place an object on a shelf above your head	1	2	3	4	5
Do heavy household chores (wash floors, wash walls)	1	2	3	4	5
Garden	1	2	3	4	5
Make a bed	1	2	3	4	5
Carry a shopping bag or briefcase	1	2	3	4	5
Carry a heavy object (over 5 kg or 10 lb)	1	2	3	4	5
Change a light bulb overhead	1	2	3	4	5
Wash or blow-dry your hair	1	2	3	4	5
Wash your back	1	2	3	4	5
Put on a pullover sweater	1	2	3	4	5
Use a knife to cut food	1	2	3	4	5
Recreational activities requiring little effort (card playing, knitting)	1	2	3	4	5

*This DASH Outcome Measure is not to be reproduced or copied in any way. For more information and to download the DASH Outcome Measure, visit www.dash.iwh.on.ca

DASH – (DISABILITIES OF THE ARM, SHOULDER AND HAND) QUESTIONNAIRE (Hudak *et al.* 1996) – *continued*

	No difficulty	Mild difficulty	Moderate difficulty	Severe difficulty	Unable
Recreational activities in which you take some force or impact through your arm, shoulder or hand (e.g. golf, hammering, tennis)	1	2	3	4	5
Recreational activities in which you move your arm freely (e.g. playing frisbee, badminton, etc.)	1	2	3	4	5
Manage public transport and driving car	1	2	3	4	5
Sexual activities	1	2	3	4	5

	Not at all	Slightly	Moderately	Quite a bit	Extremely
During the *past week*, **to what extent has your arm, shoulder or hand problem** interfered with your normal social activities with family, friends, neighbours or groups? (circle number)	1	2	3	4	5

	Not limited at all	Slightly limited	Moderately limited	Very limited	Unable
During *the past week* were you limited in your work or other regular activities as a result of your arm, shoulder or hand problems? (circle number)	1	2	3	4	5

Please rate the severity of the following symptoms in the last week (circle number)

	None	Mild	Moderate	Severe	Extreme
Arm, shoulder or hand pain	1	2	3	4	5
Arm, shoulder or hand pain when you performed any specific activity	1	2	3	4	5
Tingling (pins and needles) in your arm, shoulder or hand	1	2	3	4	5
Weakness in your arm, shoulder or hand	1	2	3	4	5
Stiffness in your arm, shoulder or hand	1	2	3	4	5

DASH – (DISABILITIES OF THE ARM, SHOULDER AND HAND) QUESTIONNAIRE (Hudak *et al.* 1996) – *continued*

	No difficulty	Mild difficulty	Moderate difficulty	Severe difficulty	So much difficulty that I can't sleep
During the past week, how much difficulty have you had sleeping because of the pain in your arm, shoulder or hand? (circle number)	1	2	3	4	5

	Strongly disagree	Disagree	Neither agree nor disagree	Agree	Strongly agree
I feel less capable, less confident or less useful because of my arm problem (circle number)	1	2	3	4	5

MICHIGAN HAND OUTCOMES QUESTIONNAIRE (Chung et al. 1998)*

Instructions This survey asks for your views about your hands and your health. This information will help keep track of how you feel and how well you are able to do your usual activities. Answer *every* question by marking the answer as indicated. If you are unsure about how to answer a question, please give the best answer you can.

I. The following questions refer to the function of your hand(s)/wrist(s) *during the past week.* (Please circle one answer for each question.)

A. The following questions refer to your *right* hand/wrist.

	Very good	Good	Fair	Poor	Very poor
1 Overall, how well did your *right* hand work?	1	2	3	4	5
2 How well did your right fingers move?	1	2	3	4	5
3 How well did your right wrist move?	1	2	3	4	5
4 How was the strength in your right hand?	1	2	3	4	5
5 How was the sensation (feeling) in your right hand?	1	2	3	4	5

B. The following questions refer to your *left* hand/wrist.

	Very good	Good	Fair	Poor	Very poor
1 Overall, how well did your *left* hand work?	1	2	3	4	5
2 How well did your left fingers move?	1	2	3	4	5
3 How well did your left wrist move?	1	2	3	4	5
4 How was the strength in your left hand?	1	2	3	4	5
5 How was the sensation (feeling) in your left hand?	1	2	3	4	5

II. The following questions refer to the ability of your hand(s) to do certain tasks *during the past week*. (Please circle one answer for each question.)

A. How difficult was it for you to perform the following activities using your *right hand?*

	Not at all difficult	A little difficult	Somewhat difficult	Moderately difficult	Very difficult
1 Turn a door knob	1	2	3	4	5
2 Pick up a coin	1	2	3	4	5

*Reprinted from the *Journal of Hand Surgery* **23A**, Chung et al., Reliability and validity testing of the Michigan hand outcomes questionnaire, 575–87, © 1998 American Society for Surgery of the Hand.

MICHIGAN HAND OUTCOMES QUESTIONNAIRE
(Chung et al. 1998) – continued

		Not at all difficult	A little difficult	Somewhat difficult	Moderately difficult	Very difficult
3	Hold a glass of water	1	2	3	4	5
4	Turn a key in a lock	1	2	3	4	5
5	Hold a frying pan	1	2	3	4	5

B. How difficult was it for you to perform the following activities using your *left hand?*

		Not at all difficult	A little difficult	Somewhat difficult	Moderately difficult	Very difficult
1	Turn a door knob	1	2	3	4	5
2	Pick up a coin	1	2	3	4	5
3	Hold a glass of water	1	2	3	4	5
4	Turn a key in a lock	1	2	3	4	5
5	Hold a frying pan	1	2	3	4	5

C. How difficult was it for you to perform the following activities using *both of your hands?*

		Not at all difficult	A little difficult	Somewhat difficult	Moderately difficult	Very difficult
1	Open a jar	1	2	3	4	5
2	Button a shirt/blouse	1	2	3	4	5
3	Eat with a knife/fork	1	2	3	4	5
4	Carry a grocery bag	1	2	3	4	5
5	Wash dishes	1	2	3	4	5
6	Wash your hair	1	2	3	4	5
7	Tie shoelaces/knots	1	2	3	4	5

III. The following questions refer to how you did in your *normal work* (including both housework and school work) during the *past 4 weeks.* (Please circle one answer for each question.)

		Always	Often	Sometimes	Rarely	Never
1	How often were you unable to do your work because of problems with your hand(s)/wrist(s)?	1	2	3	4	5

MICHIGAN HAND OUTCOMES QUESTIONNAIRE
(Chung *et al.* 1998) – *continued*

	Always	Often	Sometimes	Rarely	Never
2 How often did you have to shorten your work day because of problems with your hand(s)/wrist(s)?	1	2	3	4	5
3 How often did you have to take it easy at your work because of problems with your hand(s)/wrist(s)?	1	2	3	4	5
4 How often did you accomplish less in your work because of problems with your hand(s)/wrist(s)?	1	2	3	4	5
5 How often did you take longer to do the tasks in your work because of problems with your hand(s)/wrist(s)?	1	2	3	4	5

IV. The following questions refer to how much *pain* you had in your hand(s)/wrist(s) *during the past week.* (Please circle one answer for each question.)

1 How often did you have pain in your hand(s)/wrist(s)?
1 Always
2 Often
3 Sometimes
4 Rarely
5 Never

If you answered *never* to *question IV-1* above, please skip the following questions and go to the next page.

2 Please describe the pain you have in your hand(s)/wrist(s).
1 Very mild
2 Mild
3 Moderate
4 Severe
5 Very severe

	Always	Often	Sometimes	Rarely	Never
3 How often did the pain in your hand(s)/wrist(s) interfere with your sleep?	1	2	3	4	5
4 How often did the pain in your hand(s)/wrist(s) interfere with your daily activities (such as eating or bathing)?	1	2	3	4	5
5 How often did the pain in your hand(s)/wrist(s) make you unhappy?	1	2	3	4	5

MICHIGAN HAND OUTCOMES QUESTIONNAIRE
(Chung et al. 1998) – continued

V.

A. The following questions refer to the appearance (look) of your *right* hand during the past week. (Please circle one answer for each question.)

		Strongly agree	Agree	Neither agree nor disagree	Disagree	Strongly disagree
1	I was satisfied with the appearance (look) of my *right* hand.	1	2	3	4	5
2	The appearance (look) of my right hand sometimes made me uncomfortable in public.	1	2	3	4	5
3	The appearance (look) of my right hand made me depressed.	1	2	3	4	5
4	The appearance (look) of my right hand interfered with my normal social activities.	1	2	3	4	5

B. The following questions refer to the appearance (look) of your *left* hand during the past week. (Please circle one answer for each question.)

		Strongly agree	Agree	Neither agree nor disagree	Disagree	Strongly disagree
1	I was satisfied with the appearance (look) of my *left* hand.	1	2	3	4	5
2	The appearance (look) of my left hand sometimes made me uncomfortable in public.	1	2	3	4	5
3	The appearance (look) of my left hand made me depressed.	1	2	3	4	5
4	The appearance (look) of my left hand interfered with my normal social activities.	1	2	3	4	5

VI.

A. The following questions refer to your satisfaction with your *right* hand/wrist during the past week. (Please circle one answer for each question.)

		Strongly agree	Agree	Neither agree nor disagree	Disagree	Strongly disagree
1	Overall function of right hand.	1	2	3	4	5
2	Motion of the fingers in your right hand.	1	2	3	4	5
3	Motion of your right wrist.	1	2	3	4	5

MICHIGAN HAND OUTCOMES QUESTIONNAIRE
(Chung et al. 1998) – continued

	Strongly agree	Agree	Neither agree nor disagree	Disagree	Strongly disagree
4 Strength of your right hand.	1	2	3	4	5
5 Pain level of your right hand.	1	2	3	4	5
6 Sensation (feeling) of your right hand.	1	2	3	4	5

B. The following questions refer to your satisfaction with your **left** hand/wrist during the past week. (Please circle one answer for each question.)

	Strongly agree	Agree	Neither agree nor disagree	Disagree	Strongly disagree
1 Overall function of left hand.	1	2	3	4	5
2 Motion of the fingers in your left hand.	1	2	3	4	5
3 Motion of your left wrist.	1	2	3	4	5
4 Strength of your left hand.	1	2	3	4	5
5 Pain level of your left hand.	1	2	3	4	5
6 Sensation (feeling) of your left hand.	1	2	3	4	5

Please provide the following information about yourself. (Please circle one answer for each question.)

1 **Are you right or left handed?**
   a Right handed
   b Left handed
   c Both

2 **Which hand gives you the most problem?**
   a Right hand
   b Left hand
   c Both

3 **Have you changed the type of job you did before you had problems with your hand(s)?**
   a Yes
   b No

Please describe the type of job you did **before** you had problems with your hand(s).

4 **What is your gender?**
   a Male
   b Female

MICHIGAN HAND OUTCOMES QUESTIONNAIRE
(Chung et *al.* 1998) – *continued*

5 **What is your ethnic background?**
  a   White
  b   Black
  c   Hispanic
  d   Asian or Pacific islander
  e   American Indian or Alaskan native
  f   Other (please specify)

6 **What is the highest level of education you received?**
  a   Less than high school graduate
  b   High school graduate
  c   Some college
  d   College graduate
  e   Professional or graduate school

7 **What is your family income, including wages, disability payment, retirement income, and welfare?**
  a   <$10,000
  b $10,000–$19,000
  c $20,000–$29,999
  d $30,000–$39,999
  e $40,000–$49,999
  f $50,000–$59,999
  g $60,000–$69,999
  h   >$70,000

8 **Is your injury covered by Workers' Compensation?**
  a   Yes
  b   No

HAND SURGERY – PATIENT EVALUATION MEASURE
(Macey and Burke 1995)*

Instructions These questions are about how you have been treated at the hospital, and how your hand is now. There are no right or wrong answers. For each question, give your answer by placing a circle around the number which shows best how things are for you.

For example:

The PAIN in my hand is:

non-existent   1   2   3   4   ⑤   6   7   unbearable

this circle indicates that the pain is
quite bad, but is not unbearable.

PART ONE: TREATMENT

1   Throughout my treatment I have seen the same doctor:
every time   1   2   3   4   5   6   7   **not at all**

2   When the doctor saw me, he or she knew about my case:
very well   1   2   3   4   5   6   7   **not at all**

3   When I was with the doctor, he or she gave me the chance to talk:
as much as I wanted to   1   2   3   4   5   6   7   **not at all**

4   When I did talk to the doctor, he or she listened and understood me:
very much   1   2   3   4   5   6   7   **not at all**

5   I was given information about my treatment and progress:
all that I wanted   1   2   3   4   5   6   7   **not at all**

PART TWO: HOW YOUR HAND IS NOW

1   The FEELING in my hand is now:
normal   1   2   3   4   5   6   7   **abnormal**

2   When my hand is cold and/or damp, the PAIN is now:
non-existent   1   2   3   4   5   6   7   **unbearable**

3   Most of the time, the PAIN in my hand is now:
non-existent   1   2   3   4   5   6   7   **unbearable**

4   The duration my PAIN is present is now:
never   1   2   3   4   5   6   7   **all the time**

5   When I try to use my hand for fiddly things, it is now:
skilful   1   2   3   4   5   6   7   **clumsy**

6   Generally, when I MOVE my hand, it is:
flexible   1   2   3   4   5   6   7   **stiff**

7   The GRIP in my hand is now:
strong   1   2   3   4   5   6   7   **weak**

HAND SURGERY – PATIENT EVALUATION MEASURE – *continued*

8 For everyday ACTIVITIES, my hand is now:
   no problem   I   2   3   4   5   6   7   **useless**

9 For WORK, my hand is now:
   no problem   I   2   3   4   5   6   7   **useless**

10 When I look at the appearance of my hand, I feel:
   unconcerned   I   2   3   4   5   6   7   **embarrassed and self-conscious**

11 Generally, when I think about my hand, I feel:
   unconcerned   I   2   3   4   5   6   7   **very upset**

PART THREE: OVERALL ASSESSMENT

1 Generally, my treatment at the hospital has been:
   very satisfactory   I   2   3   4   5   6   7   **very unsatisfactory**

2 Generally, my hand is now:
   very satisfactory   I   2   3   4   5   6   7   **very unsatisfactory**

3 Bearing in mind my original injury or condition, my hand is now:
   better than I expected   I   2   3   4   5   6   7   **worse than I expected**

Thank you very much for your help

18

Pelvic and acetabular fractures
Philip J. Chapman-Sheath and Keith M. Willett

INTRODUCTION

Injury to the pelvis and acetabulum are relatively common events, and occur across all age groups from the child and young adult as a result of high-energy trauma, to the elderly and infirm population, often as a result of lower energy falls. The pelvis supports the axial skeleton and protects the abdominal and pelvic viscera and neurovascular structures. The acetabulum plays an integral role in stance and gait. Disruption of the pelvic ring is a serious injury that has high levels of associated morbidity and mortality. In contrast, acetabular fractures have lower levels of mortality but high levels of associated morbidity, due to the limitation of motion, pain and secondary degeneration that result from long-term disruption of the acetabular articular congruity. Outcome measures for pelvis and acetabular fractures are therefore discussed separately.

Information for the chapter comprises all papers cited on a search of the Medline database since 1966 to the present day, containing the text acetabulum, pelvis, fracture or outcome measure and certain historical papers that are referenced within those papers.

Established outcome measures for pelvic fractures are poorly defined and rarely validated. There are no commonly accepted outcome measures in use today worldwide, and individual centres utilize different outcomes based on clinical and radiological features. Clinical outcome measures that are frequently chosen include mortality, morbidity, pain scores, level of function, gait or occasionally, specific scoring systems based on a combination of the above.

Fractures of the acetabulum should be considered as a quite separate and distinct entity. Outcome measures for these are again based on clinical and radiological features and in addition, include scoring systems that have been modified from total hip arthroplasty outcomes. These arthroplasty outcome measures, although widely utilized in current clinical practice for the purpose of acetabular fracture outcome measurement, were not designed for that role and therefore have not been rigorously validated and scrutinized.

The purpose of the chapter is three-fold. First, to discuss the key complications of the injuries and treatments that are likely to influence outcome and to ascertain their incidence, to guide power analysis calculations in study design. Second, to establish whether validated and appropriate outcome measures exist for these two distinct types of injury. Third, to assist future investigators attempting to compare and contrast the available data and to provide information on which outcome measures to choose for each injury.

It will be for the reader to determine whether the outcome measures and scoring systems previously chosen are sensitive for the specific complications, recognizing that few are validated and few are cross-referenced.

PELVIC FRACTURE

Mortality

Use of the overall mortality for the assessment of pelvic fractures is a valid comparative outcome

Table 18.1: Mortality in pelvic fracture

Death rate (%)	No. of patients	Reference	Fracture type
0–17	37	Latenser (1991)	All fractures
2–14	79	McMurtry (1980)	All fractures
3–11	255	Alost (1997)	<65 years 3% / >65 years 11%
5–17	1254	Ismail (1996)	Children 5% / adults 17%
5.5	407	Huittinen (1972)	All fractures
6.8	163	Slatis (1972)	Type C fractures
7.6	236	Poole (1991)	All fractures
7.8	141	Torode (1985)	Children
8	348	Poole (1994)	All fractures
8.6	210	Burgess (1990)	All fractures
12	50	Holdsworth (1948)	Posterior fractures
12	60	Leung (2001)	Age > 60 years
12	604	Rothenberger (1978)	Operated fractures
12.5–36.4	111	Eastridge (1997)	All fractures
13	39	Van-Veen (1995)	Unstable fractures
13.4	3260	Gansslen (1996)	All fractures
15	216	Biffl (2001)	All fractures
16	175	Fox (1990)	All fractures
16–25	1179	Brenneman (1997)	All fractures
19	103	Gustavo-Parreira (2000)	All fractures
26	39	Jones (1997)	Open fractures
29.6	58	Pohlemann (1994)	All fractures; operated

measure that can be utilized for different fracture series and between different treatments. The weakness is in determining the contribution of the pelvic injury to that overall mortality. Ideally, the total spectrum of injuries and the proportion of each injury group should be fully defined in each study and not simply allocated a number from one of the many injury scoring systems, such as the injury severity score (ISS). Studies have confirmed that by using such a system, patients who score the same overall trauma score will have quite different injuries to different body systems which may not all contribute to the overall mortality. All patients should be followed up over a reasonable time course, and consensus appears to favour greater than one year. The use of mortality as an outcome measure is highly reliable if the above factors are considered and in addition, if there is a complete data set. The use of mortality as an outcome measure in pelvic fractures associated with severe trauma therefore, would appear useful.

The studies outlined in Table 18.1 have all utilized mortality as the outcome measure in pelvic fractures, although they all vary in the groups studied and the associated injuries. Although they cannot be utilized as a comparative group for all future studies, they do provide a guide to previously determined mortality rates in specific fracture groups.

Morbidity

Numerous components of morbidity have been studied within pelvic fracture series. They include injuries to other body systems as well as the musculoskeletal system. Many studies have simply identified one outcome of morbidity to record and have not used any standardized method of recording or analysing the data. Accordingly, there are no validated and standardized morbidity outcome measures currently available. Studies which have attempted to use morbidity as an outcome measure, together with details of the composition of the group sampled are listed in Table 18.2. Specific analysis and detailed discussion is lacking in most of these studies, however, and

Table 18.2: Morbidity in pelvic fracture

	Morbidity (%)	No. of patients	Reference	Fracture types
Vascular injury	8	53	Semba (1983)	Unstable malgaigne
	11	64	Cole (1996)	Operated type C
	23	312	Gansslen (1996)	Complex fractures
Sphincteric	2.5	494	Tile (1988)	All fractures
	17	35	Oliver (1996)	B & C fractures
	21	255	Copeland (1997)	Women: all fractures
	21	407	Huittinen (1972)	All fractures
	26	58	Pohlemann (1996)	Operated unstable fractures
	37	64	Cole (1996)	Operated type C
	50	53	Semba (1983)	Unstable
Neurological	5.5	494	Tile (1988)	All fractures
	17	35	Oliver (1996)	B & C fractures
	18	65	Raf (1966)	Unstable malgaigne
	21	83	Reilly (1996)	Unstable fractures
	24	312	Gansslen (1996)	Complex fractures
	27	111	Eastridge (1997)	All fractures
	30	64	Cole (1996)	Operated type C
	32	407	Huittinen (1972)	All fractures
	32–40	58	Pohlemann (1994)	Operated unstable fractures
	35	46	Tornetta (1996)	Operated type C
	36	53	Semba (1983)	Unstable malgaigne
	42	26	Henderson (1989)	All fractures
	47	21	Ragnarsson (1993)	Sacroiliac disruption
	48	163	Slatis (1972)	Type C #
	64	28	Weis (1984)	SI joint EMG changes
Visceral	4–17	196	Colapinto (1980)	Urogenital trauma
	14.4	111	Eastridge (1997)	Abdominal: all fractures
	20	312	Gansslen (1996)	Complex fractures
	26.1	111	Eastridge (1997)	Thoracic: all fractures
	47	53	Semba (1983)	Unstable malgaigne
Sexual function	2	21	Ragnarsson (1993)	Sacroiliac disruption
	12.5	58	Pohlemann (1994)	Operated unstable fractures
	29	64	Cole (1996)	Operated type C
	39	123	McCarthy (1995)	Sexual pleasure
	40	37	Van den Bosch (1999)	Unstable operated fractures
	43	255	Copeland (1997)	Women: displaced fractures
	45	123	McCarthy (1995)	Sexually attractive

Table 18.2: Morbidity in pelvic fracture – *continued*

	Morbidity (%)	No. of patients	Reference	Fracture types
Infection	1.3–6.7	2561	Gansslen (1996)	All fractures
	11.4	44	Brenneman (1997)	Open fractures
	18–27	15	Goldstein (1986)	Early vs. late fixation
	28	246	Woods (1998)	Open fractures
Length discrepancy	1	21	Ragnarsson (1993)	Sacroiliac disruption
	4	155	Tile (1988)	>2.5 cm short
	27	15	Van Gulik (1987)	1–2.5 cm short
	29	31	Van den Bosch (1999)	>1 cm
General complications	36	103	Gustavo-Parreira (2000)	All fractures

often the mere presence of an injury is stated without qualification as to the grade or severity of injury.

Note should be made of the usefulness of each of the factors listed in the table as an outcome measure. The presence or absence of vascular injury can be used as a valid outcome measure of pelvic fracture, but no study has quantified the degree or extent of injury. The presence of sphincteric injury includes the urogenital and gastrointestinal tract, but few studies include quantifiable data or manometric assessment values. Neurological injury is described in these studies in terms of limp, pain and loss of function again without standardized quantifiable – and therefore reproducible – assessment. Indeed, as with an assessment of sexual function, the previous two outcome measures of sphincteric injury and neurological function are highly subjective assessments which are enquiry-dependent and therefore maybe subject to substantial recording bias. The individual weighting of each complication on the overall subjective morbidity has not been determined in studies to date. The following lists, however, provide useful guidance to study designers for detection of contributing factors and their incidence.

PAIN

The incidence of pain as an outcome measure for pelvic fractures is less useful than those studies utilizing a validated pain score, which are subjective patient-based outcome measures. These have been shown to be both reproducible and reliable in previous studies. They can be utilized in addition to standard validated psychometric testing, such as the validated SF-36 questionnaire. They are all, however, prone to high inter-study and inter-patient variability, and also cannot alone be used for the assessment of final outcome, as the function score may not correlate with pain score. Many studies have merely quoted the incidence of pain in the study population of patients with pelvic fractures, and those listed in Table 18.3 provide some idea as to both the number of patients and the type of fractures studied.

Gait

Several studies reported in the literature have utilized a measure of gait as the outcome measure for pelvic fractures. None of the specific scores or measurement systems is routinely or widely utilized however, and most are used by one or few institutions. The studies detailed in Table 18.4 are therefore isolated studies with no direct means of comparison. The majority of the studies suffer from the fact that the analysis of gait is subjective and difficult to quantify. These methods of assessment lack the reproducibility and sensitivity of modern computerized gait analysis techniques, but are of course much cheaper and available

Table 18.3: Pain in pelvic fracture

Proportion in pain (%)	No. of patients	Reference	Fracture type
5	22	Slatis (1980)	All fractures
11	58	Pohlemann (1994)	Type B fractures
17	163	Slatis (1972)	Type C fractures
27	53	Semba (1983)	Unstable malgaigne
31	29	Tornetta (1996)	Operated unstable fractures
31	26	Henderson (1989)	All fractures
33–52	65	Raf (1966)	All fractures
34	17	Schwarz (1998)	Paediatric
40	248	Tile (1988)	All fractures
41.4	58	Pohlemann (1996)	Operated unstable fractures
43	21	Ragnarsson (1993)	Sacroiliac disruption
40–85	114	Fell (1995)	All fractures: conservative
50	26	Henderson (1989)	All fractures
60	37	Van den Bosch (1999)	Operated unstable fractures
66	58	Pohlemann (1994)	Type C fractures
71	155	Tile (1988)	Type B fractures

Table 18.4: Gait assessment in pelvic fracture

	Incidence (%)	No. of patients	Reference	Fracture type
Impaired gait	10	22	Slatis (1980)	All fractures
	12	65	Raf (1966)	Unstable malgaigne
	16	37	Latenser (1991)	Unstable operated early
	19	21	Ragnarsson (1993)	Sacroiliac disruption
	24	29	Tornetta (1996)	Unstable fractures
	31	53	Semba (1983)	Unstable malgaigne
	32	168	Slatis (1972)	Type C fracture
	60	37	Latenser (1991)	Unstable operated early
Limp	32	26	Henderson (1989)	All fractures
	69	42	Pennal (1980)	All fractures
Walking ability	52–80	88	Upperman (2000)	Paediatric
Timed Test-Patient led	Medical patients	NA	Butland (1982)	Not tested
Shuttle walking test	Medical patients	NA	Singh (1992)	Not tested
Energy consumption	Not recorded	NA	Roberts (1990)	Unspecified

NA = not available.

to the majority of researchers. They also fail to correlate with patient function. There are no good qualitative assessments of gait function applied to the patient with pelvic injury.

Scoring systems

The inherent problem with the use of most scoring systems for the assessment of outcomes is that they are composite scores. They comprise an amalgamation of scores based on clinical and radiological criteria. In addition, the clinical data comprise both subjective patient-based data (known to be reliable) and subjective clinician-based data. Composite scores have the disadvantage already mentioned for the ISS in that two patients may have identical scores overall, but have different scores for each criteria. There is little reason to assume that scores allocated within criteria are proportional, or that they may be summed in any meaningful way with a score given for another criteria. None of the scoring

systems is considered a standardized outcome measure, and none has been adequately validated for use as such. A study of the literature reveals numerous scoring systems, and these are outlined in Table 18.5.

Radiology

Both radiography and computed tomography (CT) have been utilized as an outcome measure of pelvic fractures. Both have been shown to be reliable at showing displacement of fracture fragments, but only CT has proved to be reliable and sensitive enough to identify fracture non-union and to measure malunions.

No standardized outcome measure has been used, and each centre still uses its own system of analysis – which makes direct and valid comparison between the groups difficult. Studies utilizing radiographic outcome assessment of pelvic fractures, and the groups which were measured, are listed in Table 18.6.

Table 18.5: Scoring systems in pelvic fracture

	Incidence (%)	No. of patients	Reference	Fracture type
Return to work	38	26	Henderson (1989)	All fractures
	38	42	Pennal (1980)	All fractures
	50	40	Keating (1995)	Operated type C
	50	15	Browner (1987)	Operated type C
	56	50	Holdsworth (1948)	All fractures
	65	64	Cole (1996)	Type C fractures
	67	46	Tornetta (1995)	Operated type C
	68	37	Van den Bosch (1999)	Unstable operated fractures
	71	21	Ragnarsson (1993)	Sacroiliac disruption
	71	103	Pennal (1980)	All fractures
	76	31	Hakim (1996)	Unstable fractures operated
	78	80	Miranda (1996)	All fractures: non-operative/exfix
	83	29	Tornetta (1996)	Unstable fractures: operated
	96	22	Slatis (1980)	Unstable fractures

Table 18.5: Scoring systems in pelvic fracture – *continued*

	Mean score	Score range	Patients	Reference	Fracture type
Majeed outcome score	78.6 (SD unknown)	0 (poor)–100 (good)	37	Van den Bosch (1999)	Unstable fractures
Pelvis outcome score	5.7 (SD = 1.1)	2 (poor)–7 (excellent)	28	Pohlemann (1996)	Operated type B
	4.9 (SD = 1.2)	2 (poor)–7 (excellent)	30	Pohlemann (1996)	Operated type C
Sickness impact profile	9.34 (SD = 7.5)	0 (good)–100 (poor)	31	Hakim (1996)	Unstable fracture
Oswestry questionnaire	13.26 (SD = 15.4)	0 (good)–100 (poor)	31	Hakim (1996)	Unstable fracture
SF-36 physical function	61 (SD unknown)	0 (poor)–100 (good)	64	Cole (1996)	Operated type C
	63 (SD = 27)	0 (poor)–100 (good)	27	Brenneman (1997)	Open fractures
	64 (SD = 27)	0 (poor)–100 (good)	46	Oliver (1996)	Unstable operated
	67 (SD unknown)	0 (poor)–100 (good)	37	Van den Bosch (1999)	Unstable operated
	82 (SD = 20)	0 (poor)–100 (good)	123	McCarthy (1995)	All fractures: women
	Not stated	0 (poor)–100 (good)	80	Miranda (1996)	All fractures: exfix
Patient outcome grading	29 (SD = 7)	0 (poor)–40 (good)	64	Cole (1996)	Operated type C
Iowa pelvic score	89	0 (poor)–100 (good)	80	Miranda (1996)	All fractures: exfix

Table 18.6: Radiographic assessment of pelvic fracture

Non-union Incidence (%)	No. of patients	Reference	Group measured	Radiographic assessment
2	64	Cole (1996)	Operated type C #	Yes
3.5	494	Tile (1988)	All fractures	Yes
Not recorded	218	Tile (1982)	All fractures	Yes
Not recorded	32	Pennal (1980)	All fractures	Yes

Table 18.6: Radiographic assessment of pelvic fracture – *continued*

Malunion Incidence (%)	No. of patients	Reference	Group measured	Displacement
13–36	42	Majeed (1990)	All fractures	>2 mm vertical/ >1 cm symphysis
14	21	Ragnarsson (1993)	Sacroiliac disruption	>5 mm displaced
18	163	Slatis (1972)	Type C #	Hemipelvic dislocation
25	46	Tornetta (1995)	Operated type C fractures	Displacement > 4 mm
32	22	Slatis (1980)	Operated type C fractures	Sacroiliac joint displacement
34	218	Tile (1982)	All fractures	Leg length > 2.5 cm
38	65	Raf (1966)	Unstable malgaigne	>5 mm displaced
48	40	Keating (1995)	Operated type C fractures	Not specified
50	58	Pohlemann (1996)	Operated unstable fractures	>5 mm displaced
58	26	Henderson (1986)	All fractures	Displacement > 1 cm
64	103	Pennal (1980)	All fractures	Not specified
Not recorded	53	Semba (1983)	Unstable: conservative	> 1 cm displacement

A summary of clinical outcome scoring systems for pelvic fracture is provided in Tables 18-A1.1–18-A1.3.

ACETABULAR FRACTURES

Scoring systems

Several scoring systems have been developed to assess the outcome of acetabular fractures, while others have been adapted from outcome measures for hip arthroplasty. Some of the scoring systems attempt to score the outcome following acetabular fracture by means of purely clinical scores – usually based on multiple factors reported by the clinician and patient. These usually include an assessment of pain, functional ability, range of movement and some method of gait assessment. Additionally, scoring systems may also incorporate a score for the radiological outcome rated by the clinician, others are purely based on radiological criteria. Those using radiological criteria are based on plain radiographs, and to date none has routinely utilized CT scan or magnetic resonance technologies.

There is increasing evidence that patient-based outcome measures, by means of patients' reporting of symptoms, are generally more reliable than those based on clinician scores. There are few studies available that have attempted to use such scoring systems, and indeed there are few specific systems available for use in orthopaedic trauma patients (Tables 18.7–18.10). The recent development of a Musculoskeletal Functional Assessment Score has added a validated and reliable scoring system for general orthopaedic patients, including trauma cases

Table 18.7: Acetabular fracture: Clinical scoring systems based on clinician's evaluation

Clinical scores	Satisfactory (%)	Mean score	Score components	Range	Group studied	Reference
Mobility index	Not studied	Not stated	Passive ROM	0 (poor)–100 (good)	Post THR	Gade (1947)
	Not studied	Not stated	Passive ROM/Pain/Function	Not specified	Post THR	Sheperd (1954)
Merle d'Aubigne	74	Not stated	Pain/ROM/Gait and X-ray	<13 (poor)–18 (excellent)	All fractures – operated	Deo (2001)
	76	16 (range 5–18)	Pain/ROM/Gait	<13 (poor)–18 (excellent)	All fractures – operated	Matta (1996)
	76	Not stated	Pain/ROM/Gait	<13 (poor)–18 (excellent)	All fractures	de Ridder (1994)
	84	Not stated	Pain/ROM/Gait	<13 (poor)–18 (excellent)	All fractures – operated	Matta (1994)
	85	Not stated	Pain/ROM/Gait	<13 (poor)–18 (excellent)	All fractures – operated	Rice (2002)
Acetabular fracture	86		Not known	X	All fractures	Kebaish (1991)
Toronto hip score	Not stated	14.5	Pain/Mobility/Gait	0 (poor)–18 (excellent)	Displaced fractures	Pennal (1980)
	Not stated	16.5	Pain/Mobility/Gait	0 (poor)–18 (excellent)	Undisplaced fractures	Pennal (1980)
	31.5	Not stated	Clinical/Radiograph	0 (poor)–18 (excellent)	All fractures	Matta (1988a,b)
Harris hip score	Not studied	Not studied	Pain/Function/ROM/Deformity	0 (poor)–100 (good)	Post THR	Harris (1969)

Table 18.7: Acetabular fracture: Clinical scoring systems based on clinician's evaluation – *continued*

Clinical scores	Satisfactory (%)	Mean score	Score components	Range	Group studied	Reference
	75	Not stated	Pain/Function/ROM/ Deformity	0 (poor)–100 (good)	All fractures – operated	Wright (1994)
	77.4	Not stated	Pain/Function/ROM/ Deformity	0 (poor)–100 (good)	All fractures – operated	Liebergall (1999)
Iowa hip score	Not studied	Not studied	Pain/Function/ROM/ Deformity	0 (poor)–100 (good)	Post THR	Larson (1963)
	80	Not stated	Pain/Function/ROM	Excellent–Poor	All fractures	Matta (1986a, b)
Functional assessment	Not studied	22 (range 0–57)	Physical/Psychological/ Social	0 (good)–100 (poor)	All fractures – operated	Borrelli (2002)
Gait analysis	Complex	Complex	Kinetic/Temporal/ Kinematic	Complex analysis	All fractures – operated	Borrelli (2002)
Other hip scores	53	Not stated	Questionnaire	Excellent–Poor	All fractures – operated	Ragnarsson (1992)
	64–74	Not stated	Not known	Excellent–Poor	All fractures	Chen (2000)
	76	Not stated	Clinical grading	Excellent–Poor	All fractures	Letournel (1980)
	76	Not stated	AO Documentation form	Unknown	All fractures	Leutenegger (1999)
	80	Not stated	Pain/ROM/Gait/Work/ Function	Excellent–Poor	All fractures	Rowe (1961)
	Not studied	Not studied	Pain/Movement/ Walking	0 (poor)–18 (excellent)	Post THR	Judet (1952)
	Not studied	Not studied	Pain/Function/ROM	6 per category	Bilateral hip pathology	Lazansky (1967)
Return to work	71	Not studied	Not analysed	Not analysed	All fractures	Pennal (1980)

THR = total hip replacement.

Table 18.8: Acetabular fracture: Combined clinical and radiological scoring systems

Acceptable (%)	Reference	Score components	Maximum score	Group studied
Not studied	Epstein (1973)	Pain/ROM/Gait/Radiograph	Excellent–Poor	All fractures
26.7	Upadhyay (1981)	Pain/ROM/Gait/Radiograph	Excellent–Poor	Posterior dislocation
39	Stewart (1954)	Pain/Function/ROM/XR changes	Excellent–Poor	Operated fracture
67	Stewart (1954)	Pain/Function/ROM/XR changes	Excellent–Poor	Conservative fracture
55	Carnesale (1975)	Pain/Function/ROM/XR changes	Good–Poor	All fractures
74	Deo (2001)	Pain/ROM/Gait/XR	Excellent–Poor	All fractures – operated

Table 18.9: Acetabular fracture: Radiological scoring systems

	Incidence (%)	Displacement	No. of patients	Group studied	Reference
Residual displacement	10	<3 mm satisfactory	119	All fractures – operated	Matta (1994)
	10	<3 mm satisfactory	268	All fractures	Matta (1986a,b)
	13	<3 mm satisfactory	87	All fractures – operated	Wright (1994)
	17	Anatomical reduction	15	All fractures – operated	Borrelli (2002)
	18	Anatomical reduction	73	All fractures – operated	Chen (2000)
	20	Anatomical reduction	201	All fractures – operated	Rice (2002)
	25	Anatomical/congruous	93	All fractures	Rowe (1961)
	26	Anatomical reduction	39	All fractures – conservative	Chen (2000)
	26	<3 mm satisfactory	127	Complex fractures – operated	Helfet (1994)
	27	<1 mm = anatomical	51	All fractures	de Ridder (1994)
	27	Perfect reduction	582	All fractures	Letournel (1980)
	29	Anatomical reduction	255	All fractures – operated	Matta (1996)
	30	<1 mm = anatomical	60	All fractures – operated	Liebergall (1999)
	33	<3 mm satisfactory	43	All fractures – operated	Hull (1997)
	37	<1 mm = anatomical	59	All fractures – operated	Ragnarsson (1992)
	64	Unspecified	103	All fractures	Pennal (1980)

Table 18.9: Acetabular fracture: Radiological scoring systems – *continued*

	Acceptable (%)	Displacement	No. of patients	Group studied	Reference
XR Scoring Criteria	73	Anatomical/congruous	15	All fractures – operated	Borrelli (2002)
	75	Anatomical/congruous	93	All fractures	Rowe (1961)
	80	Anatomical/congruous	201	All fractures – operated	Rice (2002)
	84	<3 mm satisfactory	119	All fractures – operated	Matta (1994)
	90	<3 mm satisfactory	268	All fractures	Matta (1986a, b)

Table 18.10: Acetabular fracture: Morbidity of treatment

	Incidence (%)	No. of patients	Reference	Group studied
Infection	0	127	Helfet (1994)	Complex fractures – operated
	3	105	Matta (1986a,b)	All fractures
	3	119	Matta (1994)	All fractures – operated
	4	79	Deo (2001)	All fractures – operated
	5	255	Matta (1996)	All fractures – operated
	5	51	de Ridder (1994)	All fractures
	5.6	582	Letournel (1980)	All fractures – operated
	6	93	Rowe (1961)	All fractures
	9	64	Matta (1986a, b)	All fractures
	36	55	Carnesale (1975)	All fractures – operated
Neurological	2	119	Matta (1994)	All fractures – operated
	3.4	255	Matta (1996)	All fractures – operated
	5	105	Matta (1986a, b)	All fractures
	8.8	60	Liebergall (1999)	All fractures – operated
	19	64	Matta (1986a, b)	All fractures
	10	51	de Ridder (1994)	All fractures
	13	242	Epstein (1974)	All fractures
	13	128	Stewart (1954)	Fracture dislocations
	17	93	Rowe (1961)	All fractures
	22	27	Urist (1948)	All fractures
	23	79	Deo (2001)	All fractures – operated
	36	127	Helfet (1994)	Complex fractures – operated

Table 18.10: Acetabular fracture: Morbidity of treatment – *continued*

	Incidence (%)	No. of patients	Reference	Group studied
Heterotopic ossification	2	127	Helfet (1994)	Complex fractures – operated
	5–30	270	Pennal (1980)	All fractures – worse operated
	5	103	Matta (1996)	All fractures – operated
	5.3	94	Schafer (2000)	All fractures – operated
	7	105	Matta (1986a, b)	All fractures
	9	119	Matta (1994)	All fractures – operated
	9	79	Deo (2001)	All fractures – operated
	10	51	Leutenegger (1999)	All fractures
	10	51	de Ridder (1994)	All fractures
	15	60	Liebergall (1999)	All fractures – operated
	15	93	Rowe (1961)	All fractures
	18	582	Letournel (1980)	All fractures – operated
	19	112	Chen (2000)	All fractures
	30	55	Carnesale (1975)	All fractures – operated
	37	201	Rice (2002)	All fractures – operated
	53	15	Borrelli (2002)	All fractures – operated
	59	27	Urist (1948)	All fractures
	86	87	Wright (1994)	All fractures – operated
Osteoarthrosis	5	255	Matta (1996)	All fractures – operated
	5.4–31	582	Letournel (1980)	All fractures – operated
	16	112	Chen (2000)	All fractures
	17–80	127	Helfet (1994)	Complex fractures – operated
	22	201	Rice (2002)	All fractures – operated
	26	93	Rowe (1961)	All fractures
	27	51	Leutenegger (1999)	All fractures
	38	59	Ragnarsson (1992)	All fractures – operated
	43	60	Liebergall (1999)	All fractures – operated
	44	27	Urist (1948)	All fractures
	47	87	Wright (1994)	All fractures – operated
	49–71	128	Stewart (1954)	Fracture dislocations
	58–89	81	Upadhyay (1981)	Posterior fracture dislocation
	79	103	Pennal (1980)	All fractures
	100	55	Romness (1990)	All fractures
	100	101	Armstrong (1948)	Fracture dislocations

Table 18.10: Acetabular fracture: Morbidity of treatment – *continued*

	Incidence (%)	No. of patients	Reference	Group studied
Conversion to THR	0	127	Helfet (1994)	Complex fractures – operated
	1.7	119	Matta (1994)	All fractures – operated
	4	51	de Ridder (1994)	All fractures
	6	255	Matta (1996)	All fractures – operated
	7.5	60	Liebergall (1999)	All fractures – operated
	7.7	201	Rice (2002)	All fractures – operated
	5.4	93	Rowe (1961)	All fractures
	11	55	Carnesale (1975)	All fractures – operated
	11	79	Deo (2001)	All fractures – operated
	11	87	Wright (1994)	All fractures – operated
	19–100	43	Hull (1997)	All fractures – operated
Arthrodesis	1.7	87	Wright (1994)	All fractures – operated
	2.2	93	Rowe (1961)	All fractures
	4	255	Matta (1996)	All fractures – operated
Avascular necrosis	2	60	Liebergall (1999)	All fractures – operated
	2.7	112	Chen (2000)	All fractures
	3	255	Matta (1996)	All fractures – operated
	4	127	Helfet (1994)	Complex fractures – operated
	4.4	51	Leutenegger (1999)	All fractures
	5	51	de Ridder (1994)	All fractures
	5.6	582	Letournel (1980)	All fractures – operated
	5.7	27	Urist (1948)	All fractures
	8	79	Deo (2001)	All fractures – operated
	9	64	Matta (1986a, b)	All fractures
	11	55	Romness (1990)	All fractures
	21	128	Stewart (1954)	Fracture dislocations
	23	87	Wright (1994)	All fractures – operated
Non-union	0	127	Helfet (1994)	Complex fractures – operated
	0.7	582	Letournel (1980)	All fractures – operated
Associated injuries	61	93	Rowe (1961)	All fractures
	82	79	Deo (2001)	All fractures – operated
	87	60	Liebergall (1999)	All fractures – operated
	87	51	de Ridder (1994)	All fractures
Muscular weakness	27–50	15	Borrelli (2002)	All fractures – operated

(Martin *et al.* 1996; Engelberg *et al.* 1996). This outcome instrument comprising 100 self-reported health items has been recently utilized, for the first time, to assess the outcome following acetabular fractures (Borelli *et al.* 2002).

COMPLICATIONS

High-energy acetabular fractures are associated with a multitude of complicating factors affecting the bones, soft tissues and neurovascular elements. In terms of the acetabulum and femoral head, complications may include late-onset osteoarthrosis, non-union, malunion, severity and degree of avascular necrosis and the rate of conversion to total hip replacement or fusion. The surrounding ligamento-capsular, neurological and muscular structures can be affected by heterotopic ossification, nerve injury and weakness.

Details of acetabular clinical and radiological outcome measures and scoring systems are listed in Tables 18-A2.1–18-A2.8, Fig. 18A2.1 and Tables 18-A3.1–18-A3.3.

SUMMARY

Injuries to the pelvis and acetabulum should be considered as totally separate injuries, and as such should be assessed using separate outcome measures. The chapter outlines the types and incidence of major complications for each of these injuries and may, therefore, be of use when attempting to calculate power analyses prior to embarking on future studies. The second aim of the chapter – to establish whether validated and appropriate outcome measures exist – has revealed that, indeed, few are currently available. Recent advances in the design and utilization of patient-based outcome measures have yielded reliable and validated outcome tools but, to date, few have been applied to either of our fracture types. The third aim of the chapter, in assisting investigators to compare and contrast previous results and study conclusions, has demonstrated the type of outcome

measures and the values determined by previous studies, and this should both direct the reader to the relevant literature and also provide them with some – albeit semi-quantitative – means of comparing the study results.

The appendices at the end of the chapter serve to provide actual details of several commonly encountered outcome measure scoring systems, that may be useful to the reader, first in understanding the previous study methodology and second, to act as a source of outcome tools for future studies. As is evident, many of these outcome measures are based on previous versions from earlier studies and therefore may be subject to the same limitations – namely that the majority are unvalidated and rely purely on clinician's assessment data.

REFERENCES

Pelvic fracture

Alost, T., and Waldrop, R. D. (1997): Profile of geriatric pelvic fractures presenting to the emergency department. *Am J Emerg Med* **15**, 576–8.

Biffl, W. L., Smith, W. R., Moore, E. E., Gonzalez, R. J., Morgan, S. J., Hennessey, T., Offner, P. J., Ray, C. E., Francoise, R. J., and Burch, J. M. (2001): Evolution of a multidisciplinary clinical pathway for the management of unstable patients with pelvic fractures. *Ann Surg* **233**, 843–50.

Brenneman, F. D., Katyal, D., Boulanger, B. R., Tile, M., and Redelmeier, D. A. (1997): Long term outcomes in open pelvic fractures. *J Trauma* **42**, 773–7.

Browner, B., Cole, D., and Graham, M. (1987): Delayed posterior internal fixation of unstable pelvic fractures. *J Trauma* **27**, 998–1006.

Burgess, A. R., Eastridge, B. J., Young, J. W. R., Ellison, T. S., Ellison, P. S., Poka, A., Bathon, G. H., and Brumback, R. J. (1990): Pelvic ring disruptions: effective classification system and protocols. *J Traum-Inj Infect Crit Care* **30**, 848–56.

Butland, R. J. A., Gross, E. R., Pang, J., Woodcock, A. A., and Geddes, D. M. (1982): Two, six and twelve minute walking tests in respiratory disease. *Br Med J* **284**, 1604–8.

Colapinto, V. (1980): Trauma to the pelvis: urethral injury. *Clin Orthop* **151**, 46–55.

Cole, J. D., Blum, D. A., and Ansel, L. J. (1996): Outcome after fixation of unstable posterior pelvic ring injuries. *Clin Orthop* **329**, 160–79.

Copeland, C. E., Bosse, M. J., McCarthy, M. L., MacKenzie, E. J., Guzinski, G. M., Hash, C. S., and Burgess, A. R. (1997): Effect of trauma and pelvic fracture on female genitourinary, sexual and reproductive function. *J Orthop Trauma* **11**, 73–81.

Eastridge, B. J., and Burgess, A. R. (1997): Pedestrian pelvic fractures: 5 year experience of a major urban trauma centre. *J Trauma* **42**, 695–700.

Engelberg, R., Martin, D. P., Agel, J., Obremsky, W., Coronado, G., and Swiontkowski, M. F. (1996): Musculoskeletal Functional Assessment instrument: criterion and construct validity. *J Orthop Res* **14**, 182–92.

Fell, M., Meissner, A., and Rahmanzadeh. (1995): Longterm outcome after conservative treatment of pelvic ring injuries and conclusions for current management. *Zentralbl Chir* **120**, 899–904.

Fox, M. A., Mangiante, E. C., Fabian, T. C., Voeller, G. R., and Kudsk, K. A. (1990): Pelvic fractures: an analysis of factors affecting prehospital triage and patient outcome. *South Med J* **83**, 785–8.

Gansslen, A., Pohlemann, T., Paul, C., Lobenhoffer, P., and Tscherne, H. (1996): Epidemiology of pelvic ring injuries. *Injury* **27** (Suppl.1), S-A13.

Gustavo-Parreira, J., Coimbra, R., Rasslan, S., Olivera, A., Fregonese, M., and Mercadante, M. (2000): The role of associated injuries on outcome of blunt trauma patients sustaining pelvic fractures. *Injury* **31**, 677–82.

Hakim, R. M., Gruen, G. S., and Delitto, A. (1996): Outcomes of patients with pelvic ring fractures managed by open reduction and internal fixation. *Phys Ther* **76**, 286–95.

Henderson, R. (1989): The long term results of non-operatively treated major pelvic disruption. *J Orthop Trauma* **3**, 41–7.

Henderson, R., and Nepola, J. (1986): Anterior-posterior traumatic pelvic disruption: an evaluation of the long term orthopaedic complications. *Orthop Trans* **10**, 440.

Holdsworth, F. W. (1948): Dislocations and fracture-dislocations of the pelvis. *J Bone Joint Surg* **30-B**, 461–6.

Huittinen, V. M., and Slatis, P. (1972): Nerve injury in double vertical pelvic fractures. *Acta Chir Scand* **138**, 571–5.

Ismail, N., Bellemare, J. F., Mollitt, D. L., DiScala, C., Koeppel, B., and Tepas, J. J. (1996): Death from pelvic fracture: children are different. *J Paediatr Surg* **31**, 82–5.

Jones, A. L., Powell, J. N., Kellam, J. F., McCormack, R. G., Dust, W., and Wimmer, P. (1997): Open pelvic fractures. A multicenter retrospective analysis. *Orthop Clin North Am* **28**, 345–50.

Keating, J., Blachut, P., and O'Brien, P. (1995): Vertically unstable pelvic fractures – the outcome of iliosacral screw fixation of the posterior lesion. *Orthop Trans* **19**, Abstract.

Latenser, B. A., Gentilello, L. M., Tarver, A. A., Thalgott, J. S., and Batdorf, J. W. (1991): Improved outcome with early fixation of skeletally unstable pelvic fractures. *J Trauma* **31**, 28–31.

Leung, W. Y., Ban, C. M., Lam, J. J., Ip, F. K., and Ko, P. S. (2001): Prognosis of acute pelvic fractures in elderly patients: retrospective study. *Hong Kong Med J* **7**, 139–45.

Majeed, S. A. (1989): Grading the outcome of pelvic fractures. *J Bone Joint Surg* **71-B**, 304–6.

Majeed, S. A. (1990): External fixation of the injured pelvis – the functional outcome. *J Bone Joint Surg* **72-B**, 612–14.

McCarthy, M. L., MacKenzie, E. J., Bosse, M. J., Copeland, C. E., Hash, C. S., and Burgess, A. R. (1995): Functional status following orthopaedic trauma in young women. *J Trauma* **39**, 828–36.

McMurtry, R., Walton, D., Dickinson, D., Kellam, J., and Tile, M. (1980): Pelvic disruption in the polytraumatised patient: a management protocol. *Clin Orthop* **151**, 22–30.

Miranda, M., Riemer, B., Butterfield, M., and Burke, C. (1996): Pelvic ring injuries: a long term functional outcome study. *Clin Orthop* **329**, 152–9.

Oliver, C., Twaddle, B., Agel, J., and Routt, M., Jr. (1996): Outcome after pelvic ring fractures: evaluation using the medical outcomes short form SF-36. *Injury* **27**, 635–41.

Pennal, G., and Massiah, K. (1980): Nonunion and delayed union of fractures of the pelvis. *Clin Orthop* **151**, 124–9.

Pohlemann, T., Bosch, U., Gansslen, A., and Tscherne, H. (1994): The Hanover experience in management of pelvic fractures. *Clin Orthop* **305**, 69-80.

Pohlemann, T., Gansslen, A., Schellwald, O., Culemann, U., and Tscherne, H. (1996): Outcome after pelvic ring injuries. *Injury* **27**, 831–8.

Poole, G. V., and Ward, E. F. (1994): Causes of mortality in patients with pelvic fractures. *Orthopaedics* **17**, 691–6.

Poole, G. V., Ward, E. F., Muakkassa, F. F., Hsu, H. S., Griswold, J. A., and Rhodes, R. S. (1991): Pelvic fracture from major blunt trauma. Outcome is determined by associated injuries. *Ann Surg* **213**, 532–8.

Raf, L. (1966): Double vertical fracture of the pelvis. *Acta Chir Scand* **131**, 298–305.

Ragnarsson, B., Olerud, C., and Olerud, S. (1993): Anterior square plate fixation of sacroiliac disruption. *Acta Orthop Scand* **64**, 138–42.

Roberts, P., and Carnes, S. (1990): The Orthopaedic Scooter: an energy saving aid for assisted ambulation. *J Bone Joint Surg* **72-B**, 620–1.

Rothenberger, D. A., Fischer, R. P., Strate, R. G., Velasco, R., and Pery, J. F. (1978): The mortality associated with pelvic fractures. *Surgery* **84**, 356–61.

Schwartz, N., Posch, E., Mayr, J., Fischmeister, F. M., Schwartz, A. F., and Ohner, T. (1998): Long term results of pelvic ring fractures in children. *Injury* **29**, 431–3.

Semba, R., Yasukawa, K., and Gustillo, R. (1983): Critical analysis of results of 53 malgaigne fractures of pelvis. *J Trauma* **23**, 535–7.

Singh, S. J., Morgan, M. D. L., Scott, S., Walters, D., and Hardman, A. E. (1992): Development of a shuttle walking test of disability in patients with chronic airways obstruction. *Thorax* **47**, 1019–24.

Slatis, P., and Huittinen, V. M. (1972): Double vertical fractures of the pelvis. *Acta Chir Scand* **138**, 799–807.

Slatis, P., and Karaharju, E. (1980): External fixation of unstable pelvic fractures: experiences in 22

patients treated with a trapezoid compression frame. *Clin Orthop* **151**, 73–9.

Tile, M. (1982): *Disruption of the Pelvic Ring*. Presentation: Combined Meeting of English Speaking Orthopaedic Surgeons, South Africa.

Tile, M. (1988): Pelvic ring fractures: should they be fixed? *J Bone Joint Surg* **70-B**, 1–12.

Tornetta, P., and Matta, J. (1995): Long term follow up of operatively treated posterior pelvic ring disruptions. *Orthop Trans* **19**, Abstract.

Tornetta, P., and Matta, J. (1996): Outcome of operatively treated unstable posterior pelvic ring disruptions. *Clin Orthop* **329**, 186–93.

Tornetta, P., Dickson, K., and Matta, M. (1996): Outcome of rotationally unstable pelvic ring injuries treated operatively. *Clin Orthop* **329**, 147–51.

Torode, I., and Zieg, D. (1985): Pelvic fractures in children. *J Paediatr Orthop* **5**, 76–84.

Upperman, J. S., Gardner, M., Gaines, B., Schall, L., and Ford, H. R. (2000): Early functional outcome in children with pelvic fractures. *J Paediatr Surg* **35**, 1002–5.

Van den Bosch, E. W., Van der Kleyn, R., Hoegervorst, M., and Van Vugt, A. B. (1999): Functional outcome of internal fixation for pelvic ring fractures. *J Trauma* **47**, 365–71.

Van Gulik, T., Raaymakers, E., and Broekhuizen, A. (1987): Complications and late therapeutic results of conservatively managed unstable pelvic ring disruptions. *Neth J Surg* **39**, 175–8.

Van-Veen, I. H., Van-Leeuwen, A. A., Van-Popta, T., Van-Luyt, P. A., Bode, P. J., and Van-Vugt, A. B. (1995): Unstable pelvic fractures – a retrospective analysis. *Injury* **26**, 81–5.

Weis, E. B., Jr. (1984): Subtle neurological injuries in pelvic fractures. *J Trauma* **24**, 983–5.

Acetabular fractures

Armstrong, J. (1948): Traumatic dislocation of the hip. *J Bone Joint Surg* **30-B**, 430.

Borrelli, J. G. C., Ricci, W., Wagner, J., and Engsberg, J. (2002): Functional outcome after isolated acetabular fractures. *J Orthop Trauma* **16**, 73–81.

Carnesale, P. S. M., and Barnes, S. (1975): Acetabular disruption and central fracture-dislocation of the hip. *J Bone Joint Surg* **57-A**, 1054–9.

Chen, C. C. F., Chuang, T., and Lo, W. (2000): Treatment of acetabular fractures: 10-year experience. *Zhonghua Yi Xue Za Zhi (Taipei)* **63**, Abstract 384–90.

de Ridder, V., Kingma, L., and Hogervorst, M. (1994): Results of 75 consecutive patients with an acetabular fracture. *Clin Orthop* **305**, 53–7.

Deo, S. T. S., Pandey, R., El-Saied, G., Willett, K., and Worlock, P. (2001): Operative treatment of acetabular fractures in Oxford. *Injury* **32**, 581–6.

Epstein, H. (1973): Traumatic dislocations of the hip. *Clin Orthop* **92**, 114–21.

Gade, H. (1947): A contribution to the surgical management of osteoarthritis of the hip joint: a clinical study. *Acta Chir Scand* **120** (Suppl.), 37–45.

Goldstein, A., Phillips, T., and Sclafani, S. (1986): Early open reduction and internal fixation of the disrupted pelvic ring. *J Trauma* **26**, 325–33.

Harris, W. (1969): Traumatic arthritis of the hip after dislocation and acetabular fractures: treatment by mold arthroplasty. *J Bone Joint Surg* **51-A**, 737–55.

Helfet, D. S. G. (1994): Management of complex acetabular fractures through single nonextensile exposures. *Clin Orthop* **305**, 58–68.

Hull, J. R. S., Stockley, I., and Elson, R. (1997): Surgical management of fractures of the acetabulum: the Sheffield experience 1976–1994. *Injury* **28**, 35–40.

Judet, R. J. J. (1952): Technique and results with the acrylic femoral head prosthesis. *J Bone Joint Surg* **34-B**, 173–80.

Kebaish, A. R. A., and Rennie, W. (1991): Displaced acetabular fractures: long-term follow-up. *J Trauma* **31**, 1539–42.

Larson, C. (1963): Rating scale for hip disabilities. *Clin Orthop* **31**, 85–93.

Lazansky, M. (1967): A method for grading hips. *J Bone Joint Surg* **49-B**, 644–51.

Letournel, M. (1980): Acetabulum fractures. *Clin Orthop* **151**, 81–106.

Leutenegger, A., and Ruedi, T. (1999): Fractures of the acetabulum and pelvic ring: epidemiology and clinical outcome. *Swiss Surg* **5**, 47–54.

Liebergall, M. M. R., Low, J., Goldvirt, M., Matan, Y., and Segal, D. (1999): Acetabular fractures. Clinical outcome of surgical treatment. *Clin Orthop* **366**, 205–16.

Martin, D. P., Engelberg, R., Agel, J., Snapp, D., and Swiontkowski, M. F. (1996): The development of a musculoskeletal extremity health status instrument: the Musculoskeletal Functional Assessment instrument. *J Orthop Res* **14**, 173–81.

Matta, J. (1994): Operative treatment of acetabular fractures through the ilioinguinal approach. *Clin Orthop* **305**, 10–19.

Matta, J. (1996): Fractures of the acetabulum: accuracy of reduction and clinical results in patients managed operatively within three weeks after the injury. *J Bone Joint Surg* **78-A**, 1632–45.

Matta, J., Anderson, L. M., Epstein, H., and Hendricks, P. (1986a): Fractures of the acetabulum: a retrospective analysis. *Clin Orthop* **205** 231–40.

Matta, J., Mehne, D. K., and Roffi, R. (1986b): Fractures of the acetabulum: early results of a prospective study. *Clin Orthop* **205**, 241–50.

Merle d'Aubigne, R., and Postel, M. (1954): Functional results of hip arthroplasty with acrylic prosthesis. *J Bone Joint Surg* **36-A**, 451–75.

Pennal, G. D. J., Garside, H., and Plewes, J. (1980): Results of the treatment of acetabular fractures. *Clin Orthop* **151**, 115–23.

Ragnarsson, B. M. B. (1992): Arthrosis after surgically treated acetabular fractures. A retrospective study of 60 cases. *Acta Orthop Scand* **63**, 511–14.

Reilly, M., Zinar, D., and Matta, M. (1996): Neurologic injuries in pelvic ring fractures. *Clin Orthop* **329**, 28–36.

Rice, J. K. M., Dolan, M., Cox, M., Khan, H., and McElwain, J. (2002): Comparison between clinical and radiologic outcome measures after reconstruction of acetabular fractures. *J Orthop Trauma* **16**, 82–6.

Romness, D. L. D. (1990): Total hip arthroplasty after fracture of the acetabulum. *J Bone Joint Surg* **72-B**, 761–4.

Rowe, C. R., and Lowell, J. D. (1961): Prognosis of fractures of the acetabulum. *J Bone Joint Surg* **43-A**, 30–59.

Schafer, S. S. L., Anglen, J., and Childers, M. (2000): Heterotopic ossification in rehabilitation patients who have had internal fixation of an acetabular fracture. *J Rehabil Res Dev* **37**, 389–93.

Sheperd, M. M. (1954): Assessment of function after arthroplasty of the hip. *J Bone Joint Surg* **30-B**, 354–63.

Stewart, M. M. L. (1954): Fracture-dislocation of the hip. *J Bone Joint Surg* **36-A**, 315–41.

Upadhyay, S. M. A. (1981): The long-term results of traumatic posterior dislocation in the hip. *J Bone Joint Surg* **63-B**, 548–51.

Urist, M. (1948): Fracture-dislocation of the hip joint. *J Bone Joint Surg* **30-A**, 699–727.

Woods, R., O'Keefe, G., Rhee, P., Routt, M., and Maier, R. (1998): Open pelvic fracture and faecal diversion. *Arch Surg* **133**, 281–6.

Wright, R. B. K., Christie, M., and Johnson, K. (1994): Acetabular fractures: long-term follow-up of open reduction and internal fixation. *J Orthop Trauma* **8**, 397–403.

APPENDIX

CLINICAL OUTCOME SCORING SYSTEMS FOR PELVIC FRACTURE

Table 18-A1.1: Final Disability Index

• Return to pre-injury occupation	• 50% permanent disability
• Return to sedentary occupation	• Totally disabled

Reprinted from Pennal, G., and Massiah, K. (1980): Nonunion and delayed union of fractures of the pelvis. *Clin Orthop* 151, 124–9.

Table 18-A1.2: Majeed Pelvic Outcome Score

Pain – 30 points		Sexual intercourse – 4 points	
Intense, continuous at rest	0–5	Painful	0–1
Intense with activity	10	Painful if prolonged or awkward	2
Tolerable, but limits activity	15	Uncomfortable	3
With moderate activity, abolished by rest	20	Free	4
Mild, intermittent, normal activity	25	**Standing – 36 points**	
Slight, occasional or no pain	30	A *Walking aids (12)*	
Work – 20 points		Bedridden or almost	0–2
No regular work	0–4	Wheelchair	4
Light work	8	Two crutches	6
Change of job	12	Two sticks	8
Same job, reduced performance	16	One stick	10
Same job, same performance	20	No sticks	12
Sitting – 10 points		B *Gait unaided (12)*	
Painful	0–4	Cannot walk or almost	0–2
Painful if prolonged or awkward	6	Shuffling small steps	4
Uncomfortable	8	Gross limp	6
Free	10	Moderate limp	8

Table 18-A1.2: Majeed Pelvic Outcome Score – *continued*

Slight limp	10	Limited with sticks, difficult without	
Normal	12	prolonged standing possible	6
C Walking distance (12)		One hour with a stick limited without	8
Bedridden or few metres	0–2	One hour without sticks slight pain or limp	10
Very limited time and distance	4	Normal for age and general condition	12

Reprinted from Majeed, S. A. (1989): Grading the outcome of pelvic fractures. *J Bone Joint Surg* **71-B**, 304–6, with permission.

Table 18-A1.3: Patient Outcome Grade

Category	Description	Points
Functional pain	*Pain secondary to physical activity*	
	None	5
	Pain only with strenuous activity	4
	Mild pain with stair climbing, lifting, mowing or other moderately strenuous activities	3
	Moderate pain with start up of activities and intermittent radicular pain	2
	Pain with sitting or standing longer than 1 hour, requires frequent position changes	1
	Chronic severe pain regardless of activity	0
Subjective pain	*Average of resting and ambulation scores on a scale of 1 (no pain) to 10 (severe pain)*	
	1–2 points	4
	3–4 points	3
	5–6 points	2
	7–8 points	1
	9–10 points	0
Narcotic use	*Narcotic use > 12 weeks postoperatively*	
	No	1
	Yes	0
Activity status	*Ability to resume previous work, household, or recreational activities*	
	Without limitations	10
	With some discomfort	8
	With limitations such as tires more easily or cannot lift as much as before injury	6
	With marked limitations requiring change in work status to part time, sedentary, or with restrictions; requires assistance with household activities or avoids strenuous recreational activities	4
	Unable to resume any previous work, household, or recreational activities; cannot drive and requires assistance with stairs or with shopping	2
	Unable to resume any previous work, household, or recreational activities and requires assistance with activities of daily living	0

Table 18-A1.3: Patient Outcome Grade – *continued*

Category	Description	Points
Physical examination	*Gait*	
	Normal gait	4
	Antalgic gait or limp	3
	Requires assistive device [cane]	2
	Requires assistive device [walker; occasionally uses wheelchair]	1
	Nonambulatory	0
	Trendelenberg	
	Negative	1
	Positive	0
	Tenderness	
	No sacral or pubic tenderness	2
	Sacral or pubic tenderness	1
	Sacral and Pubic tenderness	0
	Lower extremity muscle group strength flexion/extension	
	Bilateral thigh flexion and extension = 5/5	1
	Thigh flexion or extension < 5/5	0
	Abduction/adduction	
	Bilateral thigh abduction and adduction = 5/5	1
	Thigh abduction or adduction <5/5	0
	Range of motion	
	Normal hip and trunk range of motion	1
	Trunk flexion <90°, hip flexion <90° or >20° difference in hip internal or external rotation when compared with contralateral side	0
Pelvic radiographs (AP, inlet, and outlet views)	*Posterior (normal Sacroiliac joint space = 4 mm)*	
	Displacement ≤0.5 cm without Sacroiliac joint reactive changes	6
	Displacement ≤0.5 cm with Sacroiliac joint reactive changes	5
	Displacement >0.5 cm and ≤1.0 cm	4
	Displacement >1.0 cm	2
	Nonunion	0
	Anterior (normal pubic symphysis space = 0.5 cm)	
	Displacement ≤0.5 cm	4
	Displacement >0.5 cm and ≤1.0 cm	3
	Displacement >1.0 cm and ≤2.0 cm	1
	Displacement >2.0 cm	0

Reprinted from Cole, J. D., Blum, D. A., and Ansel, L. J. (1996): Outcome after fixation of unstable posterior pelvic ring injuries. *Clin Orthop* **329**, 160–79.

ACETABULAR CLINICAL OUTCOME MEASURES AND SCORING SYSTEMS

Table 18-A2.1: Musculoskeletal Function Assessment (MFA) Questionnaire (Total = 100)

Self care	(18)
Sleep/rest	(6)
Hand/fine motor	(6)
Mobility	(19)
Housework	(9)
Employment/work	(3)
Leisure/recreation	(4)
Family relationships	(10)
Cognition/thinking	(4)
Emotional adjustment	(21)

Reprinted from Martin, D. *et al.* (1996): The development of a musculoskeletal extremity health status instrument: the Musculoskeletal Functon Assessment instrument. *J Orthop Res* **14**, 173–81, with permission from the Orthopaedic Research Society.

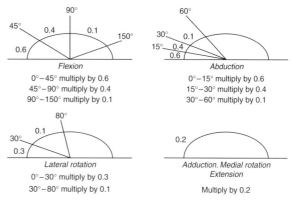

Flexion
0°–45° multiply by 0.6
45°–90° multiply by 0.4
90°–150° multiply by 0.1

Abduction
0°–15° multiply by 0.6
15°–30° multiply by 0.4
30°–60° multiply by 0.1

Lateral rotation
0°–30° multiply by 0.3
30°–80° multiply by 0.1

Adduction. Medial rotation Extension
Multiply by 0.2

Figure 18-A2.1 Mobility Index.

Reprinted from Gade, H. (1947): A contribution to the surgical management of osteoarthritis of the hip joint: a clinical study. *Acta Chir Scand* **120**(Suppl.) 37–45.

Table 18-A2.2: Merle d'Aubigne and Postel Outcome Score

Score	Pain	Mobility	Ability to walk
0	Intense/permanent	Ankylosis bad position	None
1	Severe night	No movement/slight deformity	With crutches
2	Severe walking	Flexion <40°	With stick
3	Tolerable limits activity	Flexion 40–60°	One stick, <1 hour
4	Mild walking none resting	Flexion 60–80°	Short periods unaided
5	Mild inconstant pain	Flexion 80–90°	Slight limp, unaided
		Abducts >15°	
6	No pain	Flexion >90°	Normal
		Abducts >30°	

Very Good (>16)–Poor (<7)
Reprinted from Merle d'Aubigne, R. and Postel, M. (1954): Functional results of hip arthroplasty with acrylic prosthesis. *J Bone Joint Surg* **36-A**, 451–75.

Table 18-A2.3: Epstein Clinical Hip Score

Excellent	Good
All of the following:	No pain
No pain	Free motion (75 per cent of normal hip)
Full range of hip motion	No more than a slight limp
No limp	Minimum roentgenographic changes
No roentgenographic evidence of progressive changes	
Fair	**Poor**
Any one or more of the following:	Any one or more of the following:
Pain, but not disabling	Disabling pain
Limited motion of the hip; no adduction deformity	Marked limitation of motion or adduction deformity
Moderate limp	Redislocation
Moderately severe roentgenographic changes	Progressive roentgenographic changes

Reprinted from Epstein, H. (1973): Traumatic dislocations of the hip. *Clin Orthop* **92**, 114–21.

Table 18-A2.5: Judet Hip Score

	Pain	Movement	Walking
1	Severe night	Fixed bad position	Impossible
2	Severe walking	Fixed good position	Short distances
3	Moderate, light work	0–70°	Restricted <1 hour, stick
4	Pain relieved resting	70–140°	Long distance, stick
5	Slight/inter-mittent, work	140–200°	No stick, limps
6	Absent	200–300°	Normal

Reprinted from Judet, R. (1952): Technique and results with the acrylic femoral head prosthesis. *J Bone Joint Surg* **34-B**, 173–80, with permission.

Table 18-A2.6: Lazansky Hip Score (Total = 6.0)

Pain, Right + Left	(12)
Function	(21)
Mobility, Right + Left	(67)

Total score = 100, converted via multiplication factors to range between 1.0 and 6.0
Excellent = 5.5–6.0 to Very Poor = 1.0–1.5
Reprinted from Lazansky, M. (1967): A method for grading hips. *J Bone Joint Surg* **49-B**, 644–51, with permission.

Table 18-A2.4: Harris Hip Score (Total = 100)

Pain	(44)
Function	(47)
ROM	(5)
Absence of deformity	(4)

Reprinted from Harris, W. (1969): Traumatic arthritis of the hip after dislocation and acetabular fractures: treatment by mold arthroplasty. *J Bone Joint Surg* **51-A**, 737–55, with permission.

Table 18-A2.7: Larson Hip Disability Rating Scale (Total = 100)

Function	(35)
Pain	(35)
Gait	(10)
Absence of deformity	(10)
ROM	(10)

Reprinted from Larson, C. (1963): Rating scale for hip disabilities. *Clin Orthop* **31**, 85–93, with permission.

Table 18-A2.8: Matta Clinical Grading Criteria

	Pain	Ambulation	ROM (%)
6	None	Normal	95–100
5	Slight/Intermittent	Slight limp	80–95
4	Mild walking, none rest	Stick long distance	70–80
3	Moderate, able to walk	Limited with support	60–70
2	Severe, walking	Very limited	<50
1	Severe, prevents walking	Bedridden	–

Excellent = 18 to Poor <13
Reprinted from Matta, J. (1996): Fractures of the acetabulum: accuracy of reduction and clinical results in patients managed operatively within three weeks after the injury. *J Bone Joint Surg* **78-A**, 1632–45, with permission.

ACETABULAR RADIOLOGICAL OUTCOME MEASURES AND SCORING SYSTEMS

Table 18-A3.1: Acetabular fracture: Rowe Grading System

Excellent	Good	Fair	Poor
Clinical			
No symptoms; no medication; full motion; no limp; no support; sustained activities; all sports; returned to original job	Minor complaints; no medication; 25 per cent limitation of motion; no limp; no support; sustained activities; all sports; returned to original job	Discomfort intermittent; relieved by rest and salicylates; mild sciatic-nerve symptoms; 50 per cent limitation of motion; intermittent limp; occasional support; adjustment of work in original job	Constant pain; frequent medication; disturbing sciatic-nerve symptoms; 75 per cent limitation of motion; constant limp; activities limited; full-time support; not able to work
Anatomical			
Normal joint space: no head changes	Fractured fragments have healed with a smooth congruous articulating surface; no head changes; less-than-normal anatomy; adequate joint space; mild myositis ossificans	Mild-to-moderate narrowing of the joint space; early arthritic changes and osteophyte formation; mild changes in contour of the ferroral head; moderate myositis ossificans	Very narrow joint space; advanced arthritic changes; sclerosis and spur formation; definite avascular necrosis of the femoral head with cystic changes; advanced myositis ossificans

Reprinted from Rowe, C. R., and Lowell, J. D. (1961): Prognosis of fractures of the acetabulum. *J Bone Joint Surg* **43-A**, 30–59.

Table 18-A3.2: Acetabular fracture: Epstein Radiological Grading Score

Excellent (normal)

All of the following:

Normal relationship between the femoral head and the acetabulum

Normal articular cartilaginous space

Normal density of the head of femur

No spur formation

No calcification in the capsule

Fair (moderate changes)

Normal relationship between the femoral head and the acetabulum

Any one or more of the following:

Moderate narrowing of the cartilaginous space

Mottling of the head, areas of sclerosis, and decreased density

Moderate spur formation

Moderate to severe capsular calcification

Depression of the subchondral cortex of the femoral head

Good (minimum changes)

Normal relationship between the femoral head and the acetabulum

Minimum narrowing of the cartilaginous space

Minimum de-ossification

Minimum spur formation

Minimum capsular calcification

Poor (severe changes)

Almost complete obliteration of the cartilaginous space

Relative increase in density of the femoral head

Subchondral cyst formation

Formation of sequestra

Gross deformity of the femoral head

Severe spur formation

Acetabular sclerosis

Reprinted from Epstein, H. (1973): Traumatic dislocations of the hip. *Clin Orthop* **92**, 114–21.

Table 18-A3.3: Acetabular fracture: Matta Radiological Grading Criteria

Excellent:	Essentially normal roentgenogram
Good:	Mild spur formation on femoral head or acetabulum
	Mild joint narrowing
	Mild sclerosis
Fair:	Mild mottling of femoral head
	Mild subluxion of femoral head
	Moderate spur formation on femoral head or acetabulum
	Moderate joint narrowing
	Moderate sclerosis
Poor:	Any collapse of femoral head
	Any subchondral cysts
	Moderate–severe mottling of femoral head
	Moderate–severe subluxation of femoral head
	Severe spur formation on femoral head or acetabulum
	Severe joint narrowing
	Severe sclerosis

Reprinted from Matta, J. (1996): Fractures of the acetabulum: accuracy of reduction and clinical results in patients managed operatively within three weeks after the injury. *J Bone Joint Surg* **78-A**, 1632–45.

19

Femoral head and neck and the hip joint
Martyn J. Parker and Andrew Pearson

INTRODUCTION

The effect of treatment for a hip condition may be assessed by a substantial number of outcome measures. These vary from subjective assessment (e.g. pain), objective assessment (e.g. range of movement), and radiographic changes through to composite measures such as hip scores. The outcome measures used will be dictated by the nature of the condition being studied and the general health of the patient. For example, the assessment of those patients after an elective hip replacement is more likely to be practical in a follow-up clinic, and long-term follow-up is feasible. Conversely, for the elderly frail patient who sustains a hip fracture, repeated clinic follow-up visits are impractical and long-term follow-up is affected by the high underlying mortality in this group of patients.

The different outcomes that may be used can be considered under the following headings:

- Mortality
- Pain
- Hip movements and deformity
- Functional outcomes
- Hip scores
- General health indicators
- Radiological assessment
- Survival analysis
- Cost–benefit analysis

MORTALITY

Whilst this outcome has less relevance to those conditions associated with a low mortality, for other conditions such as hip fracture this can be considered as a key outcome measure. Mortality is certainly a definite outcome measure, but variations in reported figures may be due to a number of reasons related to data collection. These include:

- Is it a consecutive series of patients or a selected series?

- What is the definition of cases to be included within the series? For example, patients between certain age ranges, or with a certain type of condition.

- How many cases were lost to follow-up? It is incorrect to assume that the mortality in those lost to follow-up is the same as in the whole group.

- What is the time period to consideration of mortality? Is it hospital mortality, three, six or 12 months after surgery, or long-term?

- Are the deaths related to the hip condition or to other causes? It may be more appropriate to look at any specific cause of death, for example pulmonary embolism.

PAIN

Pain is the most relevant of all outcome measures for hip conditions. However, as pain is a subjective measure, it can be heavily influenced by how it is recorded, or who collects the information. Numerous methods for describing pain in hip conditions exist, including a variety of pain scores and visual analogue scales. One of the most frequently used pain scores for the hip is that of Charnley (1972), which has six grades (Table 19.1). When considering hip conditions – and particularly that of uncemented arthroplasty – it may be necessary to consider pain in the thigh separate from pain in the hip.

Table 19.1: Charnley hip score. Reprinted from Charnley (1972)

Pain

1. Severe and spontaneous
2. Severe on attempting to walk. Prevents all activity
3. Tolerable, permitted limited activity
4. Only after some activity. Disappears quickly with rest
5. Slight or intermittent pain on starting to walk but getting less with normal activity
6. No pain

Movement

1. 0–30°
2. 60°
3. 100°
4. 160°
5. 210°
6. 260°

Walking

1. Few yards or bedridden. Two crutches or sticks
2. Time and distance very limited with or without sticks
3. Limited to one stick (less than 1 hour). Difficulty without a stick. Able to stand without a stick.
4. Long distances with one stick. Limited without a stick
5. No stick, but a limp
6. Normal

HIP MOVEMENTS AND DEFORMITY

The measurement of hip movement, shortening and deformity is a component of many of the hip scoring systems. To be meaningful, hip movements need to be compared with either a normal contralateral hip, or with those movements of the hip recorded prior to treatment. As many hip conditions are bilateral, pre-treatment movements are to be preferred. However, this is not possible for certain conditions such as traumatic hip conditions. Measurement of hip flexion may be as accurate in assessing outcome as a more comprehensive assessment of hip movements (Bryant *et al.* 1993).

FUNCTIONAL OUTCOMES

These include numerous aspects of function that may be influenced by disorders of the hip. Those that have been used for hip arthroplasty include:

- Walking ability (distance, speed).
- Use of walking aids.
- Work/level of activity/occupation.
- Ability to undertake various activities of daily living (e.g. go up stairs, tying shoelaces, put socks on and off, pick object from the floor).

Also relevant for some conditions such as hip fracture will be the ability to return to the same residential status and perform basic and advanced activities of daily living. A standardized system of recording basic data for the outcome after hip fracture has been devised (SAHFE; Standardised Audit of Hip Fracture in Europe), and this enables valid comparison to be made between centres (Parker *et al.* 1998). The assessment of mobility after hip fracture may be made by using the definitions of SAHFE; alternatively, a composite mobility score may be used (Parker and Palmer 1993). Other functional outcome scores that have been used for hip fractures are those based on activities of daily living such as the Barthel index (Mahoney and Barthel 1965) and that of Katz and colleagues (Katz *et al.* 1963).

HIP SCORES

These may be based on clinical or radiological criteria, or a combination of the two. There are a large number of different hip scoring systems, and most of these have undergone a number of modifications. The score may use a number of different factors, which may be either subjective (e.g. pain), objective (e.g. range of movement), or radiological. These are then added together to give a final score. This number may be manipulated statistically, but as the scores do not resemble normal distributions this is of dubious validity. Alternatively, arbitrary levels are set so as to define those hips that are considered to be either excellent, good, fair or poor.

One of the earliest systems used was that of Merle d'Aubigne and Postel (1954), which was based on that of Fergusson and Howarth (1931). This simple scoring system, which is similar to that of Robert and Jean Judet (Judet and Judet 1952), rated the three items of pain, range of hip movement and walking ability from grade 1 to 6; the three numbers obtained are added together to determine a final score. Charnley (1972) proposed a modification to the Merle d'Aubigne score system, whereby pain, hip movements and walking are scored on a scale of 0 to 6 (see Table 19.1), with movement being the sum of the ranges of movement in the three standard directions. Charnley did not combine the pain, mobility and walking scores to obtain a total score, but this assessment system has since been widely used.

The Harris hip score (Harris 1969) was first described using a series of young predominantly male patients who had sustained an acetabular fracture. Factors assessed were pain (scored 0 to 44), function (total score 0 to 47), range of motion (score 0 to 5) and absence of deformity (score 0 to 4). Function is derived from the presence of a limp, the use of walking aids, and activities. Larson (Larson 1963; Johnston and Larson 1969) described the Iowa hip score, which uses a 100-point rating scale. In this system, 35 points were allocated for pain assessment, 35 for function, 10 for gait, 10 for freedom from deformity, and 10 for range of motion.

Kavanagh and Fitzgerald (1985) described the Mayo hip scoring system, which included both clinical and radiological criteria to give a single number on a scale of 0 to 100. The clinical criteria contributed 80 points, and the radiological criteria 20 points. The radiological criteria were included as it was felt that they helped to predict the long-term outcome. The clinical criteria used were pain (40 points), function (20 points) and mobility and muscle power (20 points). For the radiological criteria, 10 points were awarded for the acetabulum and 10 for the femur. With this system, an excellent result scored 90–100, good scored 80–89, fair scored 70–79, and poor scored less than 70. The Mayo hip score has the advantage that, as the range of movement is not quantified exactly, the clinical data can be collected by using a questionnaire. The Harris, Iowa and Mayo hip scores have all been validated. Other scoring systems which have been described include those of Gade (1947), Shepherd (1954), Stinchfield *et al.* (1957), Danielsson (1964), Goodwin (1968), Wilson *et al.* (1972), Salvati and Wilson (1973), Amstutz *et al.* (1984) and Pellicci *et al.* (1985).

The Western Ontario and McMaster Universities (WOMAC) is a 24-item index divided into three sections of pain (5 items), stiffness (2 items) and physical function (17 items). It has recently been extensively used in patients with arthritis of the hip or knee (Bellamy *et al.* 1988; McConnell *et al.* 2001). In a comparison of the WOMAC, Harris score and SF-36 (Söderman and Malchau 2001) all three were found to be valid, reproducible and reliable. Some studies on outcome scores and their findings are listed in Table 19.2. The Oxford hip score (Dawson 1996) has more recently been used in the UK (Table 19.2)

In order to rectify some of the problems of numerous different measurement methods, a unifying system of reporting results has been suggested (Johnston *et al.* 1990). This incorporates most of the factors involved in the various different scores. Parameters included were pain, levels of work and activities, walking capacity and patient satisfaction. Physical examination included range of movement and limb shortening. These authors also described a radiographic evaluation for both cemented and uncemented implants. The considerable information collected enables most of the previously described

Table 19.2: Studies determining outcome scores and their findings

Outcome measure	Study design	Description — Subjects, intervention, outcomes, inclusion and exclusion criteria	Validity — Methodology, rigor, selection, bias	Results	Comment
Bellamy et al. (1988). Validation study of **WOMAC**: a health status instrument for measuring clinically important patient-relevant outcomes following total hip or knee arthroplasty in osteoarthritis.	Prospective	**Patients:** n = 30 with primary OA of the hip or knee **Intervention:** Assessed day before surgery and then at 6 weeks, 3 months and 6 months post-operatively by same interviewer **Inclusion and exclusion criteria:** All patients ambulatory, unrestricted by any co-morbidity, for primary surgery, attend the orthopaedic clinic	**Randomization:** N/A **Selection:** 30 consecutive patients, 14M, 16F **Rigor:** Compared to Doyle, Lequesne, Bradburn indexes and social component of the McMaster health index questionnaire.	**Reliability:** Reliability coefficient >0.80 **Validity:** Validity confirmed for pain, stiffness and physical function.	WOMAC is a reliable, valid and responsive multi-dimensional, self-administered questionnaire.
Söderman and Malchau (2000) Validity and reliability of Swedish **WOMAC** osteoarthritis index: a self-administered disease-specific questionnaire vs. generic instruments [SF-36 and Nottingham Health Profile (NHP)]	Retrospective	**Patients:** n = 58 at 2–10 years following THA **Intervention:** All patients filled in WOMAC, SF-36 and NHP scores and repeated at 4 weeks.	**Randomization:** Yes	**Reliability and Validity:** All three tests were found to be highly reliable and valid.	The use of WOMAC after THA is to be encouraged.

Fitzpatrick et al. (2000). The value of short and simple measures to assess outcomes for patients of total hip replacement surgery. **Oxford Hip Score**	Survey of patients undergoing primary THA before operation and 3 and 12 months after surgery	**Patients:** n = 7151 in 143 hospitals in three NHS English regions. **Intervention:** Patient-completed questionnaires, surgeons' questionnaire and ASA classification for 5038 patients.	**Randomization:** No **All patients accounted for:** Yes **Potential for bias:** Older patients and those with major health problems were more likely not to complete the form.	**Reliability:** Reliability coefficient 0.88. **Validity:** Validity is confirmed, despite the relatively small number of questions in the score.	
Dawson et al. (1996) Questionnaire on the perceptions of patients about total hip replacement. **Oxford Hip Score**	20 patients attending an out-patient clinic interviewed regarding their hips resulted in a questionnaire. Prospective study developed from this questionnaire.	**Patients:** n = 220 consecutive, early 1994 **Intervention:** Patients completed the questionnaire pre-operatively and at 6 months post-operatively, as well as the SF-36.	**Randomization:** N/A	**Reliability:** Reliability coefficient >0.8 **Validity:** The results compared well with the proven SF-36, especially regarding physical function and pain.	A short practical valid and reliable questionnaire which is sensitive to clinically important changes.
Alonso et al. (2000). The pain and function of the hip **(PFH)** scale: a patient-based instrument for measuring outcome after total hip replacement.	Prospective	**Patients:** n = 131 **Intervention:** Patients completed the questionnaire and NHP questionnaire pre-THA, and at 3 and 12 months post-operatively.	**Randomization:** N/A **All patients accounted for:** Yes	**Reliability:** Reliability coefficient 0.8 **Validity:** Not demonstrated, but stated by authors.	Comparison with the Harris hip score or WOMAC might have been appropriate.

hip scores to be calculated. This standardized assessment has subsequently been validated (Katz *et al.* 1995) and adopted by the Société Internationale de Chirurgie Orthopédique et de Traumatologie (SICOT) and the American Academy of Orthopaedic Surgeons (Liang *et al.* 1991).

Hip scores for other conditions have also been described. Epstein (1974) described a scoring system for fracture dislocations of the hip. This was subsequently modified by Matta and Merrit (1988) by incorporating some of the features of the Merle D'Aubinge system. Tonnis (1987) described a scoring system based on pain and hip movements for congenital dislocation of the hip, while Catterall (1971) described a grading system for Perthes' disease. Two scoring systems for slipped upper femoral epiphysis using both clinical and radiological criteria have been described (Hall 1957; Gunn and Angel 1978).

Different hip scores produce very different results such that it is not possible to compare results by using the scores obtained (Andersson 1972; Callaghan *et al.* 1990). In addition, different authors may obtain different results using the same scores (Thomas and Bannister 1991). Another problem is that, ideally, the score should be measured pre-operatively, to determine the change in score that has occurred. This precludes the use of the system for conditions such as hip fractures, unless the pre-fracture score is estimated retrospectively, though this may introduce further errors, especially if the score incorporates hip movements. Others hip scores have assumed that hip function was normal prior to treatment; an example is the Harris hip score which is described for use after acetabular fractures (Harris 1969). Another problem with hip scores is that they cannot be used equally for all age groups. For example, a scoring system that would represent the needs of a young man with a slipped capital epiphysis will in no way represent those of an elderly person with a hip fracture. A more recent statistical evaluation of 13 different hip scores found the results of the different scores to be inconsistent. Consequently, the suggestion was made that the hip scores be reduced to three key factors of pain, walking ability and hip flexion (Bryant *et al.* 1993).

For hip fracture patients, the hip scores previously described have been used, but with questionable value (Parker and Maheshwer 1997). Many other simpler scores have been used, including that of Kyle *et al.* (1979), who defined an excellent result as being patients with a normal range of movement, minimal limp and no pain; 'good' were patients with a normal range of movement, a limp and occasional mild pain; 'fair' were patients with a limited range of movement, a limp, moderate pain and who used two sticks; and 'poor' were patients who had pain on any motion or were confined to a wheelchair or who were non-ambulatory. Using hip scores for hip fracture patients makes no allowance for the function pre-fracture. For example, a patient who prior to sustaining a hip fracture walked with a Zimmer frame about the house and following treatment has identical mobility with a completely pain-free hip, would be graded as having a 'fair' result out of a possible range of 'excellent', 'good', 'fair' and 'poor' using the Salvati and Wilson score (Salvati and Wilson 1973).

GENERAL HEALTH INDICATORS

A number of more general outcome scores have been used for assessing various hip conditions. These include the lower extremity measure (LEM) score (Jagal *et al.* 2000), functional recovery score (Zuckerman *et al.* 2000a, b) the short form-36 (McHorney *et al.* 1993) and the Nottingham Health profile (Hunt and McEwen 1980). The short form-36 is the most commonly used of these measures and version 2 has recently been released.

RADIOLOGICAL ASSESSMENT

Numerous methods exist for assessing different aspects of hip pathologies. In addition, some of the hip scores described earlier incorporate a radiographic assessment such as that of Johnston and Larson (1969) and the Mayo hip score for hip arthroplasty (Kavanagh and Fitzgerald 1985).

Total hip replacement

A number of different methods have been used to assess the radiographic features after arthroplasty. For the femoral component, Gruen *et al.* (1979) divided the femoral stem into thirds, as viewed on both antero-posterior and lateral radiographs. These areas were then analysed for acrylic cement fracture and radiolucency at the stem–cement and cement–bone interface. Radiographs were evaluated chronologically to assess loosening as manifested by progressive changes in the width or length of the radiolucent zones; the appearance of sclerotic bone reaction; widening of the acrylic cement fracture gap; and fragmentation of the cement and gross movement of the femoral component.

DeLee and Charnley (1976) described a method of quantifying radiological demarcation of cemented sockets in total hip replacement. The width of the radiolucent zone around the cement was measured on radiographs without correction for the 10 per cent magnification. The width was divided into four groups: <0.5 mm; <1 mm; <1.5 mm; and >1.5 mm. As the width varied, the widest dimension was recorded. In addition to the width of demarcation, its distribution around the circumference of the socket was categorized into three zones:

- Type I being lateral to a vertical line drawn through the centre of the acetabulum

- Type III being below a horizontal line to run through the centre of the acetabulum; and

- Type II being the remainder.

The radiographs were also assessed for migration of the socket. Two types of movement were described, namely subsidence and tilting of the socket.

Acetabular fractures (See also Chapter 18)

The scoring systems of Epstein (1974) and Matta *et al.* (1986) included an assessment of radiographic criteria. Letournel (1980) divided acetabular fracture

reductions into perfect and imperfect. The imperfect reductions were subdivided into groups with the head centred, with protrusio, with loss of parallelism, and with development of the secondary congruent centre medial to the normal acetabulum. Matta and Merrit (1988) subsequently described a method of assessing reduction whereby a displacement of >3 mm on any of the three standard X-radiography views was considered unsatisfactory, a displacement of ≤3 mm was rated satisfactory, and an anatomic reduction was referred to as displacement of ≤1 mm.

Heterotrophic ossification

Booker and colleagues (Booker *et al.* 1973) classified heterotrophic bone formation into four groups from an antero-posterior radiographic viewpoint:

- Class 1: Islands of bone within soft tissues about the hip.

- Class 2: Bone spurs from the pelvis or proximal end of the femur, leaving at least 1 cm between opposing bone surfaces.

- Class 3: Bone spurs from the pelvis or proximal end of the femur, reducing the space between opposing bone surfaces to <1 cm.

- Class 4: Apparent bone ankylosis of the hip.

Maloney *et al.* (1991) later modified this assessment method.

Avascular necrosis

Radiographic assessment of avascular necrosis has been described using a number or methods, including the classifications of Ficat (1985), Marcus (Marcus *et al.* 1973) or Myers (1983). Other authors just determine whether collapse occurs (Myers 1978). Ficat (1985) also described a way of assessing outcome which combined pain, range of movement and radiological criteria, and provided an overall result which was graded as 'very good', 'good', 'fair' or 'failure'. With the advent of magnetic resonance imaging (MRI) and computed tomography (CT) scanning, Steinberg's modification of Ficat's original classification has become widely used:

- Stage 0: Radiograph, MRI and bone scan normal.

- Stage 1: Normal radiograph, abnormal MRI and/or bone scan.

- Stage 2: Abnormal radiograph showing cystic or sclerotic changes in the femoral head.

- Stage 3: Subchondral collapse – crescent sign.

- Stage 4: Flattening of the femoral head.

- Stage 5: Joint narrowing with or without acetabular involvement.

- Stage 6: Advanced degenerative changes.

Developmental dysplasia of the hip

A number of radiological criteria have been used to assess developmental dysplasia of the hip. In older children and adults, the centre edge angle of Wiberg (Wiberg 1939) assesses acetabular cover. In dysplastic hips, this angle is <20°. The acetabular head index (Heyman and Herdon 1950) is also used for assessing head coverage in congenitally dislocated and dysplastic hips, although it was initially described for assessing Perthes' disease.

In 1941, Severin (1941) described a classification of radiological results:

- Type 1: Normal head and centre-edge angle.

- Type 2: Abnormal head, normal centre-edge angle.

- Type 3: Residual dysplasia with reduced centre-edge angle.

- Type 4: Subluxation.

- Type 5: Subluxation severe with 'wandering acetabulum'.

- Type 6: Complete dislocation.

Perthes' disease

Radiological measures are used as predictors of clinical outcome for Perthes' disease. The shape of the head of the femur can be assessed using a template of concentric circles outlined on a transparent material (Moes et al. 1977). To be classified as spherical, the surface of the head must follow the same circle on the template within a variation of 2 mm in both the frontal and lateral views. If it does not, then the head is considered to be irregular. Head irregularity has been shown to correlate with the late development of arthritis, and the reliability of this measurement has been confirmed (Lauritzen 1975). The radius quotient, which is also known as the head size ratio, is a method of quantifying the abnormal shape of the femoral head (Meyer 1966).

Other radiological classifications made at presentation have been described for Perthes' disease, including the classifications of Catterall (1971) and Salter and Thompson (1984). Heyman and Herdon (1950) developed the acetabular head index for the assessment of cover after Perthes' disease, while Meyer (1966) and Moes (1980) each introduced a number of other ways to assess the radiological outcome. These included the epiphyseal quotient and the joint surface quotient, both of which are ratios comparing the abnormal to the normal.

Slipped capital femoral epiphysis

Slip severity can be classified radiographically by several methods. These are based on either the amount of capital displacement, or on the angular measurement of the epiphysis relative to either the femoral neck or shaft (Cohen et al. 1986). The classifications divide the slip into mild, moderate and severe. In a mild slip, the epiphysis is displaced less than one-third of the neck width, or if the head-neck angle is less than 30°; in a moderate slip the displacement is between one-third and one-half of the neck width, or the head-neck angle is between 30° and 50°; in a severe slip the displacement is more than one-half of the neck width, or the head-neck angle is greater than 50°. The head-shaft angle is the most commonly used classification.

Although most assessments are performed on plain radiographic views, CT scanning can be used for more quantitative accuracy. Carney *et al.* (1991), in a long-term follow-up of 155 hips over a mean of 41 years, showed that all outcome measures worsened with an increase in the severity of the slip or if any attempt had been made at reduction. Loder *et al.* (1993) described a clinical classification for the severity of slipped upper capital femoral epiphysis, dividing patients into either a stable slip that can achieve weight-bearing, or an unstable slip which cannot bear weight (even with support) due to pain. This assessment indicates that none of the 55 patients with stable slips developed osteonecrosis, whereas 50 per cent in the unstable group did.

Hip fracture

For intracapsular fractures treated by internal fixation, a number or radiographic criteria for adequate reduction have been defined (Garden 1961; Parker and Pryor 1993). The radiographic assessment after arthroplasty will be dependent on the implant used. An assessment for the technical adequacy of the Austin Moore prosthesis has been described (Pryor 1990). For trochanteric fractures treated by internal fixation, criteria for correct fracture reduction and implant positioning have been described (Parker and Pryor 1993; Baumgaertner and Solberg 1997).

SURVIVAL ANALYSIS

Survival analysis was first used to report the long-term results of hip replacements (Dobbs 1980), and has since been used in numerous similar studies. The proportion of the cases reviewed for each year postoperatively that do not fail is determined. For each year, the cumulated proportions surviving are plotted against the time (in years) since surgery was carried out. Details of the calculations with corrections for intermittent sampling have been described (Carr *et al.* 1993). The three main problems with survival analysis are: the outcome of patients who are lost to follow-up; analysis with small numbers; and the definition of failure.

For each year a number of patients will have died and some may be lost to follow-up. A fundamental assumption in survival analysis is that the group of withdrawals has the same failure rate as the group that has not been withdrawn. This is probably a valid assumption for the patients who die, but it is less likely to be valid for those patients who are not followed-up, though there is some evidence to support this assumption (Dorey and Amstutz 1989). It is essential that the number of patients lost to follow-up is included with the survival analysis, and this may be done either numerically or graphically (Carr *et al.* 1993; Murray *et al.* 1993).

With regard to the small numbers involved, in survival analysis it is common that only a small number of patients are followed for long periods. Therefore, the confidence limits are likely to be large at the end of the follow-up. Survival curves may give a false impression unless they include stand-ard errors or confidence limits (Lettin *et al.* 1991). It is important that some indication of errors is included, and these are probably best calculated with the equation of Peto *et al.* (1977).

A fixed end-point needs to be chosen in the analysis for the definition of failure, which is usually revision of the prosthesis. Another end-point may be the development of a particular radiological sign. The decision to revise an implant will depend on many factors, including the fitness of the patient, the length of the waiting list, and how aggressive the surgeon is. A revision is therefore not necessarily a good criterion on which to base survival analysis, even though it is easy to measure. Some authors have attempted to overcome this by including patients in severe pain, but this is difficult to quantify. Survival analysis does not take into account how well the prosthesis is functioning. For example, two prostheses with the same revision rate would, apparently, perform equally well when investigated with survival analysis, even though one caused severe thigh pain and the other did not.

COST–BENEFIT ANALYSIS

In recent years comparisons have been undertaken between different treatment methods in order to estimate their relative cost effectiveness. This may then be used to rationalize what treatment methods are appropriate and affordable within budget constraints (Kitzhaber 1993). A number of methods have been employed, but the most commonly used method has been by using Quality Adjusted Life Years (QALY). One QALY is equal to a procedure or treatment that gives an additional year of life at 100 per cent health. Therefore, the QALY calculation involves estimating for how many years a procedure will last (such as a total hip replacement), how many extra years of life a procedure may bring, and to what extent it improves the patient's quality of life. Cost per QALY can then be determined if the cost of the particular treatment under study is known. This enables different treatments to be compared in a cost–benefit analysis.

QALYs and cost per QALY have been determined for a number of orthopaedic conditions including hip replacement (Williams 1991) and for different treatment methods for hip fracture (Parker *et al.* 1992). At present, the role of such cost–benefit analyses are questionable and the calculations are based on a number of assumptions, including the estimated duration of benefit of a procedure (e.g. how long a hip replacement will last) and to what extent the procedure improves the quality of life and life expectancy. In addition, when considering cost per QALY, cost of treatments will vary between countries and also change with inflation.

SUMMARY

At present, the assessment of any hip condition is fraught with difficulties due to the large numbers of assessment systems available. Hip scores are of questionable value, and few have been validated with known degrees of intra- and inter-observer variation. The clinician should be advised to use standardized assessment tools and to report variables as individual outcome measures, thereby avoiding the errors incurred with composite scores. Survival analysis is appropriate for comparing different implants, but needs to be considered in conjunction with other assessments of outcome. It is to be expected that the radiographic parameters will continue to change and be refined.

REFERENCES

Alonso, J., Lamarca, R., and Martí-Valls, J. (2000): The pain and function of the hip (PFH) scale: a patient-based instrument for measuring outcome after total hip replacement. *Orthopedics* 23, 1273–7.

Amstutz, H. C., Thomas, B. J., Jinnah, R., Kim, W., Grogan, T., and Yale, C. (1984): Treatment of primary osteoarthritis of the hip. A comparison of total joint and surface replacement arthroplasty. *J Bone Joint Surg* 66-A, 228–41.

Andersson S, G. (1972): Hip assessment: a comparison of nine different methods. *J Bone Joint Surg* 54-B, 621–5.

Baumgaertner, M. R., and Solberg, B. D. (1997): Awareness of tip-apex distance reduces failure of fixation of trochanteric fractures of the hip. *J Bone Joint Surg* 79, 969–71.

Bellamy, N., Buchanan, W. W., Goldsmith, C. H., Campbell, J., and Stitt, L. W. (1988): Validation study of WOMAC: a health status instrument for measuring clinically important patient-relevant outcomes following total hip or knee arthroplasty in osteoarthritis. *J Orthop Rheumatol* 1, 95–108.

Booker, A. F., Bowerman, J. W., Robinson, R. A., and Riley, L. E. (1973): Ectopic ossification following total hip replacement. *J Bone Joint Surg* 55-A, 1629–32.

Bryant, M. J., Kernohan, W. G., Nixon, J. R., and Mollan, R. A. B. (1993): A statistical analysis of hip scores. *J Bone Joint Surg* 75-B, 705–9.

Callaghan, J. J., Dysart, S. H., Savory, C. F., and Hopkinson, W. I. (1990): Assessing the results of hip replacement. A comparison of five different rating systems. *J Bone Joint Surg* 72-B, 1008–9.

Carney, B. T., Weinstein, S. L., and Noble, J. (1991): Longterm follow-up of slipped capital femoral epiphysis. *J Bone Joint Surg* 73-A, 667–74.

Carr, A. J., Morris, R. W., Murray, D. W., and Pynsent, P. B. (1993): Survival analysis in joint replacement surgery. *J Bone Joint Surg* 75-B, 178–82.

Catterall, A. (1971): The natural history of Perthes' disease. *J Bone Joint Surg* 53-B, 37–53.

Charnley, J. (1972): Long term results of low friction arthroplasty of the hip performed as a primary intervention. *J Bone Joint Surg* 54-B, 61–76.

Cohen, M. S., Gelberman, R. H., and Griffin, P. P. (1986): Slipped capital femoral epiphysis: Assessment of epiphyseal displacement and angulation. *J Paediatr Orthop* 6, 259–64.

Danielsson, L. G. (1964): Incidence and prognosis of coxarthrosis. *Acta Orthop Scand* 66S, 1–114

Dawson, J., Fitzpatrick, R., Carr, A., and Murray, D. (1996): Oxford Hip Score: questionnaire on the perceptions of patients about total hip replacement. *J Bone Joint Surg* 78-B, 185–90.

DeLee, I. G., and Charnley (1976): Radiological demarcation of cemented sockets in total hip replacement. *Clin Orthop* 121, 20–31.

Dobbs, H. S. (1980): Survival of total hip replacement. *J Bone Joint Surg* 62-B, 168–73.

Dorey, F., and Amstutz, H. C. (1989): The validity of survivorship analysis in total joint arthroplasty. *J Bone Joint Surg* 71-A, 544–8.

Epstein, H. C. (1974): Posterior fracture dislocations of the hip. Long term follow up. *J Bone Joint Surg* 56-B, 1103–34.

Fergusson, A. B., and Howarth, M. B. (1931): Slipping of the upper femoral epiphysis. *JAMA* 97, 1867–72.

Ficat, R. P. (1985): Idiopathic bone necrosis of the femoral head – early diagnosis and treatment. *J Bone Joint Surg* 67-B, 3–9.

Fitzpatrick, R., Morris, R., Hajat, S., Reeves, B., Murray, D. W., *et al.* (2000): Oxford Hip Score: the value of short and simple measures to assess outcomes for patients of total hip replacement surgery. *Qual Health Care* 9, 146–50.

Gade, H. G. (1947): A contribution to the surgical management of osteoarthritis of the hip joint. A clinical study. *Acta Chir Scand* 1205, 37–45.

Garden, R. (1961): Low-angle fixation in fractures of the femoral neck. *J Bone Joint Surg* 43-B, 647–63.

Goodwin, R. A. (1968): The Austin Moore prosthesis in fresh femoral neck fractures – a review of 611 post-operative cases. *J Orthop Surg* 10, 40–3.

Gruen, T. A., NcNeis, G. M., and Amstutz, H. C. (1979): Modes of failure of cemented stem type femoral components. *Clin Orthop* 141, 17–27.

Gunn, D. M., and Angel, I. C. (1978): Replacement of the femoral head by open operation in severe adolescent slipping of the upper femoral epiphysis. *J Bone Joint Surg* 60-B, 394–403.

Hall, J. E. (1957): The results of the treatment of slipped upper femoral epiphysis. *J Bone Joint Surg* 39, 659–73.

Harris, W. H. (1969): Traumatic arthritis of the hip after dislocation in acetabular fractures treatment by mold arthroplasty. *J Bone Joint Surg* 51-A, 737–55.

Heyman, C. E., and Herdon, C. E. (1950): Legg Calve Perthes' disease: method for the measurement of roentgenographic result. *J Bone Joint Surg* 32-A, 767–8.

Hunt, S. M., and McEwen, J. (1980): The development of a submissive health indicator. *Social Health Illness* 2, 231–46.

Jagal, S., Lakhani, Z., and Schatzer, J. (2000): Reliability, validity, and responsiveness of the lower extremity measure for patients with a hip fracture. *J Bone Joint Surg* 82-A, 955–62.

Johnston, R. C., Fitzgerald, R. H., Harris, W. H., Pass, R., Muller, M. E., and Sledge, C. B. (1990): Clinical and radiographical evaluation of total hip replacements. *J Bone Joint Surg* 72-A, 161–8.

Johnston, R. C., and Larson, C. B. (1969): Results of treatment of hip disorders with cup arthroplasty. *J Bone Joint Surg* 51-A, 1461–76.

Judet, R., and Judet, J. (1952): Technique and results with the acrylic femoral head prosthesis. *J Bone Joint Surg* 34-B, 1973–80.

Katz, J. N., Phillips, C. B., Poss, R., Harrast, J. J., Fossel, A. H., Liang, M. H., and Sledge, C. B. (1995): The validity and reliability of a total hip arthroplasty outcome evaluation questionnaire. *J Bone Joint Surg* 77-A, 1528–34.

Katz, S., Ford, A. B., Moskowitz, R. W., Jackson, B. A., and Jaffe, M. W. (1963): Studies of illness in the aged. The index of ADL: a standardized measure of biological and psychosocial function. *JAMA* 18, 914–19.

Kavanagh, B. F., and Fitzgerald, R. H. (1985): Clinical and roentgenographic assessment of total hip arthroplasty. A new hip score. *Clin Orthop* 193, 133–40.

Kitzhaber, J. A. (1993): The Oregon Health Plan; a process for reform. *J Bone Joint Surg* 75, 1074–9.

Kyle, R. F., Gustino, R. B., and Prenner, R. F. (1979): Analysis of 622 intertrochanteric fractures. *J Bone Joint Surg* 64-A, 206–21.

Larson, C. B. (1963): Rating scale for hip disabilities. *Clin Orthop* 31, 85–93.

Lauritzen (1975): Legg Calve Perthes' disease – a comparative study. *Acta Orthop Scand* 159S, 1–137.

Letournel, E. (1980): Acetabular fractures: classification of management. *Clin Orthop* 151, 81–106.

Lettin, A. W., Ware, H. S., and Morris, R. W. (1991): Survivorship analysis and confidence intervals. *J Bone Joint Surg* 73-B, 729–31.

Liang, M. H., Katz, J. N., Phillips, C., Sledge, C., and Cats-Baril, W. (1991): The total hip arthroplasty outcome evaluation form of the American academy of orthopaedic surgeons. *J Bone Joint Surg* 73-A, 639–46.

Loder, R. T., Arbor, A., and Richards, B. S. (1993): Acute slipped capital femoral epiphysis: the importance of physeal stability. *J Bone Joint Surg* 75-A, 1134–40.

Mahoney, F. I., and Barthel, D. W. (1965): Functional evaluation: the Barthel index. *Maryland State Med J* 14, 61–5.

Maloney, W. I., Krushell, R. I., Jasty, M., and Harris, W. H. (1991): Incidence of heterotopic ossification after total hip replacement: effect of the type of fixation of the femoral component. *J Bone Joint Surg* 73-A, 191–3.

Marcus, N. D., Enneking, W. E., and Massam, R. A. (1973): The silent hip in idiopathic aseptic necrosis. Treatment by bone grafting. *J Bone Joint Surg* 55-A, 1351–66.

Matta, J. M., Anderson, L., Epstein, H., and Hendrick, P. (1986): Fractures of the acetabulum. A retrospective analysis. *Clin Orthop* 205, 230–40.

Matta, J. M., and Merrit, P. O. (1988): Displaced acetabular fractures. *Clin Orthop* 230, 83–97.

McConnell, S., Kolopack, P., and Davis, A. M. (2001): The Western Ontario and McMaster Universities Osteoarthritis Index (WOMAC): a review of its utility and measurement properties. *Arthritis Rheum* 45, 453–61.

McHorney, C. A., Ware, J. E., and Raczek, A. E. (1993): The MOS 36-item Short-Form Health Survey (SF-36): II. Psychometric and clinical test of validity in measuring physical and mental health constructs. *Med Care* 3, 247–63.

Merle d'Aubigne, R., and Postel, M. (1954): Functional results of hip arthroplasty with acrylic prosthesis. *J Bone Joint Surg* 36-A, 451–75.

Meyer, J. (1966): Treatment of Legg Calve Perthes' disease. *Acta Orthop Scand* 86S, 9–111.

Moes, K. (1980): Method of measuring in Legg Calve Perthes' disease with special regard to prognosis. *Clin Orthop* 150, 103–9.

Moes, K., Hjorth, L., Ulfeld, T. M., Christiansen, E. R., and Jensen, A. (1977): Legg Calve Perthes' Disease: the late occurrence of coxarthrosis. *Acta Orthop Scand* 169S, 7–39.

Murray, D. W., Carr, A. J., and Bulstrode, C. (1993): Survival analysis of joint replacements. *J Bone Joint Surg* 75-B, 697–704.

Myers, M. H. (1978): The treatment of osteonecrosis of the hip with fresh osteochondral allografts and with the muscle pedicle graft technique. *Clin Orthop* 130, 202–9.

Myers, M. H. (1983): Surgical treatment of osteonecrosis of the femoral head. In: *Instructional Course Lectures*. The American Academy of Orthopaedic Surgeons. St Louis. C V Mosby, Volume 32, pp. 260–5.

Parker, M. J., Currie, C. T., Mountain, J. A., and Thorngren, K.-G. (1998): Standardised Audit of Hip Fracture in Europe (SAHFE). *Hip International* 8 (10), 15.

Parker, M. J., and Maheshwer, C. B. (1997): Hip score of no value for assessing the results of proximal femoral fracture treatment. *Int Orthop* **21**, 262–4.

Parker, M. J., Myles, J. W., Anand, J. K., and Drewett, R. (1992): Cost-benefit analysis of hip fracture treatment. *J Bone Joint Surg* **74-B**, 261–4.

Parker, M. J., and Palmer, C. R. (1993): A new mobility score for predicting mortality after hip fracture. *J Bone Joint Surg* **75-B**, 797–8.

Parker, M. J., and Pryor, G. A. (1993): *Hip Fracture Management*. Blackwell Scientific Publications, Oxford.

Pellicci, P. M., Wilson, P. D., Sledge, C. B., Salvati, E. A., Ranawat, C. S., Poss, R., and Callaghan, J. J. (1985): Long term results of revision total hip replacement. *J Bone Joint Surg* **67-A**, 513–16.

Peto, R., Pike, M. C., Armitage, P., Breslow, N. E., Cox, D. R., Howard, S. V., Mantel, N., McPherson, K., Peto, I., and Smith, P. G. (1977): Design and analysis of randomised clinical trials requiring prolonged observation of each patient. *Br J Cancer* **35**, 1–39.

Pryor, G. A. (1990): A study of the influence of technical adequacy on the clinical result of Moore hemiarthroplasty. *Injury* **21**, 361–5.

Salter, R. B., and Thompson, G. H. (1984): Legg Calve Perthes. The prognostic significance of the subchondral fracture in the two group classification of femoral head involvement. *J Bone Joint Surg* **66-A**, 479.

Salvati, E. A., and Wilson, P. D. (1973): Long-term results of femoral-head replacement. *J Bone Joint Surg* **55-A**, 516–24.

Severin, E. (1941): Contribution to the knowledge of congenital dislocation of the hip joint. Late results of closed reduction and arthrographic studies of recent cases. *Acta Chir Scand* **84**, (Suppl.) 63, 1–142.

Shepherd, M. M. (1954): Assessment of function after arthroplasty of the hip. *J Bone Joint Surg* **36-B**, 354–63.

Söderman, P., and Malchau, H. (2000): Validity and reliability of Swedish (WOMAC) osteoarthritis index: a self-administered disease-specific questionnaire vs. generic instruments (SF36 and NHP). *Acta Orthop Scand* **71**, 39–46.

Söderman, P., and Malchau, H. (2001): Is the Harris hip score system useful to study the outcome of total hip replacement? *Clin Orthop* **384**, 189–97.

Stinchfield, F. E., Cooperman, B., and Shea, C. E. (1957): Replacement of the femoral head by Judet or Austin Moore prosthesis. *J Bone Joint Surg* **39-A**, 1043–58.

Thomas, D. I., and Bannister, G. C. (1991): Exchange arthroplasty best for infected total hip replacement. *Hip International* **1**, 17–20.

Tonnis, D. (1987): *Congenital Dysplasia and Dislocation of the Hip in Children and Adults*. Springer-Verlag, Berlin.

Wiberg, G. (1939): Studies on the dysplastic acetabular and congenital subluxation of the hip joint: with special reference to the complication of osteoarthritis. *Acta Surg Scand* **83S**, 58.

Williams, A. (1991): Setting priorities in health care: an economist's view. *J Bone Joint Surg* **73-B**, 365–7.

Wilson, P. D., Amstutz, H. C., Czerniecki, A., Salvati, E. A., and Mendes, D. G. (1972): Total hip replacement with fixation by acrylic cement. *J Bone Joint Surg* **54-A**, 207–36.

Zuckerman, J. D., Koval, K. J., Aharonoff, G. B., Hiebert, R., and Skovron, M. L. (2000a): A functional recovery score for elderly hip fracture patients I. Development. *J Orthop Trauma* **14**, 20–5.

Zuckerman, J. D., Koval, K. J., Aharonoff, G. B., and Skovron, M. L. (2000b): A functional recovery score for elderly hip fracture patients: II. Validity and reliability. *J Orthop Trauma* **14**, 26–30.

20

Tibial and femoral shafts

Badri Narayan, Raman V. Kalyan and David R. Marsh

INTRODUCTION

The measurement of outcome following diaphyseal fractures in the lower limbs takes place on three levels:

- The measurement of long-bone fracture healing *per se*, which is appropriately covered in this chapter because these are the injuries in which it is most often problematic. This would include the attainment of surgical objectives such as union (as well as the speed with which that is achieved) and the occurrence of complications such as malunion or infection.

- The measurement of lower-limb function. Instruments which quantify this have been developed primarily to assess the joints adjacent to the long bones rather than the shafts themselves.

- The inclusion of ambulatory capacity as a component of overall musculoskeletal function or generic health status.

It is interesting to note that, although they are interdependent and inseparable, the three levels are ranked in descending order of what surgeons would regard as the challenge facing them, but in ascending order of what is important to the patient in a holistic sense. Therefore, although the first level is that on which we have to strive to improve surgical technique, the proof of efficacy of our advances rests on their reflection in patient-centred outcomes. Furthermore, the pay-off to the patient of investment in the rehabilitation and holistic elements of

the trauma team may be as great, or greater than investment in the surgical element.

As with all outcome measurement, the results on all three levels cannot be properly interpreted without evaluation of the severity of injury, since the latter determines the outcome of treatment more than anything else. This chapter will therefore start with consideration of how femoral and tibial shaft fractures may be classified in terms of their severity. We will then consider measures of bone healing (including surgical complications), followed by regional and generic measures of outcome. In order not to clutter the text, many of the scoring systems are detailed in Appendix Tables 20-A.1 to 20-A.7 (see pp. 294–300).

ASSESSMENT OF SEVERITY OF FEMORAL AND TIBIAL SHAFT FRACTURES

The classic papers of Ellis (1958) and Nicoll (1964) both used the same three elements in grading the severity of tibial fractures: degree of displacement; comminution; and the magnitude of the soft-tissue wound. Since then, these elements have remained the three cardinal components, though various authors have differed in the importance they attach to each one.

Fracture displacement

Sarmiento and colleagues (Sarmiento *et al.* 1995) and Marsh (1998) both found displacement of the fracture ends, as seen on the presenting radiograph, to be a strong predictor of outcome in conservatively treated tibial shaft fractures. Ilizarov (1992), in his treatise on fine-wire fixation, agreed with this point. On the other hand, Gaston *et al.* (1999) found displacement to be irrelevant to the outcome in a series of similar fractures treated by intramedullary (IM) nailing. To the extent that displacement does indicate severity, the basis on which it does so is likely to be the stripping of the soft-tissue envelope from the bone surface.

Fracture comminution

The AO school (Müller *et al.* 1990) maintain that displacement is not relevant, arguing that X-radiographs taken in hospital may not represent the degree of displacement at the time of injury. These authors emphasized comminution of the fracture; the degree of comminution on the radiograph of course reflects the amount of energy absorbed by the bone. They based their morphological classification on that of Johner and Wruhs (1983), with three groups – A, B and C – representing the degree of comminution, and each group subclassified as 1, 2 and 3 representing morphological pattern as determined by injury mechanism, in ascending order of direct violence. The AO classification of long-bone fractures was subsequently adopted by the Orthopaedic Trauma Association in 1991, with the avowed purpose of enhancing uniformity of comparison of different forms of treatment.

Comminution-based classifications combine two points. The first point is a measure of the energy of injury, as evidenced by the degree of breaking-up of the bone. The second point is a description of morphological features with therapeutically significant consequences, such as axial instability. Recent attempts to develop the first aspect into an energy-based measure of fracture severity have involved techniques for calculating the total area of fracture surfaces from computed tomography (CT) images (Beardsley *et al.* 2002), but this approach has not yet been developed for routine use.

The AO classification does not perform well in terms of either reliability or validity. Johnstone *et al.* (1993) showed 10 radiographs of fractures of different long-bone segments to 18 observers and found poor inter-observer reliability: on average, only 32 per cent of observers agreed with the final consensus classification. Incorrect answers were given by 66 per cent of observers with previous experience of the AO classification and 69 per cent of inexperienced observers. The authors submitted that a 'consensus classification' was more appropriate than attempted individual classification of fractures.

Swiontkowski *et al.* (2000) questioned the validity of the AO classification as a measure of severity, on the basis of its poor prediction of outcome. In 200 patients with isolated lower-limb fractures, outcome at 6 and 12 months differed only between type C fractures and the rest. The paper in discussion looked at clinical outcomes of fractures of the entire lower limb, from the proximal femur to the distal tibia; and the type C fractures in question included not only those with diaphyseal comminution, but also severe articular fractures. However, the authors suggested that fracture pattern in purely diaphyseal fractures – that is, simple A-type, wedge B-type and the fragmented C-type – was unlikely to affect patient outcome. It must be borne in mind though that the entire patient population was treated in Level I trauma centres, and outcomes between the various subsets of diaphyseal fractures may well vary between different centres.

Despite its questionable validity, the AO-OTA classification has been more or less accepted as providing at least some degree of uniformity for purposes of peer review and for aggregating case series. It may also provide a framework for treatment planning. However, the role of this purely morphological classification system as a predictor of outcome remains doubtful.

Winquist and Hansen (1980) classified the comminution patterns of femoral shaft fractures in order to provide a guide for intramedullary nailing technique. They identified five degrees of stability – segmental and four grades of comminuted fracture (types I–IV). Fractures of grades I and II were considered to be axially and rotationally stable following

IM nailing; grades III and IV require interlocking screws. Although the Winquist classification is widely used to describe comminution both in femoral and tibial shaft fracture, it has not so far been subject to the same rigorous examination of its reliability and validity as the AO classification.

Soft-tissue injury

Damage to the soft tissues adjacent to the fracture is recognized as being a key determinant of outcome, through loss of vascularity, susceptibility to microbial invasion and, probably, inflammatory mediators. As with comminution, measurement of severity is difficult. Methods for quantitating blood flow are only experimental, and clinical practice and research depend on subjective, ordinal scales of damage to muscle, skin and subcutaneous tissue. The well-known Gustilo-Anderson classification (Gustilo and Anderson 1976; Gustilo et al. 1984) was initially shown to be predictive of complications such as infection and amputation and is the de-facto standard. It must be applied after debridement of the fracture, but even then shows poor to moderate reliability (Brumback and Jones 1994). Recent advances in the medical and surgical management of open fractures may well render the distinction between the Grade 2, 3A and the less severe 3B fractures somewhat superfluous as a means of predicting the same complications. On the other hand, all surgeons know that the more severe 3B fractures are a completely different proposition, with a much worse outlook.

Krettek et al. (2001) used the Hannover Fracture Scale (HFS-98) in the prospective evaluation of 87 open long-bone fractures (see Appendix; Table 20-A.1). The HFS-98, which is an advanced version of the original Hannover Fracture Scale, attempts to provide an ordinal scale for the quantification of soft-tissue injury in open fractures. The authors reported a correlation between an increasing HFS score and a worse Gustilo grade, and therefore suggested that the HFS-98 be used in all open fractures to provide a practical and standardized method to evaluate open fractures. The advantage of a numerical score is enticing, as the Gustilo 3A and 3B fractures represent a wide spectrum of injury severity. However, further independent validation of the HFS-98 as a means of evaluating outcome in open fractures is awaited.

The Gustilo grade is only relevant to open fractures, whereas soft tissues are clearly also damaged in closed fractures. Tscherne's grading system (see Appendix; Table 20-A.2) applies to closed as well as open fractures, and represents a measure of the energy absorbed by the soft tissues. Some authors have reported that it predicts outcome somewhat better than the Gustilo grade (Gaston et al. 1999).

Energy of injury

The very least categorization of injury severity that must be reported along with measures of outcome in any series is that into high- and low-energy injury mechanisms. An example of the dangers of failing to do this is an early publication on the treatment of pilon fractures (Ruedi and Allgower 1979), which argued the case for early open reduction and internal fixation. The series consisted of predominantly low-energy injuries, but the message was that this form of treatment was good for pilon fractures in general. Many infected non-unions of high-energy pilon fractures resulted from uncritical acceptance of this idea.

Bauer et al. (1962) first attempted to grade the causative energy as either 'high' or 'low'. High-energy fractures include all those where a motor-vehicle, or motorcycle is involved, falls from a height of more than 2 metres, and fractures caused by blows from heavy objects. Low-energy fractures include those caused by falls at ground level or from a low level, injuries from sport, and those in which motor vehicles are not involved. Using this classification in a prospective study of 100 non-operatively treated fractures of the tibial shaft, Oni et al. (1988) found a very significant correlation between energy of injury and speed of healing.

It would seem logical therefore that fracture energy – using either the simple classification of Bauer or the more refined Tscherne classification – be included as a stratification variable in the reporting of any study analysing outcomes after tibial and femoral fractures.

Mangled extremity scores

The decision of whether or not to salvage a severely injured limb and attempt to reconstruct it has traditionally been made on an intuitive basis, often based on the treating surgeon's past experiences with that type of injury. There is a demand for a scoring system to help decide what type of injury can be salvaged, taking into account the function of the salvaged limb as opposed to a prosthetic replacement. The mere preservation of the limb should not nowadays be considered a therapeutic success.

Several scores, of varying degrees of complexity, have appeared over the past few years (Table 20.1). Of these schemes, the Mangled Extremity Severity Score (MESS) (Johansen *et al.* 1990) remains the most popular (see Appendix; Table 20-A.3), perhaps because of its simplicity, or perhaps the catchiness of the acronym! A fundamental criticism of many of the published studies is that they judge the scores on the basis of their ability to predict the decisions taken by the surgeons involved; they do not question whether those decisions were correct. Few studies use the functional outcome of reconstruction or amputation as their validating criterion.

An ideal score should be sensitive (i.e. a limb needing an amputation should always have a score above the threshold described in the score), and specific (i.e. all salvageable limbs should have a score below the threshold described in the score). Most scores described for limb salvage have been derived from retrospective data, and the five most popular are the subject of an independent, prospective appraisal in the ongoing LEAP trial (Lower Extremity Assessment Project), under the aegis of the National Institutes of Health, USA.

Table 20.1: Comparison of the commonly used Extremity Severity Scores (after Bosse *et al.* 2001, with permission)

	MESS[1]	LSI[2]	PSI[3]	NISSA[4]	HFS-97[5]
Age	+			+	
Shock	+			+	+
Warm ischaemia time	+	+	+	+	+
Bone injury		+	+		+
Muscle injury		+	+		
Skin injury		+			+
Nerve injury		+		+	+
Deep vein injury		+			
Skeletal/soft-tissue injury	+			+	
Contamination				+	+
Time to treatment			+		

[1] Mangled Extremity Severity Score (Johansen *et al.* 1990).
[2] Limb Salvage Index (Russell *et al.* 1991).
[3] Predictive Salvage Index (Howe *et al.* 1987).
[4] Nerve Injury, Ischemia, Soft-Tissue Injury, Skeletal Injury, and Age of Patient Score (McNamara *et al.* 1994).
[5] Hannover Fracture Scale-1997 (Sudkamp *et al.* 1993).

Bosse *et al.* (2001) published a critical evaluation on the prospective use of the five scores mentioned in Table 20.1, as part of the LEAP project. In summary, the authors found that each of the scores offered varying degrees of sensitivity and specificity, depending on whether the injury was open or closed, or whether there was an associated ischaemia. However, none was sufficiently sensitive or specific to be consistently helpful in decision-making for limb salvage. These authors concluded that the scores had limited usefulness, and should be used with caution by the treating surgeon who must decide the fate of a lower extremity with a high-energy injury.

BONE HEALING AND COMPLICATIONS

However much they accept the importance of a holistic view of fracture patients and their outcomes, surgeons will always regard the primary goal of their efforts as being the achievement of bone union without complications. *Assurance of healing* is to be distinguished from *speed of union*, and the former would generally be regarded as more important in high-energy injuries. The need for secondary intervention to achieve union is also an important outcome of the primary treatment. None of these concepts can be utilized without a definition of fracture union and a means of establishing that it has occurred.

This subsection deals first with the measurement, including progress of fracture healing in the tibia and femur. This is followed by a discussion on the two important complications of fracture treatment, malunion and infection.

Measures of fracture healing (and non-union)

The identification of completion of union across a femoral or tibial diaphyseal fracture, though superficially simple, remains a vexed issue.

CLINICAL CRITERIA

Sarmiento *et al.* (1984) specified criteria for the judgement of union:

- the ability of the patient to bear weight without pain;
- the absence of clinically detectable movement across the fracture; and
- visible bridging callus across the fracture on plain radiographs.

While these criteria are applicable to non-operative treatment of tibial fractures, the first two cannot be used in fractures treated by fixation, either internal or external.

MECHANICAL CRITERIA

A fully united fracture will be stable to bending and/or torsion. The ability to resist such a force will remain the 'gold standard' of a healed fracture for purposes of experimental study in animal models, but is obviously difficult to carry out in the clinical setting. A bending stiffness of 15 Nm per degree in the sagittal plane was described as being diagnostic of union across a tibial fracture treated by external fixation (Richardson *et al.* 1994). This particular instrumented method of diagnosing union cannot be applied to fractures treated by any method other than half-pin external fixation or conservatively and is very difficult to apply to a femoral fracture.

Kay *et al.* (1992) and Marsh (1998) also used bending strength to assess union across non-operatively treated tibial shaft fractures, and reported good correlation between mechanical behaviour and the state of healing of tibial fractures.

It is tempting to try to reproduce manually a bending force corresponding to 15 Nm per degree in the out-patient setting to check for union across tibial fractures, but an attempt to do this proved consistently unsuccessful (Webb *et al.* 1996).

RADIOLOGICAL CRITERIA

The judgement of union from radiographs forms the mainstay of clinical practice; unfortunately, this remains a contentious issue. The correlation between radiological appearances and mechanical strength of a fracture was addressed in experimental osteotomies by Panjabi *et al.* (1985), who reported that best single predictor of mechanical strength was cortical continuity.

However, others (Hammer *et al.* 1985) compared mechanical testing in human tibial fractures (using a sling to measure deflection) with radiographs, and suggested that there was poor correlation between mechanical strength of the fracture and radiological appearances across it. A five-point scale (Table 20.2) was produced to assess progress of healing, based on the presence of callus and the visibility of the fracture line.

Sharrard (1990), in a report which discussed the role of electromagnetic stimulation in the treatment of delayed union of tibial fractures, emphasized that absence of movement in a tibial fracture was not necessarily associated with a healed appearance on radiographs. An orthopaedic surgeon and a radiologist assessed progress towards union of tibial diaphyseal fractures using slightly different criteria, and there seemed to be broad agreement in the interpretation of healing. Interestingly, the radiologist placed more emphasis on continuity of cortices, and the orthopaedic surgeon on continuity of cancellous bone.

Other authors (Lane and Sandhu 1987; Tower *et al.* 1993) have also produced scoring systems to evaluate fracture callus. Panjabi and colleagues (Panjabi *et al.* 1989), in another experimental study, found significant inconsistency when clinicians

attempted to assess healing (and therefore, the mechanical strength) across an osteotomy based on radiographs alone.

In a recent study, Whelan *et al.* (2002) examined inter-observer and intra-observer variation in the assessment of healing of tibial fractures. Orthopaedic surgeons achieved moderate inter-observer reliability (kappa 0.6) when using the criteria of Hammer (Hammer *et al.* 1985). Interestingly, almost the same amount of agreement (kappa 0.65) was reached when surgeons evaluated the same radiographs using an 'overall rating' – this was a non-ordinal system based on the considered (and probably largely instinctive) judgement of healing, and subdivided into 'healed', 'probably healed', 'indeterminate', 'probably not healed', 'not healed', without the use of definite criteria for allocation into each group. The highest inter-observer agreement (kappa 0.75) was regarding the determination of the number of cortices bridged by callus. The authors considered this finding significant. On the other hand, intra-observer agreement was highest for overall impression of healing (kappa 0.89), and rather surprisingly, least for the Hammer scale (kappa 0.76).

Since the surgeons' 'overall impression' of fracture healing was as reliable in this study as using the criteria of Hammer *et al.* (1985), the authors questioned the need for having any rating system for fracture healing beyond an overall assessment. In view of the findings of others (Panjabi *et al.* 1985), who proved that cortical continuity was the

Table 20.2: Assessment of fracture healing on radiographs. Reprinted from Hammer *et al.* (1985)

	Radiological assessment		
Grade	Callus formation	Fracture line	Stage of union
1	Homogeneous bone structure	Obliterated	Achieved
2	Massive callus. Bone trabeculae crossing fracture site	Barely discernible	Achieved
3	Apparent callus. Bridging of fracture line	Discernible	Uncertain
4	Trace of callus. No bridging of fracture line	Distinct	Not achieved
5	No callus formation	Distinct	Not achieved

best predictor of mechanical strength, the authors suggested that measurement of number of cortices bridged was the most reliable measure to assess fracture healing.

The findings of the above study apply to a vast majority of tibial fractures treated by IM nailing, but may not be applicable to fractures treated by external fixation, which heal largely by endosteal callus. With the advent of digital radiography, it is hoped that quantitative methods of estimating endosteal and periosteal healing will be produced, and the correlation between 'radiological', 'mechanical', and 'clinical' union established.

Malunion

While it is the ideal goal of treatment of a tibial or femoral fracture to return the bone to its exact anatomical alignment, this is not always easily achieved, or may come with a high price in terms of invasiveness of the surgery. It is therefore imperative that a treating surgeon is aware of what constitutes 'acceptable' alignment of the limb after fracture, and what degree of deformity would reliably be predicted to be deleterious to long-term function of the limb.

The clinical evidence is conflicting. For tibial fractures, Merchant and Dietz (1989) suggested that deformity greater than 5° was associated with radiographic changes in the ankle, but Kristinsen et al. (1989), in the same year, presented data showing no radiographic changes with deformity up to 10°. Later, van der Schoot et al. (1996) reported a significant relationship between tibial malunion and the risk of degenerative changes in the knee and ankle.

These publications discuss degrees of malunion purely in terms of the angle of the deformity, without description of deviation of the mechanical axis, which depends also on the location of the fracture in the shaft and any translational malalignment, and which must be the real basis for any deleterious consequences for neighbouring joints. For example, varus malalignment of a proximal tibial fracture causes a more marked shift of the mechanical axis and consequent increase in medial compartmental loading than a similar degree of varus malalignment in a distal tibial fracture.

Traditionally, malunion has been divided into that occurring in the coronal plane (valgus/varus), sagittal plane (procurvatum/recurvatum), and transverse plane (internal or external rotation). In addition, shortening across a fracture can also be considered a deformity in the longitudinal plane. Fractures of course, do not malunite across a single anatomical plane, but in an 'oblique' plane.

While very little has been published concerning the consequences of femoral shaft malunion, many papers have addressed tibial malunion. The differing thresholds for significance of a tibial malunion, collected from 10 different studies (Lindsey and Blair 1996) are shown in Table 20.3.

Shortening across the fracture, with its perceived effects on gait, aesthetics, and long-term effects on the lumbar spine has fairly strict criteria for degree of acceptability. Most authors accept a shortening of no more than 10 mm.

The acceptable degree of deformity may well be dependent on the individual patient's functional expectations and demands, and this reinforces the need for the use of patient-orientated measures of outcome, rather than clinician-derived outcomes. It is suggested that any publication on malunion following tibial shaft fractures should include data derived from long-leg radiographs taken in the erect position (for example, see Tuten et al. 1999) in order to provide a true representation of the mechanical axis.

Infection

The identification of infection in bone depends on the application of clinical judgement and the appropriate use of investigations such as technetium scanning, labelled scans, and magnetic resonance imaging and/or CT. The use of molecular diagnostic methods, such as polymerase chain reaction (PCR) techniques (Hoeffel et al. 1999), is still in the realm of research.

In an attempt to reduce ambiguity in definition, The Surgical Infection Study Group (Peel and Taylor 1991) produced standardized definitions of

Table 20.3: Criteria traditionally used to diagnose a tibial malunion (after Lindsey and Blair 1996, reproduced with permission from the American Academy of Orthopaedic Surgeons)

Authors	Varus	Valgus	Anterior/ Posterior	Rotation	Shortening
Bone and Johnson (1986)		5		15–20	10
Bostman (1983)	5	5			10
Collins et al. (1990)	5	5	5–10		10
Haines et al. (1984)	4	4		5	13
Jensen et al. (1977)	8	8	15		20
Johner and Wruhs (1983)	5	5	10	10	
Nicoll (1964)	10	10	10	10	20
Puno et al. (1991)	10	10	20		20
Trafton (1988)	5	5	10	10	20
Van der Werken and Marti (1983)				15–20	

postoperative infection:

- A 'minor' infection is defined as discharge of pus from the wound, without lymphangitis or deep tissue destruction.

- A 'major' infection is defined as 'purulent discharge accompanied by painful or complete dehiscence of the fascial layers of the wound, or by spreading cellulites and lymphangitis that requires antibiotic therapy'.

- 'Early' postoperative infection in bone is defined by the presence of pain at rest, a fever of greater than 38°C persisting for more than 48 hours, supported by the isolation of bacteria from cultures where available.

- 'Late' postoperative infection is indicated by the presence of pain at rest, a persisting elevation of the erythrocyte sedimentation rate (ESR) greater than 30 mm above the preoperative level, radiological changes in bone indicative of infection, and the isolation of bacteria from cultures where available.

- Infection after implant surgery is indicated by the presence of one or more of the following: pain, persistent pyrexia greater than 38°C for 48 hours, local signs of inflammation where the implant is superficial, radiological signs where the implant involves, or is adjacent to bone, and an elevated white cell count.

However, the Public Health Laboratory Service (2000), as part of the Nosocomial Infection National Surveillance Group has chosen to classify postoperative infection into three different types:

- 'Superficial infection' is defined as that involving only the skin and subcutaneous tissues of the incision.

- 'Deep infection' involves the fascial or muscle layers of the incision.

- 'Organ or space infections' involve any area other than the incision opened or manipulated during the procedure.

Interpretation of infection requires considerable judgement and thought, and the amount of inter-observer variation in diagnosis has been documented (Platt et al. 2001). The above definitions can also be quite difficult to apply in implant-related orthopaedic infections, where the symptoms and signs are often more subtle. This unfortunately detracts from their use in orthopaedic literature.

Table 20.4: Classification of tibial osteomyelitis (after May *et al.* 1989)

Type	Description	Expected rehabilitation
I	Intact tibia and fibula	6–12 weeks
II	Intact tibia with bone graft needed for support	3–6 months
III	Tibial defect less than 6 cm, intact fibula	6–12 months
IV	Tibial defect more than 6 cm, intact fibula	12–18 months
V	Tibial defect more than 6 cm, fibula not usable	>18 months

OSTEOMYELITIS

Bony infection, whether as a consequence of injury or related to surgical intervention, is a dreaded complication. The classification of bony infection may be useful if it can be used as a guide to treatment or prognosis. In this context, the classical classifications of Waldvogel *et al.* (1970), while being descriptive, have no therapeutic or prognostic significance.

Others (May *et al.* 1989) developed a classification system for osteomyelitis of the tibia after debridement (Table 20.4). This classification provided a guideline for selecting the type of skeletal reconstruction, including probable time for rehabilitation.

This classification is of course applicable only to infections involving the tibia, is based on the probability of using the fibula as a donor to replace tibial loss, and has therefore not found wide favour.

The most modern classification for bony infection was proposed by Cierny *et al.* (1985), and incorporates the segmental location of infection within a bone (Table 20.5). The physiology of the host, which has a major role to play in infection, is included by subdividing hosts into different classes based on either local or systemic compromise.

Although the Cierny-Mader classification has not been validated, it offers a method of classification that is applicable throughout the skeleton, is easy to understand, and includes systemic factors that play an important role in the body's defence against infection.

Table 20.5: Classification system for osteomyelitis. Reprinted from Cierny *et al.* (1985)

Stage	Anatomic type
I	Medullary osteomyelitis
II	Superficial osteomyelitis
III	Localized osteomyelitis
IV	Diffuse osteomyelitis

Physiological class	Feature
A	Normal
Bl	Local compromise[*]
Bs	Systemic compromise[§]
Bls	Both
C	Treatment worse than disease

[*]Chronic lymphoedema; venous stasis; major vessel compromise; arteritis; extensive fibrosis; radiation scarring; small-vessel disease; tobacco abuse (>20 cigarettes/day).
[§]Malnutrition, renal or hepatic failure; diabetes mellitus; chronic hypoxia; immune disease; malignancy; extremes of age; immunosuppression or immune deficiency.

The treatment of diffuse osteomyelitis in a long bone involves major limb reconstructive surgery, and outcome following treatment of this nature does not lend itself to assessment by conventional scoring systems. The Toronto Extremity Salvage Score (Davis *et al.* 1996) has been tested for reliability and validity in the context of surgery in musculoskeletal tumours (Davis *et al.* 1999); its use following limb reconstruction for infected non-union requires to be tested, however.

MEASURES OF LOWER-LIMB FUNCTION

With modern-day treatment, a vast majority of femoral and tibial diaphyseal fractures heal without major morbidity and complications. However, as Benirschke *et al.* (1993) established, this does not necessarily mean that patients are happy. Outcome analysis must include – and indeed be focused on – the functional deficits that patients are often left with. The various instruments quantifying functional capacity and symptomatology must be deployed at an appropriate time, and not too soon after the fracture is treated. A final review at two years should be standard, although some issues, such as secondary osteoarthritis, may need even longer.

In the past, scoring systems (Johner and Wruhs 1983) have been used to analyse variables such as alignment of the fracture, knee and ankle function, pain and gait, and a nominal rating of 'excellent', 'good', 'fair', or 'poor' has been assigned to each. Though simple to use, this method of scoring is clearly inappropriate because a fracture may score 'excellent' on one or two variables and 'poor' in some, thus causing ambiguity in the final analysis. Interestingly, this method of analysing outcome following tibial diaphyseal fractures has been followed as late as 2001 (Toivanen *et al.* 2001).

Since the mid-1980s, there has been a proliferation of scores designed to provide numerical values for knee and ankle function following knee injury, ligamentous reconstruction, and in degenerative disease; these scoring systems have been applied to the analysis of outcome following tibial fractures.

Often, these scores are relatively insensitive to the degrees of morbidity seen after fracture in adjacent joints, leading to a ceiling effect. However, as detailed later, even a minor drop in these scores can be perceived as significant by the patient. Following tibial fracture, it is desirable to evaluate both the knee and ankle, because minor impairment in the ankle can also lead to functional disability in jobs that involve kneeling or similar movement.

Knee scores

The details of the individual components of each of the knee scores are more appropriately covered in Chapter 21. Suffice to say, all of the knee score systems are weighted for pain, function, range of motion and instability in varying proportions. It is obvious however that most isolated tibial fractures will have little, if any, effect on range of motion and instability of the knee.

The Iowa knee and ankle scores, derived from the existing Iowa Hip Score (Dietz 2001) were first described in 1989 as a means of measuring outcome following tibial shaft fractures. To the knowledge of the authors and the originators (Dietz 2001), the score has not been validated. However, this scoring system has been used in one prospective study (Toivanen *et al.* 2002) and also in three retrospective studies (Bone *et al.* 1997; Dogra *et al.* 2000, 2002) since its original description.

The fact that most united tibial fractures have a very high Iowa knee score would seem to detract from the value of using it to measure outcome. However, Dogra *et al.* (2002) noted that there was a strong correlation between the Iowa knee and ankle score and the physical and mental summary components of the SF-36, suggesting that even a minor drop in the Iowa score is associated with a global physical and functional deficit.

Validated knee scores such as the Cincinnati (Noyes *et al.* 1989), Lysholm (Lysholm and Gillquist 1982) and Tegner (Tegner *et al.* 1988) scores have also been used in the assessment of function following united tibial fractures (Tuten *et al.* 1999; Boyd *et al.* 2001). It should be borne in mind however that these knee scores have been validated for assessment of function following knee injuries and not tibial fractures *per se*. Also, the tests of validation have been performed on a group of people who are active in sports; this validation may not apply to the less homogeneous population sustaining tibial fractures.

An additional confounding factor that is, perhaps, unique to fractures is the need to evaluate function in the joint above *and* below. This can lead to a spuriously low score in *both* joints where function is measured, whereas the morbidity is actually in one joint – for example, a patient who is unable to squat because of difficulty in dorsiflexion of the *ankle* would, by definition have a lower *knee* score, because of the construct of the questionnaire.

Interestingly, Toivanen *et al.* (2002) evaluated a system for functional evaluation of the knee, based on the ability of the patient to perform activities such as one-leg jumping, duck-walking, ability to perform repeated squatting, and the ability to kneel (Table 20.6). These authors reported a good correlation between the score derived from this functional evaluation and the Lysholm and Iowa knee scores. Though the repeated performance of these tasks is not strictly a part of normal knee function, such an evaluation may well be suited to the rigorous evaluation of lower limb function following tibial fractures.

A summary of the commonly used knee scores to evaluate function after tibial diaphyseal fractures is shown in Table 20.7.

Table 20.6: Functional evaluation of the knee following tibial shaft fractures (after Toivanen *et al.* 2002)

Parameter	Score 0	1	2	3
One-leg jumping and duck-walking	Unable to perform, or intense pain			Able to perform without pain
25-repetition full squats	Unable to squat	1–10 squats without pain	11–20 squats without pain	More than 20 squats
Ability to kneel	Impossible	Less than 10 seconds without pain	10–20 seconds without pain	No time limitation

Table 20.7: Summary of the knee scores used in tibial shaft fractures

Instrument name (Reference)	What it measures	Validation	Reliability	Responsiveness	Usage	Score
Iowa Knee Score (Merchant and Dietz 1989)	Knee function	0	0	0	4	4
Lysholm Knee Score (Lysholm and Gillquist 1982)	Knee function	1	1	1	1	4
Tegner Activity Score (Tegner *et al.* 1988)	Knee function	1	1	1	1	4
Cincinnati Activity Evaluation (Noyes *et al.* 1989)	Knee function	1	1	1	1	4

Ankle scores

As alluded to earlier, the Iowa Ankle Score was developed from a model of pre-existing ankle scores and used to measure morbidity around the ankle following tibial diaphyseal fractures. Since its inception in 1989, the score has been used in four peer-reviewed publications (Merchant and Dietz 1989; Bone *et al.* 1997; Dogra *et al.* 2000, 2002). The score is yet to be validated.

Kitaoka *et al.* (1994) described a 100-point score to evaluate function of the ankle and hindfoot (the ankle and hindfoot score of the American Orthopaedic Foot and Ankle Society; AOFAS). Although this score has rapidly gained popularity, it remains to be validated. Subsequently, Tuten *et al.* (1999) used the AOFAS score to evaluate function in a series of tibial diaphyseal fractures. Unpublished data from the senior author's department in Belfast has shown excellent correlation ($r^2 = 0.92$) between the Iowa Ankle Score and the AOFAS ankle and hindfoot score after tibial pilon fractures.

Olerud and Molander (1984) reported a 100-point score to evaluate ankle function following surgical treatment of ankle fractures. To the present authors' knowledge, the only publication that has used the Olerud and Molander ankle score to evaluate ankle function after tibial diaphyseal fractures is that of Skoog *et al.* (2001). This score has not been validated, and the weighting of its components has

been subject to some criticism in the past (Simpson 1994).

A summary of the commonly used ankle scores to evaluate function after tibial diaphyseal fractures is shown in Table 20.8.

Femoral diaphyseal fractures

This subsection deals with measurement of outcome following femoral diaphyseal fractures alone. Fractures of the proximal and distal femur are discussed in Chapters 19 and 21.

Femoral shaft fractures are routinely treated by IM nailing, with an expected union rate of between 95 and 99 per cent, and infrequent malunion or infection (Wolinsky *et al.* 2001). Current debate is focussed largely on antegrade versus retrograde nailing, and reamed versus unreamed nailing. Outcomes following femoral shaft fractures have traditionally concentrated on gross issues such as mortality, length of hospital stay, whether union is achieved, at what point union is achieved, and complications of treatment (Fakhry *et al.* 1994; Smith *et al.* 1990) rather than on subtle functional problems.

Thoresen *et al.* (1985) were perhaps the first to produce a tabular form of measuring outcome (Table 20.9) following treatment of femoral shaft fractures. In common with many other systems

Table 20.8: Summary of the ankle scores used in tibial shaft fractures

Instrument name (Reference)	What it measures	Validation	Reliability	Responsiveness	Usage	Score
Iowa Ankle Score (Merchant and Dietz 1989)	Ankle function	0	0	0	3	3
AOFAS Ankle-Hindfoot Score (Kitaoka *et al.* 1994)	Ankle function	0	0	0	I	I
Olerud and Molander Score (Olerud and Molander 1984)	Ankle function	0	0	0	I	I

Table 20.9: Thoresen's criteria (Thoresen *et al.* 1985, with permission) to evaluate function after a femoral diaphyseal fracture

| Variable | Result | | | |
	Excellent	Good	Fair	Poor
Malalignment				
Varus/valgus	5	5	10	>10
Procurvatum/recurvatum	5	10	15	>15
Internal rotation	5	10	15	>15
External rotation	10	15	20	>20
Shortening (in cm)	1	2	3	>3
Range of motion (knee)				
Flexion	>120	120	90	<90
Extension deficit	5	10	15	>15
Pain or swelling	None	Sporadic, Minor	Significant	Severe

developed during that time, this system suffers from one major inadequacy – namely that a patient may fall into different groups for different criteria, thus causing ambiguity in the interpretation of the final outcome. In addition, it is felt that the differences in rotation of 5° are difficult to measure and should not be used to stratify results. Interestingly, this method of assessing outcome has been recently used in a peer-reviewed publication (Arazi *et al.* 2001).

Also during 1985, another report was published which described a scoring system to evaluate the results of femoral shaft fractures (Cheng *et al.* 1985). This system, which was very similar to that of Thoresen and colleagues, has (to the best of our knowledge) not been used in peer-reviewed papers after its initial appearance.

A more recent report (Bain *et al.* 1997) brought attention to the not insignificant morbidity around the hip following antegrade nailing. Although this study included patients who had undergone closed femoral shortening as well as nailing for fractures, the morbidity – which included heterotopic ossification and abductor weakness – was considered to be consequent on the nailing procedure rather than the injury. Hip scores combined with generic measures of outcome have not been used to assess function after femoral fractures in adults.

Assessment of the knee following treatment of femoral fractures has usually concentrated on range of motion (Thoresen *et al.* 1985). With the increasing popularity of retrograde femoral nailing, assessment of subtle functional deficits in the knee, using established scoring systems, may well be an issue in the long term following this procedure, particularly following experimental investigations (ElMaraghy *et al.* 1998) which have shown a decrease in perfusion of the cruciate ligaments following retrograde nailing. Short-term follow-up (Ostrum *et al.* 2000) has shown no increase in knee symptoms with retrograde nailing.

AMBULATION AS A COMPONENT OF GENERIC OUTCOME SCORES

Generic health status scores (see Chapter 6) are well established in the assessment of orthopaedic interventions. Many publications now combine the use of a regional disease-specific measure, and a generic measure, such as the SF-36, and studies such as those of Dogra *et al.* (2002) demonstrate the strong correlation between the two.

The principal advantage of generic scores is that they afford an estimate of the importance or salience to the patient of any deficit in locomotor function. This allows comparison with health problems in other body systems and pathologies. It also raises the possibility of the use of *only* a generic score as a 'universal' outcome measure, rather than having to use different regional scores for each anatomical area of the body.

However, the weakness of the generic instrument may be that it is less sensitive to subtle changes in regional function, and thus provides only a poor discriminator in studies of musculoskeletal outcome. Furthermore, the generic score reflects the impact of *all* the patient's problems, so that the measure of the consequences of any one injury under study is contaminated by noise. Indeed the effect of all pre-injury morbidities will be registered, although this can to some extent be mitigated by obtaining a quasi-baseline score by asking the patient, shortly after injury, to complete a questionnaire on the basis of how they felt just before the injury occurred.

This contradiction is inescapable. Measures such as the Musculoskeletal Function Assessment Questionnaire (Martin *et al.* 1997) and the Short Musculoskeletal Function Assessment Questionnaire (Swiontkowski *et al.* 1999), designed to enhance the sensitivity to musculoskeletal impairments, immediately sacrifice the advantage of comparability to disabilities produced by impairments in other body systems.

The only solution is to use a combination of disease-specific and generic scores, the former to achieve musculoskeletal sensitivity, the latter to achieve a comparative measure of holistic impact.

SUMMARY AND CONCLUSION

Outcome measures for lower-limb function following trauma are continuing to evolve. A few have been used more commonly than others, but this in itself does not mean they are necessarily better. However, the validity of the deployment of outcome measures depends critically on study design, allowing the successful incorporation of the severity of injury in the interpretation.

We agree with Littenberg *et al.* (1998), that the reporting of results following treatment of tibial fractures should ideally be in the context of a well-conducted prospective randomized trial. The use of the CONSORT® flowsheet (Moher *et al.* 2001) permits a systematic analysis of the flow of patients through such trials.

In spite of its weaknesses, the AO-OTA classification provides a basis for morphological comparison of bony injuries. For the accompanying soft-tissue injury – too often ignored – the Tscherne grading system correlates best with outcome in tibial shaft fractures. Energy of injury is a very important variable for stratification, as it correlates with time for union.

The ideal mangled extremity score should be both sensitive and specific and, to date, none has proved to be so. The LEAP study will hopefully provide more answers to this problem.

In assessing fracture healing *per se*, mechanical testing would be ideal, as interpretation of radiographs is subject to variation. However, the problem of mechanical assessment of fractures that have been nailed remains unsolved. The advent of digital radiographic techniques may help to quantify callus, following further research, and thus allow quantification of at least the bone regeneration, if not structural restitution. The minimum requirement is that criteria used for the definition of 'time to union' should be explicitly stated in all reports.

Malunion of a lower-limb fracture is only as important as its effect on function and aesthetics. Artificial figures to 'define' a malunion are often contradictory. The true consequences of a malunion – its effects on the neighbouring joints – can only be assessed by long-leg radiographs and measurement of the mechanical axis.

Outcome measures should include regional and generic measures of function, rather than one of these in isolation. Though seemingly interrelated, the use of both types of outcome will permit a more comprehensive analysis of results.

REFERENCES

Arazi, M., Ogun, T. C., Oktar, M. N., Memik, R., and Kutlu, A. (2001): Early weight-bearing after statically locked reamed intramedullary nailing of comminuted femoral fractures: is it a safe procedure? *J Trauma* 50, 711–16.

Bain, G. I., Zacest, A. C., Paterson, D. C., Middleton, J., and Pohl, A. P. (1997): Abduction strength following intramedullary nailing of the femur. *J Orthop Trauma* 11, 93–7.

Bauer, G. C. G., Edwards, P., and Widmark, P. H. (1962): Shaft fractures of the tibia: etiology of poor results in a consecutive series of 173. *Acta Chir Scand* 124, 386–95.

Beardsley, C. L., Bertsch, C. R., Marsh, J. L., and Brown, T. D. (2002): Interfragmentary surface area as an index of comminution energy: proof of concept in a bone fracture surrogate. *J Biomech* 35, 331–8.

Benirschke, S. K., Melder, I., Henley, M. B., *et al.* (1993): Closed interlocking nailing of femoral shaft fractures: assessment of technical complications and functional outcomes by comparison of a prospective database with retrospective review. *J Orthop Trauma* 7, 118–22.

Bone, L. B., and Johnson, K. D. (1986): Treatment of tibial fractures by reaming and intramedullary nailing. *J Bone Joint Surg Am* 68, 877–87.

Bone, L. B., Sucato, D., Stegemann, P. M., and Rohrbacher, B. J. (1997): Displaced isolated fractures of the tibial shaft treated with either a cast or intramedullary nailing. An outcome analysis of matched pairs of patients. *J Bone Joint Surg Am* 79A, 1336–41.

Bosse, M. J., MacKenzie, E. J., Kellam, J. F., *et al.* (2001): A prospective evaluation of the clinical utility of the lower-extremity injury-severity scores. *J Bone Joint Surg Am* 83A, 3–14.

Bostman, O. M. (1983): Rotational refracture of the shaft of the adult tibia. *Injury* 15, 93–8.

Boyd, K. T., Tippett, R. J., and Moran, C. G. (2001): Anterior knee pain after intramedullary nailing of the tibia: are knee function and work a problem in the long-term? Proceedings, Annual Meeting of the Orthopedic Trauma Association, October 18–20, 2001, San Diego, California. Volume 9, 20.

Brumback, R. J., and Jones, A. L. (1994): Interobserver agreement in the classification of open fractures

of the tibia. The results of a survey of two hundred and forty-five orthopaedic surgeons. *J Bone Joint Surg Am* 76A, 1162–6.

Cheng, J. C., Tse, P. Y., and Chow, Y. Y. (1985): The place of the dynamic compression plate in femoral shaft fractures. *Injury* 16, 529–34.

Cierny, G., Mader, J. T., and Pennick, H. (1985): A clinical staging system of adult osteomyelitis. *Contemp Orthop* 10, 17–37.

Collins, D. N., Pearce, C. E., and McAndrew, M. P. (1990): Successful use of reaming and intramedullary nailing of the tibia. *J Orthop Trauma* 4, 315–22.

Davis, A. M., Wright, J. G., Williams, J. I., Bombardier, C., Griffin, A., and Bell, R. S. (1996): Development of a measure of physical function for patients with bone and soft tissue sarcoma. *Qual Life Res* 5, 508–16.

Davis, A. M., Bell, R. S., Badley, E. M., Yoshida, K., and Williams, J. I. (1999): Evaluating functional outcome in patients with lower extremity sarcoma. *Clin Orthop* 80, 90–100.

Dietz, F. R. (2001): Origin of the Iowa Scoring System for tibial fractures. *Pers Commun* 12, 12.

Dogra, A. S., Ruiz, A. L., Thompson, N. S., and Nolan, P. C. (2000): Dia-metaphyseal distal tibial fractures – treatment with a shortened intramedullary nail: a review of 15 cases. *Injury* 31, 799–804.

Dogra, A. S., Ruiz, A. L., and Marsh, D. R. (2002): Late outcome of isolated tibial fractures treated by intramedullary nailing: the correlation between disease-specific and generic outcome measures. *J Orthop Trauma* 16, 245–9.

Ellis, H. (1958): The speed of healing after fractures of the tibial shaft. *J Bone Joint Surg Br* 40B, 42–6.

ElMaraghy, A. W., Schemitsch, E. H., and Richards, R. R. (1998): Femoral and cruciate blood flow after retrograde femoral reaming: a canine study using laser Doppler flowmetry. *J Orthop Trauma* 12, 253–8.

Fakhry, S. M., Rutledge, R., Dahners, L. E., and Kessler, D. (1994): Incidence, management, and outcome of femoral shaft fracture: a statewide population-based analysis of 2805 adult patients in a rural state. *J Trauma* 3, 255–60.

Gaston, P., Will, E., Elton, R. A., McQueen, M. M., and Court, B. (1999): Fractures of the tibia. Can their outcome be predicted? *J Bone Joint Surg Br* **81**, 71–6.

Gustilo, R. B., and Anderson, J. T. (1976): Prevention of infection in the treatment of one thousand and twenty-five open fractures of long bones: retrospective and prospective analyses. *J Bone Joint Surg Am* **58**, 453–8.

Gustilo, R. B., Mendoza, R. M., and Williams, D. N. (1984): Problems in the management of type III (severe) open fractures: a new classification of type III open fractures. *J Trauma* **24**, 742–6.

Haines, J. F., Williams, E. A., Hargadon, E. J., *et al.* (1984): Is conservative treatment of distal tibial shaft fractures justified? *J Bone Joint Surg Br* **66**, 84–8.

Hammer, R. R., Hammerby, S., and Lindholm, B. (1985): Accuracy of radiologic assessment of tibial shaft fracture union in humans. *Clin Orthop* **199**, 233–8.

Hoeffel, D. P., Hinrichs, S. H., and Garvin, K. L. (1999): Molecular diagnostics for the detection of musculoskeletal infection. *Clin Orthop* **360**, 37–46.

Howe, H. R. J., Poole, G. V. J., Hansen, K. J., *et al.* (1987): Salvage of lower extremities following combined orthopedic and vascular trauma. A predictive salvage index. *Am Surg* **53**, 205–8.

Ilizarov, G. A. (1992): Clinical studies on fracture displacement in the treatment of fractures. In: Ilizarov, G. A., and Green, S. (eds), *Transosseous Osteosynthesis*. Springer, Berlin, pp. 381–401.

Jensen, J. S., Hansen, F. W., and Johansen, J. (1977): Tibial shaft fractures: A comparison of conservative treatment and internal fixation with conventional plates or AO compression plates. *Acta Orthop Scand* **48**, 204–12.

Johansen, K., Daines, M., Howey, T., Helfet, D., and Hansen, S. T. J. (1990): Objective criteria accurately predict amputation following lower extremity trauma. *J Trauma* **30**, 568–72.

Johner, R., and Wruhs, O. (1983): Classification of tibial shaft fractures and correlation with results after rigid internal fixation. *Clin Orthop* **178**, 7–25.

Johnstone, D. J., Radford, W. J., and Parnell, E. J. (1993): Interobserver variation using the AO/ASIF classification of long bone fractures. *Injury* **24**, 163–5.

Kay, P. R., Edwards, J., Taktak, A., and Laycock, D. (1992): Measurement of fracture healing by simple bending and vibration. *J Bone Joint Surg Br* **74B** (Suppl. II), 230–1.

Kitaoka, H. B., Alexander, I. J., Adelaar, R. S., Nunley, J. A., Myerson, M. S., and Sanders, M. (1994): Clinical rating systems for the ankle-hindfoot, midfoot, hallux, and lesser toes. *Foot Ankle Int* **15**, 349–53.

Krettek, C., Seekamp, A., Kontopp, H., and Tscherne, H. (2001): Hannover Fracture Scale '98 – re-evaluation and new perspectives of an established extremity salvage score. *Injury* **32**, 317–28.

Kristensen, K. D., Kiaer, T., and Blicher, J. (1989): No arthrosis of the ankle 20 years after malaligned tibial-shaft fracture. *Acta Orthop Scand* **60**, 208–9.

Lane, J. M., and Sandhu, H. S. (1987): Current approaches to experimental bone grafting. *Orthop Clin North Am* **18**, 213–25.

Lindsey, R. W., and Blair, S. R. (1996): Closed tibial-shaft fractures: which ones benefit from surgical treatment? *J Am Acad Orthop Surg* **4**, 35–43.

Littenberg, B., Weinstein, L. P., McCarren, M., *et al.* (1998): Closed fractures of the tibial shaft. A meta-analysis of three methods of treatment. *J Bone Joint Surg Am* **80**, 174–83.

Lysholm, J., and Gillquist, J. (1982): Evaluation of knee ligament surgery results with special emphasis on use of a scoring scale. *Am J Sports Med* **10**, 150–4.

Marsh, D. (1998): Concepts of fracture union, delayed union, and non-union. *Clin Orthop* **355** (Suppl.), S22–30.

Martin, D. P., Engelberg, R., Agel, J., and Swiontkowski, M. F. (1997): Comparison of the Musculoskeletal Function Assessment questionnaire with the Short Form-36, the Western Ontario and McMaster Universities Osteoarthritis Index, and the Sickness Impact Profile health-status measures. *J Bone Joint Surg Am* **79**, 1323–35.

May, J. W., Jupiter, J. B., Weiland, A. J., and Byrd, H. S. (1989): Clinical classification of post-traumatic tibial osteomyelitis. *J Bone Joint Surg Am* **71**, 1422–8.

McNamara, M. G., Heckman, J. D., and Corley, F. G. (1994): Severe open fractures of the lower extremity: a retrospective evaluation of the Mangled Extremity Severity Score (MESS). *J Orthop Trauma* **8**, 81–7.

Merchant, T. C., and Dietz, F. R. (1989): Long-term follow-up after fractures of the tibial and fibular shafts. *J Bone Joint Surg Am* **71**, 599–606.

Moher, D., Schulz, K. F., and Altman, D. G. (2001): The CONSORT statement: revised recommendations for improving the quality of reports of parallel-group randomised trials. *Lancet* **357**, 1191–4.

Müller, M. E., Nazarian, S., Koch, P., and Schatzker, J. (1990): *The Comprehensive Classification of Fractures of Long Bones*. Springer, Berlin.

Nicoll, E. A. (1964): Fractures of the tibial shaft. *J Bone Joint Surg Br* **46B**, 373–87.

Noyes, F. R., Barber, S. D., and Mooar, L. A. (1989): A rationale for assessing sports activity levels and limitations in knee disorders. *Clin Orthop* **16**, 238–49.

Oesterne, H. J., and Tscherne, H. (1984): Pathophysiology and classification of soft-tissue injuries associated with fractures. In: Tscherne, H., and Gotzen, L. (eds), *Fractures with Soft-Tissue Injuries*. Springer-Verlag, Berlin, pp. 1–9.

Olerud, C., and Molander, H. (1984): A scoring scale for symptom evaluation after ankle fracture. *Arch Orthop Trauma Surg* **103**, 190–4.

Oni, O. O., Hui, A., and Gregg, P. J. (1988): The healing of closed tibial shaft fractures. The natural history of union with closed treatment. *J Bone Joint Surg Br* **70**, 787–90.

Ostrum, R. F., Agarwal, A., Lakatos, R., and Poka, A. (2000): Prospective comparison of retrograde and antegrade femoral intramedullary nailing. *J Orthop Trauma* **14**, 496–501.

Panjabi, M. M., Walter, S. D., Karuda, M., White, A. A., and Lawson, J. P. (1985): Correlations of radiographic analysis of healing fractures with strength: a statistical analysis of experimental osteotomies. *J Orthop Res* **3**, 212–18.

Panjabi, M. M., Lindsey, R. W., Walter, S. D., and White, A. A. (1989): The clinician's ability to evaluate the strength of healing fractures from plain radiographs. *J Orthop Trauma* **3**, 29–32.

Peel, A. L., and Taylor, E. W. (1991): Proposed definitions for the audit of postoperative infection: a discussion paper. Surgical Infection Study Group. *Ann R Coll Surg Eng* **73**, 385–8.

Platt, R., Yokoe, D. S., and Sands, K. E. (2001): Automated methods for surveillance of surgical site infections. *Emerg Infect Dis* **7**, 212–16.

Public Health Laboratory Service (2000): *Surveillance of Surgical Site Infection in English Hospitals*. Central Public Health Laboratory, London.

Puno, R. M., Vaughan, J. J., Stetten, M. L., *et al.* (1991): Long-term effects of tibial angular malunion on the knee and ankle joints. *J Orthop Trauma* **5**, 247–54.

Richardson, J. B., Cunningham, J. L., Goodship, A. E., O'Connor, B. T., and Kenwright, J. (1994): Measuring stiffness can define healing of tibial fractures. *J Bone Joint Surg Br* **76**, 389–94.

Ruedi, T. P., and Allgower, M. (1979): The operative treatment of intra-articular fractures of the lower end of the tibia. *Clin Orthop* **138**, 105–10.

Russell, W. L., Sailors, D. M., Whittle, T. B., Fisher, D. F. J., and Burns, R. P. (1991): Limb salvage versus traumatic amputation. A decision based on a seven-part predictive index. *Ann Surg* **213**, 473–80.

Sarmiento, A., Sobol, P. A., Sew, H., Ross, S. D., Racette, W. L., and Tarr, R. R. (1984): Prefabricated functional braces for the treatment of fractures of the tibial diaphysis. *J Bone Joint Surg Am* **66**, 1328–39.

Sarmiento, A., Sharpe, F. E., Ebramzadeh, E., Normand, P., and Shankwiler, J. (1995): Factors influencing the outcome of closed tibial fractures treated with functional bracing. *Clin Orthop* **315**, 8–24.

Sharrard, W. J. (1990): A double-blind trial of pulsed electromagnetic fields for delayed union of tibial fractures. *J Bone Joint Surg Br* **72**, 347–55.

Simpson, A. H. R. W. (1994): The Ankle. In: Pynsent, P. B., Fairbank, J. C. T., and Carr, A. J.

(eds), *Outcome Measures in Trauma*. Butterworth-Heinemann, Oxford, pp. 337–56.

Skoog, A., Soderqvist, A., Tornkvist, H., and Ponzer, S. (2001): One-year outcome after tibial shaft fractures: results of a prospective fracture registry. *J Orthop Trauma* **15**, 210–15.

Smith, J. S. J., Martin, L. F., Young, W. W., and Macioce, D. P. (1990): Do trauma centers improve outcome over non-trauma centers: the evaluation of regional trauma care using discharge abstract data and patient management categories. *J Trauma* **30**, 1533–8.

Sudkamp, N. P., Barbey, N., Veuskens, A., *et al.* (1993): The incidence of osteitis in open fractures: an analysis of 948 open fractures (a review of the Hannover experience). *J Orthop Trauma* **7**, 473–82.

Swiontkowski, M. F., Engelberg, R. P. M. D., and Agel, J. (1999): Short musculoskeletal function assessment questionnaire: validity, reliability, and responsiveness. *J Bone Joint Surg Am* **81**, 1245–60.

Swiontkowski, M. F., Agel, J., McAndrew, M. P., Burgess, A. R., and MacKenzie, E. J. (2000): Outcome validation of the AO/OTA fracture classification system. *J Orthop Trauma* **14**, 534–41.

Tegner, Y., Lysholm, J., Odensten, M., and Gillquist, J. (1988): Evaluation of cruciate ligament injuries. A review. *Acta Orthop Scand* **59**, 336–41.

Thoresen, B. O., Alho, E., A, Stromsoe, K., Folleras, G., and Haukebo, A. (1985): Interlocking intramedullary nailing in femoral shaft fractures. A report of forty-eight cases. *J Bone Joint Surg Am* **67**, 1313–20.

Toivanen, J. A., Honkonen, S. E., Koivisto, A. M., and Jarvinen, M. J. (2001): Treatment of low-energy tibial shaft fractures: plaster cast compared with intramedullary nailing. *Int Orthop* **25**, 110–13.

Toivanen, J. A., Vaisto, O., Kannus, P., Latvala, K., Honkonen, S. E., and Jarvinen, M. J. (2002): Anterior knee pain after intramedullary nailing of fractures of the tibial shaft: a prospective, randomized study comparing two different nail-insertion techniques. *J Bone Joint Surg Am* **84-A**, 580–8.

Tower, S. S., Beals, R. K., and Duwelius, P. J. (1993): Resonant frequency analysis of the tibia as a measure of fracture healing. *J Orthop Trauma* **7**, 552–7.

Trafton, P. G. (1988): Closed unstable fractures of the tibia. *Clin Orthop* **230**, 58–67.

Tuten, H. R., Keeler, K. A., Gabos, P. G., Zionts, L. E., and MacKenzie, W. G. (1999): Posttraumatic tibia valga in children. A long-term follow-up note. *J Bone Joint Surg Am* **81**, 799–810.

Van der Schoot, D. K., Den Outer, A. J., Bode, P. J., Obermann, W. R., and van Vugt, A. (1996): Degenerative changes at the knee and ankle related to malunion of tibial fractures 15-year follow-up of 88 patients. *J Bone Joint Surg Br* **78**, 722–5.

Van der Werken, C., and Marti, R. K. (1983): Post-traumatic rotational deformity of the lower leg. *Injury* **21**, 217–19.

Waldvogel, F. A., Medoff, G., and Swartz, M. N. (1970): Osteomyelitis: a review of clinical features, therapeutic considerations and unusual aspects. *N Engl J Med* **28**, 198–206.

Webb, J., Herling, G., Gardner, T., Kenwright, J., and Simpson, A. H. (1996): Manual assessment of fracture stiffness. *Injury* **27**, 319–20.

Whelan, D. B., Bhandari, M., McKee, M. D., *et al.* (2002): Interobserver and intraobserver variation in the assessment of the healing of tibial fractures after intramedullary fixation. *J Bone Joint Surg Br* **84**, 15–18.

Winquist, R. A., and Hansen, S. T. (1980): Comminuted fractures of the femoral shaft treated by intramedullary nailing. *Orthop Clin North Am* **11**, 633–48.

Wolinsky, P., Tejwani, N., Richmond, J. H., Koval, K. J., Egol, K., and Stephen, D. J. G. (2001): Controversies in intramedullary nailing of femoral shaft fractures. *J Bone Joint Surg Am* **83**, 1404–15.

APPENDIX

Table 20-A.1: Hannover Fracture Scale '98 (Krettek *et al.* 2001, reprinted with permission from Elsevier)

Factor	Score
Bone loss	
None	0
<2 cm	1
>2 cm	2
Skin injury	
None	0
<¼ circumference	1
¼–½ circumference	2
½–¾ circumference	3
>¾ circumference	4
Muscle injury	
None	0
<¼ circumference	1
¼–½ circumference	2
½–¾ circumference	3
>¾ circumference	4
Wound contamination	
None	0
Partly	1
Massive	2
Deperiostation	
No	1
Yes	2

Table 20-A.1: Hannover Fracture Scale '98 (Krettek *et al.* 2001, reprinted with permission from Elsevier) – *continued*

Factor	Score
Local circulation	
Normal pulse	0
Capillary pulse only	1
Ischaemia <4 hours	2
Ischaemia 4–8 hours	3
Ischaemia >8 hours	4
Systemic circulation (systolic blood pressure)	
Constantly >100 mmHg	0
Until admission <100 mmHg	1
Until operation <100 mmHg	2
Constantly <100 mmHg	3
Neurology	
Palmar-plantar 'yes'	0
Absent sensation	1
Finger-toe 'yes'	0
Active motion: no	1

Table 20-A.2: The Tscherne grading system for soft-tissue injury. Reprinted from Oesterne and Tscherne (1984)

Tscherne grade	Description	Example
0	Simple fracture configuration with little or no soft-tissue injury	Torsional injury to the tibia
1	Mild to moderately severe fracture configuration, mild to moderate soft tissue damage due to fragment pressure from within	Fracture dislocation of ankle with medial skin pressure
2	Moderately severe fracture configuration deep contaminated skin abrasion local damage to skin or muscle	Segmental bumper fracture of tibia
3	Severe or comminuted fracture configuration extensive contusion or crushing of skin or subcutaneous tissue ± degloving; destruction of muscle	Closed fracture with prolonged crush injury

Table 20-A.3: Mangled Extremity Severity Score. Reprinted from Johansen *et al.* (1990)

Factor	Score
Skeletal/soft-tissue injury	
Low-energy (stab, fracture, civilian gunshot wound)	1
Medium-energy (open or multiple fractures)	2
High-energy (shotgun or military gunshot wound, crush)	3
Very high-energy (above plus gross contamination)	4
Limb ischaemia	
Pulse reduced or absent but perfusion normal	1*
Pulseless, diminished capillary refill	2*
Patient is cool, paralysed, insensate, numb	3*
Shock	
Systolic blood pressure always >90 mmHg	0
Systolic blood pressure transiently <90 mmHg	1
Systolic blood pressure persistently <90 mmHg	2
Age	
<30 years	0
30–50 years	1
>50 years	2

*Double value if duration of ischaemia is >6 hours.

Table 20-A.4: Iowa Knee Evaluation (Merchant and Dietz 1989, with permission)

Function (35 points)

Eleven activities of daily living are listed with a value. If the patient can perform the activity easily without restriction, give full value; if the patient cannot (or could not if he/she tried) perform the activity at all, give no points; if the patient can or could perform the activity but with difficulty, give an appropriate number of points between 0 and the full value.

Does most of housework or job, which requires moving about	5
Walks enough to be independent	5
Dresses unaided (including tying shoes and putting on socks)	5
Sits without difficulty at table or toilet, including sitting down and getting up	4
Picks up objects from floor by squatting or kneeling	3
Bathes without help	3
Negotiates stairs foot over foot	3
Negotiates stairs in any manner	2
Carries objects, such as a suitcase	2

Table 20-A.4: Iowa Knee Evaluation (Merchant and Dietz 1989) – *continued*

Gets into an automobile, or public conveyance	2
Drives an automobile	1
Freedom from pain (maximum 35 points)	
Circle the value that is over-all most representative of the patient's pain; using the word descriptors.	
Scoring should not be based simply on asking the patient the word descriptors in question form.	
No pain	35
Mild pain with fatigue	30
Mild pain with weight-bearing	20
Moderate pain with weight-bearing	15
Severe pain with weight-bearing, mild or moderate at rest	10
Severe, continuous pain	0
Gait (maximum, 10 points)	
No limp, no support	10
Limp, no support	8
One cane or crutch	8
One long brace	8
One brace with crutch or crane	6
Two crutches with or without a brace	4
Cannot walk	0
Absence of deformity or stability	
No fixed flexion (FF) of more than 10° with weight-bearing (WB)	3
No FF or more than 20° with WB	2
No FF of more than 30° with WB	1
No varus or valgus of more than 10° with WB	3
No varus or valgus of more than 20° with WB	2
No varus or valgus of more than 30° with WB	1
No ligamentous instability	2
No locking, giving way, or extension lag of more than 10°	2
Range of motion (10 points)	
Total amount of flexion or extension, in degrees (normal: 150°); assign 1 point for every 15°	

Table 20-A.5: Iowa Ankle Evaluation (Merchant and Dietz 1989, with permission)

Function (40 points)	
Does housework or job without difficulty	8
Climbs stairs	
Foot over foot	6
Any manner	4
Carries heavy objects, such as a suitcase	4
Is able to run, participate in athletics, or work at heavy labour	4
Walks enough to be independent	8
Does yard work, gardening, lawn-mowing	4
Has no difficulty getting in or out of an automobile	6
Freedom from pain (40 points)	
No pain	40
Pain only with fatigue or prolonged use	30
Pain with weight-bearing	20
Pain with motion	10
Pain at rest, or continuous pain	0
Gait (10 points)	
No limp	10
Antalgic limp	8
Uses cane or one crutch	2
Uses wheelchair or cannot walk	0
Range of motion (10 points)	
Total amount of dorsiflexion and plantar flexion (normal, 30 to 70°); assign 2 points for every 20°	

Table 20-A.6: The Ankle and Hindfoot Score of the American Orthopaedic Foot and Ankle Society. Reprinted from Kitaoka *et al.* (1994)

Pain (40) points	
None	40
Mild, occasional	30
Moderate, daily	20
Severe, almost always present	0
Function (50) points	
Activity limitations, support requirement	
No limitations, no support	10
No limitation of daily activities, limitation of recreational activities, no support	7
Limited daily and recreational activities, cane	4
Severe limitation of daily and recreational activities, walker, crutches, wheelchair, brace	0
Maximum walking distance, blocks	
>6	5
4–6	4
1–3	2
<1	0
Walking surfaces	
No difficulty on any surface	5
Some difficulty on uneven terrain, stairs, inclines, ladders	3
Severe difficulty on uneven terrain, stairs, inclines, ladders	0
Gait abnormality	
None, slight	8
Obvious	4
Marked	0
Sagittal motion (flexion plus extension)	
Normal or mild restriction ($\geqslant 30°$)	8
Moderate restriction ($15–29°$)	4
Severe restriction ($<15°$)	0
Hindfoot motion (inversion plus extension)	
Normal or mild restriction (75%–100% normal)	6
Moderate restriction (25%–74% normal)	3
Marked restriction (<25% normal)	0
Ankle-hindfoot stability (AP, varus-valgus)	
Stable	8
Definitely unstable	0
Alignment (10 points)	
Good, plantigrade foot, ankle-hindfoot well aligned	10
Fair, plantigrade foot, some degree of ankle-hindfoot malalignment, no symptoms	5
Poor, non-plantigrade foot, severe malalignment, symptoms	0

Table 20-A.7: The Olerud and Molander Ankle Score. Reprinted from Olerud and Molander (1984)

Pain (25 points)	
None	25
While walking on uneven surface	20
While walking on even surface outdoors	10
While walking indoors	5
Constant and severe	0
Stiffness (10 points)	
None	10
Stiffness	0
Swelling (10 points)	
None	10
Only evenings	5
Constant	0
Stair climbing (10 points)	
No problems	10
Impaired	5
Unable	0
Running (5 points)	
Possible	5
Impossible	0
Jumping (5 points)	
Possible	5
Impossible	0
Squatting (5 points)	
No problems	5
Unable	0
Supports (10 points)	
None	10
Taping, wrapping	5
Stick or crutch	0
Work, activities of daily living (20 points)	
Same as before injury	20
Change to a simpler job/half-time	10
Disabled, or strongly impaired work capacity	0

21

The knee
Amir W. Hanna

INTRODUCTION

The development of new techniques in knee surgery has created a demand for accurate assessment of the results. Historically, empirical assessment was used to document the relative efficacy of treatment. This unscientific approach often resulted in erroneous conclusions by researchers. O'Donoghue (1955) stated that 'results from various methods have been unsatisfactory despite the rather glowing reports from the promulgator of each'.

The problem lies in the subjective interpretations of variables and a difficulty in evaluating results. Researchers – many of whom are surgeons – are subject to bias, and patients may present an optimistic assessment to please the surgeon (Anderson and Lipscomb 1986). The question then arises how to find the true outcome of treatment? Is it the clinical findings at the out-patient follow-up? Is it what the patient thinks of the knee after treatment as compared to before? Is it special tests that need to be done to put the knee under dynamic stresses to test its performance (objective functional testing)? Or is it a combination of all of these?

Some criteria mentioned in the published rating scales can not be quantified and may not reflect the clinical results. The methods of grading and formatting data also influence the assessment. Values for a variable or a category of variables are arbitrarily assigned a numeric score. Different interpretations of the relative value of the variable inevitably alter the evaluation. Many authors have provided relative or no information on how the weighting algorithms had been derived (Drake *et al.* 1994). Different methods have been used to produce the grading systems in common use; hence, some use numeric scores, some use categoric scales, and others use visual analogue scales.

The outcome scores are categorized into three main categories: those dealing with knee arthropathy; fractures around the knee; and with soft-tissue injuries of the knee.

KNEE ARTHROPATHY

Discussion and general specification of tools

The outcome tools used under this category of knee disorders deal with impairment and disabilities arising from knee arthritis in order to assess the outcome of knee replacement surgery, which has grown dramatically during the past two decades. The need to evaluate the outcome has become an important aspect of each practising surgeon to evaluate critically and objectively his or her results if trends and failures are to be noted.

Interest in measuring knee function started by producing condition-specific and site-specific outcome tools. Early instruments included assessment of pain, function, range of movement deformity, stability and muscle strength around the knee. These were thought to be the basic parameters that influence the structure and function of the knee. X-radiography was used to define the group of patients who were not yet sufficiently symptomatic clinically but showing radiological criteria of failure. These were component migration, cement or component fracture or complete radiolucent lines – that is, the at-risk group. Survival analysis on the other hand, assesses the outcome in terms of time to revision or failure as the end-point.

In most outcome scores a patient with a knee arthrodesis would score 'good' or 'excellent', which seems impractical in today's surgical practice. The ideal outcome tool should include patient subjective assessment, symptoms, clinical examination, some ancillary tests as well as assessment of complications, their grading, time of onset and duration (Miller and Carr 1993).

One of the first tools that used these parameters was the Hospital for Special Surgery (HSS) (Ranawat et al. 1976) (Fig. 21-A.1). Function was evaluated in relation to walking, stairs and transfer, with all of these being measured by a clinician. Aichroth et al. (1978) subsequently attempted to add patient satisfaction assessment (Fig. 21-A.2). Later, other scoring systems such as the New Jersey (Buechel 1982) (Fig. 21-A.3) and the Lequesne index of severity (Lequesne 1989) were also developed.

Konig et al. (1989) realized that, using the HSS, patients' scores gradually decline years after knee replacement surgery, and that this was related to patient ageing. Knee function remained the same, while the decline was in the patients' general health and the ability to perform activities of daily living. This stimulated the modification of the HSS into the American Knee Society scoring system (KSS; Insall et al. 1989) (Fig. 21-A.4) which separated knee function from patient activities.

The difficulty lies in attempting to quantify a surgical result. From the patient's viewpoint this is best expressed in subjective terms. A technical success from the surgeon's standpoint may not necessarily have had a significant impact on a patient's quality of life. Thus, from the patient's point of view, the result is a failure.

Researchers started to use quality of life and general health questionnaires as another measure of assessing results of surgery. The WOMAC Index (site-specific/disease-specific) was used successfully (Bellamy et al. 1988), in addition to other general

health questionnaires including the Nottingham Health Profile (NHP; Hunt et al. 1981), Short Form 36 (SF-36; Ware and Hays 1988), Short-Form 12 (SF-12; Ware et al. 1996) and the Musculoskeletal Functional Assessment (MFA; Martin et al. 1996).

Roos et al. (1998) derived part of the KOOS questions from the WOMAC Osteoarthritis Index Likert version 3.0. This employed five-item scales (Bellamy et al. 1988), and covered five patient-relevant dimensions: pain; other disease-specific symptoms; activities of daily living; sport and recreation functions; and knee-related quality of life (Fig. 21-A.5). The system is intended as a measure of disabilities from knee disorders, including osteoarthritis of the knee, and has been proven to be both valid and reliable. Activity of daily living scale of knee outcome survey (ADLS of KOS) (Irrgang et al. 1998) was developed on the basis of a review of existing instruments including the Cincinnati, Lysholm, WOMAC and IKDC (Fig. 21-A.6). This was shown to be reliable, valid and responsive to change in the same study. In the same year, the Oxford Knee Questionnaire was published in a study that confirmed its validity, reliability and responsiveness to change (Dawson et al. 1998) (Fig. 21-A.7).

The use of generic outcomes questionnaires carries the risk of not being accurate. For example, Kreibich et al. (1996) believed that the SF-36 was not sensitive to the change over time for patients with knee osteoarthritis. The success of WOMAC as a disease-specific tool stimulated the development of other systems that are both disease- and site-specific and which are patient-administered. These depend mainly on the subjective assessment of function, without the need for clinical objective evaluation. This is supposed to avoid the risk of clinician bias as well as the bias of using unreliable signs.

Others (Ryd et al. 1997) stated that there was no need to validate outcome questionnaires by comparing them to 'objective ratings' by a surgeon because, they believed, that this in itself produces bias. Liow et al. (2000) showed that there was more reliability with the 'subjective' part of KSS compared to its 'objective' part.

Drake et al. (1994) identified 34 different published scoring systems which were either 'generic' or 'disease- or site-' specific. These authors felt that none of the systems had been proven to be either reliable or valid, in contrast to recently developed tools such as KOOS which had been tested for validity and reliability. In spite of the wide use of KSS in assessing knee arthroplasty, few investigations have been carried out to assess its validity. Kreibich *et al.* (1996) found that KSS and WOMAC were both responsive to change, but that SF-36 was the least responsive instrument. Others (Stucki *et al.* 1998) showed that the Lequesne index of severity was not valid in a comparison with the WOMAC index.

Lingard *et al.* (2001) subsequently demonstrated construct validity of the KSS, but believed the WOMAC and SF-36 to be more responsive measures for assessing outcomes following knee arthroplasty. Others (Dunbar *et al.* 2001) believed that SF-12 and the Oxford Knee Questionnaire represented the most useful outcome measure for knee arthroplasty, but felt that other generic outcomes – such as the Sickness Impact Profile – performed poorly.

'Best buy'

Six instruments have scored between 8 and 10 (Table 21.1), among which were WOMAC, Oxford-12 questionnaire, KSS, the Lequesne index of severity, SF-36 and SF-12. Only the KSS includes objective measures for assessment. Because most clinicians prefer subjective, self-administered tools, the best condition-specific systems were seen to be the WOMAC and Oxford-12 questionnaires, while the best generic measures were the SF-36 and SF-12.

The SF-36 has a lower sensitivity to change over time for patients with osteoarthritis of the knee (Kreibich *et al.* 1996), and it takes longer to fill all of its components than its rivals (Dunbar *et al.* 2001). The SF-12 ranked best for general health assessment in patients with knee arthropathy, while the Oxford-12 questionnaire showed the best rank for disease-specific scale for its reliability, content validity and feasibility to use. WOMAC came second in the rankings (Dunbar *et al.* 2001).

A combination of the SF-12 and Oxford-12 questionnaires seems to be the best buy. The specificity of the Oxford-12 questionnaire to knee disorders remains in question (Harcourt *et al.* 2001), though WOMAC can be used instead.

SOFT-TISSUE INJURIES

Knee ligament injuries

DISCUSSION AND GENERAL SPECIFICATION OF TOOLS

The complexity of the knee and the number of criteria used to assess the results make accurate evaluation difficult. A deficiency in the understanding of knee ligament injuries and the resultant pathological motions is reflected in the different perception of which criteria are important, and how they should be measured. Thus, if clinical examination is a good method of assessing outcome, the variability between surgeons and their clinical abilities will interfere with the results. This might be in the form of producing an appreciable difference in translation and rotation when evaluating the limits of knee motion. Even when the examiners produce the same displacement, the correct interpretation depends on accurate perception of motion. A comprehensive tool should include: grading of knee symptoms; function; an assessment of functional disability; activities of daily living; and sports and work assessments.

There is an increasing tendency to use more than one scale in the same study, and this probably reflects the large number of instruments that are available. It also suggests that there is no agreed 'gold standard'. Investigators tend to use outcome instruments in ways that differ from their original design (Höher *et al.* 1997).

The first attempt to evaluate the results of managing knee injuries was carried out by O'Donoghue (1955). While attempting to assess the results of anterior cruciate ligament (ACL) reconstruction, he devised a rating system which included an objective examination and a 100-point questionnaire to be filled in by an interviewer. The questionnaire responses were binary (10 points for yes, 0 points for no). Later on, the system was refined by adding an assessment of swelling, disability and functional assessment, and

Table 21.1: Scoring systems used for assessing results of knee arthroplasty

Tool	Year	Type	Tool domain	Method of administration	Form	A	B	C	D	Total score
HSS	1976	Disease- and site-specific	Pain, function, ROM, muscle strength, deformity	Observer-administered	Objective signs + symptoms, disability assessment	0	0	0	4	4
Knee Function assessment chart	1978	Disease- and site-specific	Patient assessment, disability, pain walking aid chair gait, alignment and deformity	Observer-administered	Objective signs + symptoms, disability assessment	0	0	0	4	4
Lequesne index of severity	1989	Disease- and site-specific		Observer-administered		1[*†]	2[a]	1	4	8
SF-36	1992	Generic	8 domains	Patient-administered	Questionnaire	2	2	2[¶]	4	10
SF-12	1994	Generic	8 domains	Patient-administered	Questionnaire	2	2	2	4	10
WOMAC	1988	Disease-specific	Physical function, pain, stiffness	Patient-administered	Questionnaire	2	2	2	4	10
KSS	1989	Disease- and site-specific	Knee score and functional score	Observer-administered	Objective signs + symptoms, disability assessment	2[b]	0[*]	2	4	8
Knee Outcome Survey (KOS)	1998	Site-specific[*]	ADL scale, sport activity scale in relation to previous 1–2 days	Patient-administered	Questionnaire	1	1	1	2	5
KOOS	1998	Site-specific[*]	Symptoms, daily activities, sports and recreational functions, quality of life time scale not specified	Patient-administered	Questionnaire	1	1	1	0	3
Oxford Knee Score[‡]	1998	Disease- and site-specific	Pain giving way and activities like walking, washing, stairs, etc. in relation to previous 4 weeks	Patient-administered	Questionnaire	2[a]	2[a]	1	4	9
MFA	1999	Generic	The dysfunction index and the bother index, etc.	Patient-administered	Questionnaire	1	1	1	4	7

A = Validity; B = Reliability; C = Responsiveness to change; D = Usage; MFA = Musculo-skeletal functional assessment questionnaire.
[‡]This tool is specific enough (Harcourt *et al.* 2001); [*]Not reliable (Liow *et al.* 2000); [*†]Not valid (Stucki *et al.* 1998); [¶]Not sensitive to change for knee disorders (Kreibich *et al.* 1996); [a]Dunbar *et al.* (2000); [b]Lingard *et al.* (2001).

grading the responses from 1 to 4 (O'Donoghue 1963). O'Donoghue observed that the results of subjective assessment were inconsistent with those of objective evaluation. Some years later, Larson (1974) developed another 100-point scale based on subjective, objective and functional categories. Functional impairment was evaluated with the criteria of walking, running, jumping and squatting.

In 1977, Marshall and colleagues developed a 50-point scale with four subcategories (Fig. 21-A.8), each of which contributed unequally to the total result: subjective parameters (22%); functional test (14%); knee stability (24%); and ligament laxity (40%) (Marshall *et al.* 1977). This system dealt partially with a binary answer system and the functional statements were under-emphasized. The Hospital for Special Surgery 100-point Knee Score (HSSKS) (Fig. 21-A.9) (Windsor *et al.* 1988) was evolved from the Marshall score, whereby the subjective parameters were greatly reduced and special criteria for sports activities were utilized. Pain, when present, leads automatically to a deduction of 10 per cent of the total score.

During the early 1980s, Lysholm and Gillquist (1982) designed a rating scale to evaluate symptoms. The Lysholm scale included the basic features of the Larson scale, but emphasized instability as a symptom representing knee ligament instability. However, thigh wasting was included in the system, which needed physical examination. Tegner and Lysholm (1985) subsequently recognized that instability does not always represent ligament laxity, and suggested that it might be incorrect to allocate 40 per cent of the points to the symptom of instability. Thus, they modified the Lysholm scale to its present version by including other symptoms such as locking and catching, and removed the item of measuring the thigh circumference (Fig. 21-A.10). In the same study, Tegner and Lysholm also introduced the Tegner activity score (Fig. 21-A.11) to grade different activities in a standardized way (Tegner and Lysholm 1985).

Also during the 1980s, Noyes *et al.* (1983) devised a scale to evaluate the results of a conservative programme for the ACL-deficient knee. They used 'subjective assessment', 'clinical examination' and 'activity modification', with each being scored

separately to refine the evaluation. The idea of separating scores originated because some criteria may have had greater long-term effects than others. The subjective rating scale analyses symptoms that occur at various levels of activity. Points were not awarded for participation in any activity that produced symptoms. These authors felt that such participation would be deleterious to the knee.

Feagin and Blake (1983) developed a questionnaire that did not add up the components to a final index. Instead, they recommended separate scores for subjective symptoms, subjective function and objective stability testing (Fig. 21-A.12), and considered instrumented testing to be more reliable and reproducible than manual testing. These authors also advocated the need for an international method for reporting results. The value of clinical examination as a measure for outcome has been debated. Lukianov *et al.* (1987) recorded clinical findings but did not include them in a final score, whilst Windsor *et al.* (1988) and Tegner and Lysholm (1985) emphasized that there were differing symptoms for different ligament deficiencies.

The Swiss Orthopaedic Society Knee Study Group (Muller *et al.* 1988) developed a system for documenting knee laxity. The evaluation form included subjective and objective evaluation and function testing (Fig. 21-A.13), and a scoring concept was introduced where the overall result could never be better than the worst category scored. Later, Noyes *et al.* (1989) revised this instrument, adding a sports activity scale and a final rating scale. Subsequently, they devised a pre- and post-injury occupational rating scale to assess return to work (Noyes *et al.* 1991).

The absence of a standardized scoring system led to the establishment of the International Knee Document Committee (IKDC) (Hefti *et al.* 1993). This created a uniform scale to evaluate outcome after ACL injury or reconstruction. It worked to achieve a standardized terminology and to establish a common evaluation form for outcome of knee function after ACL injury. The IKDC criticised the different clinical examination techniques for knee function, but agreed on the representation and relevance of the items included in the published form (Fig. 21-A.14). Many items in the IKDC form were adopted from the

Cincinnati knee rating system (Barber-Westin *et al.* 1999). The Cincinnati knee rating system was originally designed for ACL injuries, but later underwent modifications to include assessment of all the major ligaments of the knee as well as degenerative meniscal tears and patellofemoral problems. The latest completed version of the scale was published recently (Barber-Westin *et al.* 1999). This distinguished the difference between assessing the acutely injured knee and the chronic unstable knee (Fig. 21-A.15; Parts I–V).

Flandry *et al.* (1991) devised the first visual analogue scale for assessing subjective knee complaints (the Hughston self-assessment questionnaire) (Fig. 21-A.16). Other authors used generic health outcome questionnaires to assess the results of ACL surgery (Shapiro *et al.* 1996), and showed the reliability and validity of the SF-36 in this application.

The Activity of Daily Living Scale of the Knee Outcome Survey (ADLS of KOS) (Irrgang *et al.* 1998) was also shown to be reliable, valid and responsive to change in one study for assessing outcome of treating ACL-deficient knees (Marx *et al.* 2001). These authors recommended use of the scale for the study of disorders of the knee in athletic patients at the same time that KOOS was published. This claimed validity in assessing knee ligament injuries (Roos *et al.* 1998).

Mohtadi (1998) developed a subjective quality of life outcome instrument for assessing ACL-deficient knees, and demonstrated adequate reliability, validity and responsiveness for the system. The instrument measures health status and knee condition using a patient-based evaluation questionnaire in a visual analogue scales format (Fig. 21-A.17). No independent observers have assessed its validity, and some have criticized it for not allowing accurate comparison between studies. Other criticisms include difficulties in comparing symptoms, or functional limitations according to different activity levels. Others dislike the use of visual analogue scales (Barber-Westin *et al.* 1999).

The American Academy of Orthopaedic Surgeons sports knee-rating scale (1998) was included in the Musculoskeletal Outcome Data Evaluation and Management System (MODEMS) for athletic patients with disorders of the knee. This instrument has five parts with a total of 23 questions: a core section (seven questions on stiffness, swelling, pain, and function); and four sections (each of four questions) on clicking or catching on activity, giving way on activity, current activity limitations due to the knee, and pain on activity due to the knee. Although it was shown to be valid and reliable, this scale has more items than other scales and a more complicated scoring system (Marx *et al.* 2001).

Anderson *et al.* (1993) found that 38 different scoring systems had been used to evaluate the results of treating ACL injuries in 52 articles published over 10 years in the *American Journal of Sports Medicine* and the *Journal of Bone and Joint Surgery*. In a more recent review, Johnson and Smith (2001) identified more than 54 different outcome measures used for assessing ACL surgery, most of which have not been validated for use.

Some studies have evaluated the most commonly used scoring systems, particularly for assessing the results of ACL reconstruction surgery. Bollen and Seedhom (1991) studied the correlation between Cincinnati Knee Ligament Rating System and the Lysholm score by using a self-administered questionnaire form. Others (Sgaglione *et al.* 1995) compared the Hospital for Special Surgery Knee Rating system (HSS) with the Lysholm score and Cincinnati Knee Ligament Rating System, and found that while the HSS and Lysholm scores did not correlate highly with the Cincinnati system, they did correlate with each other. These authors recommended that the Cincinnati system was the best instrument to use.

More recently, Risberg *et al.* (1999) studied the Lysholm, Cincinnati and IKDC knee ligament rating systems, and determined the sensitivity of each system to change over time. To do this, they measured outcome between each follow-up at 3, 6, 12 and 24 months postoperatively, and found the Cincinnati system to be the most sensitive to change. They also concluded that IKDC (1–4) was useful for documenting a clinical examination at one consultation, but not for detecting change. They advised against the use of Lysholm score for assessing outcome after ACL reconstruction.

A recent study has shown that the Lysholm score is reliable, valid and sensitive to change over time

(Marx *et al.* 2001). Indeed, others (Johnson and Smith 2001) recommended that the Lysholm score be used as the 'gold standard'.

Barber-Westin *et al.* (1999) have demonstrated the reliability, validity and responsiveness of all the components of the Cincinnati knee rating system, while Marx *et al.* (2001) were able to demonstrate reliability, validity and responsiveness in only the subjective component of the system.

One major controversy is the inconsistent way in which the instruments have been used in published reports. For example, Höher *et al.* (1997) analysed 106 reports which used the Lysholm score, and found differences in the mode of data collection. In 92 reports (87%), an interview between the investigator and the patient was used for data collection, as proposed in the original description of the scale. However, in the other 14 reports (13%) the authors used a self-administered questionnaire that was completed by the patient alone (Höher *et al.* 1997).

The value of subjective assessment of patients' disabilities and its direct relationship to the outcome of treatment has become more evident (Flandry *et al.* 1991; Hoher *et al.* 1995; Roos *et al.* 1998). One group (Höher *et al.* 1997) found a difference in the final score between self-administered and the interviewer-based Lysholm scale, with the self-administered system scoring consistently lower. It is to be noted that most of the comparative studies were carried out against the Lysholm score. The Cincinnati system scored lower than other objective systems in all the published studies (Anderson *et al.* 1993; Bollen and Seedhom 1991; Sgaglione *et al.* 1995). In a recent study, even the subjective part of the Cincinnati system scored lower than the remainder of the self-administered tools (ADLS, MODEMS) (Marx *et al.* 2001).

BEST BUY

It appears that the Cincinnati has the most supporting evidence to be a valid scale (Table 21.2), mainly because it is comprehensive and covers all aspects regarding knee symptoms and function. The inclusion of 'objective' assessment is against its use, however. These assessments are not unreliable, and there is no evidence to support the use of the

IKDC. In spite of the popularity of the Lysholm score, the weighting of its items and the calculation of a total score by adding up unrelated domains weaken its value.

The ADLS scale – a patient-based scale for ACL injuries – has been shown to be valid and scored 9 (Table 21.2). Hence, on the basis of the standards set up for this book, it is the 'best buy'. There is still a need to evaluate the KOOS and ACL-QOL, and the use of generic quality-of-life outcome tools is not probably justified in the highly demanding athletic group of patients.

Patellofemoral disorders

DISCUSSION AND GENERAL SPECIFICATION OF TOOLS

Fewer scores have been published to assess the management of these disorders. Fulkerson *et al.* (1990) modified the Lysholm score to evaluate the results of managing patellofemoral maltracking (Fig. 21-A.18). Others (Kujala *et al.* 1993) produced a questionnaire that included items related to patellofemoral disorders (Fig. 21-A.19). The questions included were modifications of those of Oretorp *et al.*'s (1979) adoption of the Larson scale (Larson 1974) with more emphasis on anterior knee pain symptoms. Others have used other scales designed for assessing ACL-deficient knees (such as Cincinnati), and some have used a generic tool.

BEST BUY

The only valid tool in this disorder is the site-specific scale ADLS. There is a need for an assessment of the validity of the Kujala score, and additional investigations are needed to evaluate independently some of the newer disease- and/or site-specific quality-of-life outcome measures such as KOOS.

Meniscal tears

DISCUSSION AND GENERAL SPECIFICATION OF TOOLS

Mintzer *et al.* (1998) used the Lysholm score for evaluating the results of treating meniscal injuries, while Cameron and Saha (1997) used a modification

Table 21.2: Functional outcome assessment for soft tissue knee disorders and fractures

Tool	Year	Type	Original use	Method of administration	Form	A	B	C	D	Total score
HSS	1977	Disease- and site-specific	ACL	Observer-administered	Objective signs + symptoms, disability assessment	0	0	0	4	4
Lysholm	1982 modified 1985	Disease- and site-specific	ACL	Observer-administered	Objective signs + symptoms, disability assessment	2[b]	2[b]	2[b]	4	10
OAK	1987	Disease- and site-specific		Observer-administered		0	0	0	4	4
Cincinnati knee score	1984, 89, 91	Disease- and site-specific	ACL expanded for other ligament meniscal injuries, and PF disorders[a]	Observer-administered	Objective signs + symptoms, disability assessment + X-ray	2[a]	2[a]	2[a]	4	10
IKDC	1993	Disease and site-specific	Ligament injuries	Observer-administered	Objective signs + symptoms, disability assessment + X-ray + hop test	2[c]	0	0	4	6
Flandry (Hughston score)	1991	Site-specific	All knee complaints	Patient-administered	VAS Questionnaire	0	0	0	1	1
ADLS of Knee Outcome Survey	1998	Site-specific	ACL, OA and PF disorders	Patient-administered	Questionnaire	2[b]	2+b	2[b]	3	9
KOOS	1998	Site-specific	ACL, OA and PF disorders	Patient-administered	Questionnaire	1	1	1	1	4
ACL-QOL	1998	Disease- and site-specific	ACL	Patient-administered	VAS Questionnaire	1	1	1	1	4
Tapper and Hoover	1969	Disease- and site-specific	Meniscal tears	Patient-administered	Questionnaire	0	0	0	4	4
Fulkerson	1990	Disease- and site-specific	PF disorders	Observer-administered	Questionnaire	0	0	0	4	4
Kujala	1993	Disease- and site-specific	PF disorders	Observer-administered	Questionnaire	0	0	0	4	4
Rasmussen	1973	Disease- and site-specific	Tibial plateau fracture	Observer-administered	Subjective pain and walking capacity + objective signs	0	0	0	4	4

A = Validity; B = Reliability; C = Responsiveness to change; D = Usage; ACL = Anterior cruciate ligament; OA = Osteoarthritis; PF = Patellofemoral; VAS = Visual Analogue Scale. [a]Barber-Westin et al. (1999); [b]Marx et al. (2001); [c]Risberg et al. (1999).

of the Fulkerson score. The only specific outcome tool for meniscal injuries was developed by Tapper and Hoover (1969) (Fig. 21-A.20). No specific questions were published, but rather a classification of results from their original report. Radiological assessment remained part of the overall assessment. New tools such as KOOS and ADLS were shown to be valid for assessing these disorders.

BEST BUY

The use of either ADLS or KOOS is recommended for assessing the outcome of meniscal surgery.

FRACTURES AROUND THE KNEE

Very few outcome measures have been developed for fractures around the knee. The Rasmussen criteria (Rasmussen 1973) was designed to evaluate the results of treating tibial plateau fractures (Fig. 21-A.21), and this has been widely used but never validated. It combines an assessment of pain and walking capacity in addition to an objective assessment. More recently, another combined subjective-objective assessment scheme was introduced (Stokel and Sadasivan 1991) where its parameters were integrated into a 100-point scoring system. However, this system was neither properly validated nor popularized. Others have used HSS, Lysholm or the WOMAC.

BEST BUY

Until the Rasmussen criteria have been validated, a site-specific (KOOS or ADLS of KOS) or generic instrument for measuring quality of life would be the choice. A radiological scoring system can add to the accuracy of evaluation in this category.

CONCLUSIONS

For assessing the results of knee replacement, a combination of SF-12 and Oxford-12 questions/ WOMAC seems to be the best available approach. As for ligament injuries, there is as yet no ideal instrument, and further studies are required to prove

that subjective assessment using a comprehensive system such as the ADLS, KOOS or ACL-QOL (when rigorously validated) produces results that are comparable with those of the Cincinnati scoring system. For patellofemoral and meniscal disorders, a validated self-administered tool is ideal. Hence, ADLS or KOOS would be the best buy.

For fractures around the knee, a combination of objective subjective and radiological scoring system is needed for short-term follow-up. The only disease-specific instrument available are the Rasmussen criteria, though subjective assessment will suffice for long-term results. As yet, there is no best buy, but the use of the WOMAC is recommended.

Although the principle of using a universal knee outcome tool for all knee disorders is appealing, such a system is unlikely to be practicable due to the differences in demands of patients from each disease group.

REFERENCES

Aichroth, P., Freeman, M., Smillie, I. S., and Souter, W. A. (1978): A knee function assessment chart. *J Bone Joint Surg* 60B, 308–9.

American Academy of Orthopaedic Surgeons (1998): *Scoring Algorithms for the Lower Limb Outcomes Data Collection Instrument, Version 2.0.* American Academy of Orthopaedic Surgeons, Rosemont, IL.

Anderson, A. F., Federspiel, C. F., and Snyder, R. B. (1993): Evaluation of knee ligament rating systems. *Am J Knee Surg* 6, 67–74.

Anderson, A. F., and Lipscomb, A. B. (1986): Clinical diagnosis of meniscal tears. Description of new manipulative test. *Am J Sports Med* 14, 291–3.

Barber-Westin, S. D., Noyes, F. R., and McCloskey, J. W. (1999): Rigorous statistical reliability, validity, and responsiveness testing of the Cincinnati knee rating system in 350 subjects with uninjured, injured, or anterior cruciate ligament-reconstructed knees. *Am J Sports Med* 27, 402–16.

Bellamy, N., Buchanan, W., and Goldsmith, C. (1988): Validation study of WOMAC: a health status instrument for measuring clinically important patient-relevant outcomes following total hip or knee arthroplasty in osteoarthritis. *Orthop Rheumat* **1**, 95–108.

Bollen, S., and Seedhom, B. (1991): A comparison of the Lysholm and Cincinnati Knee scoring questionnaires. *Am J Sports Med* **19**, 189–90.

Buechel, F. F. (1982): A simplified evaluation system for the rating of knee function. *Orthop Rev* **11**, 97–101.

Cameron, J. C., and Saha, S. (1997): Meniscal allograft transplantation for unicompartmental arthritis of the knee. *Clin Orthop* **337**, 164–71.

Dawson, J., Fitzpatrick, R., Murray, D., and Carr, A. (1998): Questionnaire on the perception of patients about total knee replacement. *J Bone Joint Surg* **80B**, 63–9.

Drake, B. G., Callahan, C. M., Dittus, R. S., and Wright, J. G. (1994): Global rating systems in assessing knee arthroplasty outcomes. *J Arthroplasty* **9**, 409–17.

Dunbar, M. J., Robertsson, O., Ryd, L., and Lidgren, L. (2000): Translation and validation of the Oxford-12 item knee score for use in Sweden. *Acta Orthop Scand* **71**, 268–74.

Dunbar, M. J., Robertsson, O., Ryd, L., and Lidgren, L. (2001): Appropriate questionnaires for knee arthroplasty. *J Bone Joint Surg* **83B**, 339–44.

Feagin, J. A., and Blake, W. P. (1983): Postoperative evaluation and result recording in the anterior cruciate reconstructed knee. *Clin Orthop* **172**, 143–7.

Flandry, F., Hunt, J. P., Terry, G., and Hughston, J. (1991): Analysis of subjective knee complaints using visual analog scales. *Am J Sports Med* **19**, 112–18.

Fulkerson, J. P., Becker, G. J., Meany, J. A., Miranda, M., and Folcik, M. A. (1990): Anteromedial tibial tubercle transfer without bone graft. *Am J Sports Med* **18**, 490–7.

Harcourt, W. G. V., White, S. H., and Jones, P. (2001): Specificity of the Oxford knee status questionnaire. *J Bone Joint Surg* **83B**, 345–7.

Hefti, F., Muller, W., Jakob, R. P., and Staubli, H. U. (1993): Evaluation of knee ligament injuries with the IKDC form. *Knee Surg Sports Traumatol Arthrosc* **1**, 226–34.

Höher, J., Bach, T., Münster, A., Bouillon, B., and Tiling, T. (1997): Does the mode of data collection change results in a subjective knee score? *Am J Sports Med* **25**, 642–7.

Höher, J., Munster, A., Klein, J., Eypasch, E., and Tiling, T. (1995): Validation and application of subjective knee questionnaire. *Knee Surg Sports Traumatol Arthrosc* **3**, 26–33.

Hunt, S. M., McKenna, S. P., McEwen, J., Williams, J., and Papp, E. (1981): The Nottingham Health Profile: subjective health status and medial consultations. *Soc Sci Med Am* **15**, 221–9.

Insall, J. N., Dorr, L. D., Scott, R. D., and Scott, W. N. (1989): Rationale of the Knee Society clinical rating system. *Clin Orthop* **248**, 13–4.

Irrgang, J. J., Snyder-Mackler, L., Wainner, R. S., Fu, F. H., and Harner, C. D. (1998): Development of a patient-reported measure of function of the knee. *J Bone Joint Surg* **80A**, 1132–45.

Johnson, D. S., and Smith, R. B. (2001): Outcome measurement of ACL deficient knee – what's the score? *Knee* **8**, 51–7.

Konig, A., Scheidler, M., Rader, C., and Eulert, J. (1989): The need for a dual rating system in total knee arthroplasty. *Clin Orthop* **248**, 13–4.

Kreibich, D. N., Vaz, M., Bourne, R. B., Rorabeck, C. H., Kim, P., Hardie, R., Kramer, J., and Kirkley, A. (1996): What is the best way of assessing outcome after total knee arthroplasty. *Clin Orthop* **331**, 221–5.

Kujala, U. M., Jaakkola, L. H., Koskinen, S. K., Taimela, S., Hurme, M., and Nelimarkka, O. (1993): Scoring of patellofemoral disorders. *Arthroscopy* **9**, 159–63.

Larson, R. L. (1974): Rating sheet for knee function. In: Smillie, I. (ed.), *Diseases of the Knee Joint*. Churchill Livingstone, Edinburgh, p. 29.

Lequesne, M. (1989): Validation of criteria and tests. *Scand J Rheumatol Suppl* **80**, 17–27.

Lingard, E. A., Katz, J. N., Wright, E. A., Wright, R. J., and Sledge, C. B. (2001): Validity and responsiveness of the Knee Society Clinical Rating System in comparison with the SF-36 and WOMAC. *J Bone Joint Surg* **83A**, 1856–64.

Liow, R. Y. L., Walker, K., Wajid, M. A., Bedi, G., and Lennox, C. M. E. (2000): The reliability of the

American Knee Society score. *Acta Orthop Scand* **71**, 603–8.

Lukianov, A. V., Gillquist, J., Grana, W. A., and DeHaven, K. E. (1987): An anterior cruciate ligament (ACL) evaluation format for assessment of artificial or autologous anterior cruciate reconstruction results. *Clin Orthop* **218**, 167–80.

Lysholm, J., and Gillquist, J. (1982): Evaluation of knee ligament surgery results with a special emphasis on use of a scoring scale. *Am J Sports Med* **10**, 150.

Marshall, J. L., Fetto, J. F., and Botero, P. M. (1977): Knee ligament injuries: a statistical evaluation method. *Clin Orthop* **123**, 115–29.

Martin, D. P., Engelberg, R., Agel, J., Snapp, D., and Swiontkowski, M. F. (1996): Development of musculoskeletal extremity health assessment instrument: the Musculoskeletal Functional Assessment Instrument. *J Orthop Res* **14**, 173–81.

Marx, R. G., Jones, E. C., Allen, A. A., Altchchek, D. W., O'Brien, S. J., Rodeo, S. A., Williams, R. J., Warren, R. F., and Wickiewicz, T. L. (2001): Reliability, validity and responsiveness of four knee outcome scales for athletic patients. *J Bone Joint Surg* **83A**, 1459–69.

Miller, R. K., and Carr, A. J. (1993): The knee. In: Pynsent, P., Fairbank, J. and Carr, A. (eds), *Outcome Measures in Orthopaedics*. Butterworth-Heinemann, Oxford, pp. 228–39.

Mintzer, C. M., Richmond, J. C., and Taylor, J. (1998): Meniscal repair in the young athlete. *Am J Sports Med* **26**, 630–3.

Mohtadi, N. (1998): Development and validation of the quality of life outcome measure (questionnaire) for chronic anterior cruciate ligament deficiency. *Am J Sports Med* **26**, 350–9.

Muller, W., Biedert, R., Hefti, F., Jakob, R. P., Munzinger, U., and Staubli, H. U. (1988): OAK knee evaluation. A new way to assess knee ligament injuries. *Clin Orthop* **232**, 37–50.

Noyes, F. R., Barber, S. E., and Mooar, L. A. (1989): A rationale for assessing sports activity levels and limitation in knee disorders. *Clin Orthop* **246**, 238–49.

Noyes, F. R., Mooar, P. A., Matthews, D. S., and Butler, D. L. (1983): The symptomatic anterior cruciate-deficient knee. Part I: The long-term functional disability in athletically active individuals. *J Bone Joint Surg* **65A**, 154–62.

Noyes, F. R., Mooar, L. A., and Barber, S. E. (1991): The assessment of work related activities and limitations in knee disorders. *Am J Sports Med* **19**, 178–88.

O'Donoghue, D. H. (1955): Analysis of end results of surgical treatment of injuries to the ligaments of the knee. *J Bone Joint Surg* **37A**, 1–13.

O'Donoghue, D. H. (1963): A method for replacement of the anterior cruciate ligament of the knee. *J Bone Joint Surg* **45A**, 905–24.

Oretorp, N., Gillquist, J., and Liljedahl, S. O. (1979): Long-term results for non-acute anteromedial rotatory instability of the knee. *Acta Orthop Scand* **50**, 329–36.

Ranawat, C. S., Insall, J. N., and Shine, J. (1976): Duocondylar knee arthroplasty. *Clin Orthop* **120**, 76–92.

Rasmussen, P. S. (1973): Tibial condyle fractures. Impairment of knee joint stability as an indication for surgical treatment. *J Bone Joint Surg* **55A**, 1331–50.

Risberg, M. A., Holm, I., Steen, H., and Beynnon, B. D. (1999): Sensitivity to change over time for the IKDC form, The Lysholm score and the Cincinnati knee score. A prospective study of 120 ACL reconstructed patients with a 2-year follow up. *Knee Surg Sports Traumatol Arthrosc* **7**, 152–9.

Roos, E., Roos, H., Lohmander, L. S., Ekdahl, C., and Beynoon, B. (1998): Development of a self-administered outcome measure. *J Orthop Sports Phys Ther* **78**, 88–96.

Ryd, L., Karrholm, J., and Ahlvin, P. (1997): Knee scoring systems in gonarthrosis. Evaluation of interobserver variability and the envelope of bias. Score Assessment Group. *Acta Orthop Scand* **68**, 41–5.

Sgaglione, N. A., Del Pizzo, W., Fox, J. M., and Friedman, M. J. (1995): Critical analysis of knee ligament rating scales. *Am J Sports Med* **23**, 660–7.

Shapiro, E. T., Richmond, J. C., Rockett, S. E., McGrath, M. M., and Donaldson, W. R. (1996): The use of generic, patient-based health assessment (SF-36) for evaluation of patients with anterior cruciate ligament injuries. *Am J Sports Med* **24**, 196–200.

Stokel, E. A., and Sadasivan, K. K. (1991): Tibial plateau fractures: standardized evaluation of operative results. *Orthopaedics* **14**, 263–70.

Stucki, G., Sangha, O., Stucki, S., Michel, B. A., Tyndall, A., Dick, W., and Theiler, R. (1998): Comparison of the WOMAC (Western Ontario and McMaster Universities) osteoarthritis index and a self-report format of the self-administered Lequesne-Algofunctional index in patients with knee and hip osteoarthritis. *Osteoarthritis Cartilage* **6**, 79–86.

Tapper, E., and Hoover, N. (1969): Late results after meniscectomy. *J Bone Joint Surg* **51A**, 517–26.

Tegner, Y., and Lysholm, J. (1985): Rating systems in the evaluation of knee ligament injuries. *Clin Orthop* **198**, 43–9.

Ware, J., and Hays, R. (1988): Methods for measuring patient satisfaction with specific medical encounters. *J Med Care* **26**, 393–402.

Ware, J., Kosinski, M., and Keller, S. D. (1996): A 12-item short-form health survey: construction of scales and preliminary tests of reliability and validity. *Med Care* **34**, 220–3.

Windsor, R. E., Insall, J. N., and Warren, R. F. (1988): The Hospital for Special Surgery knee rating system. *Am J Knee Surg* **1**, 140–5.

Appendix

	RIGHT						LEFT					
		Post						Post				
	Pre	6m	1	2	3	4	Pre	6m	1	2	3	4
1. PAIN – 30 points												
1. No pain at any time	30											
2. No pain on walking	15											
3. Mild pain on walking	10											
4. Moderate pain on walking	5											
5. Severe pain on walking	0											
6. No pain at rest	15											
7. Mild pain at rest	10											
8. Moderate pain at rest	5											
9. Severe pain at rest	0											
2. FUNCTION – 22 points												
A1. Walking and standing unlimited	12											
2. Walking distance of 5 to 10 blocks and standing ability intermittent (more than 1/2 hour)	10											
3. Walking 1 to 5 blocks and standing ability up to 1/2 hour	8											
4. Walk less than 1 block	4											
5. Can't walk	0											
B1. Climb stairs	5											
2. Climb stairs with support	2											
3. Transfer activity	5											
4. Transfer activity with support	2											
3. ROM – 18 points												
1. 1 point for each 8° of arc of motion-maximum of 18 points												
4. MUSCLE STRENGTH – 10 points												
1. Good – Can't break quadriceps power	10											
2. Good – Can break quadriceps power	8											
3. Fair – Moves through arc of motion	4											
4. Poor – Can't move through arc of motion	0											
5. FL DEFORMITY – 10 points												
1. No deformity	10											
2. Few degrees	8											
3. 5 – 10°	5											
4. 11° or more	0											
6. INSTABILITY – 10 points												
1. N	10											
2. Mild – 0–5°	8											
3. Moderate – 6–15°	5											
4. Severe – 16° or more	0											

Remarks: Subtract 1 point for using a cane, 2 points for 1 crutch and 3 points for 2 crutches. Two points for 5° of extension lag, 3 points for 10° and 5 points for 15° or more. One point for 5° valgus and varus deformities.

Figure 21-A.1 Knee disability assessment. Developed for follow-up evaluations of total knee replacement. Reprinted from Ranawat et al. (1976).

Knee function assessment chart
(British Orthopaedic Association Research Sub-committee)

Name   Age
Hospital number   Sex
Occupation

DIAGNOSIS

DURATION OF DISEASE   General   (years)
                              Knee   (years)

SIDE

PREVIOUS KNEE OPERATIONS

OTHER JOINTS (*See Appendix*)

STATE OF OTHER KNEE   Normal
                              Slightly affected
                              Moderately affected
                              Severely affected
                              Replaced

STATE OF HIPS   RIGHT   LEFT
                              Normal
                              Slightly affected
                              Moderately affected
                              Severely affected
                              Replaced

STATE OF   RIGHT   LEFT
FEET/ANKLES   Normal
                                Slightly affected
                              Moderately affected
                              Severely affected
                              Replaced

FOLLOW-UP (months)

1. ASSESSMENT BY THE PATIENT

   A. After treatment the patient is:
      (4) Enthusiastic
      (3) Satisfied
      (2) Non-committal
      (1) Disappointed

   B. Is the patient's present disability due to the
      affected knee?
      (4) Entirely
      (3) Mainly
      (2) Partially
      (1) Scarcely at all

2. PAIN
   (4) None
   (3) Mild pain, not interfering with activities or sleep
   (2) Moderate pain, either reducing activities or
      disturbing sleep
   (1) Severe pain

3. ABILITY TO WALK
   Distance   OR   *Time*
   (5) >1 kilometre   >60 minutes
      (unlimited)
   (4) Up to 1 kilometre   30–60 minutes
   (3) Up to 50 metres   10–30 minutes
   (2) 50–100 metres   5–10 minutes
      (outdoors)
   (1) Indoors only   Indoors only
   (0) Unable   Unable

4. WALKING AID
   (4) None
   (3) Stick outside
   (2) Stick always
   (1) Two sticks/
      crutches/frame
   (0) Unable to walk

5. GAIT
   (4) Normal free swing
   (3) Slight limitation of swing
   (2) Minimal movement
   (1) Stiff knee

6. FLEXION DEFORMITY
   (5) 0 degrees
   (4) <10 degrees
   (3) 11–20 degrees
   (2) 21–30 degrees
   (1) >30 degrees

7. MAXIMUM FLEXION
   (4) >100 degrees
   (3) 81–100 degrees
   (2) 61–80 degrees
   (1) <60 degrees

8. EXTENSION LAG
   Additional to flexion contracture if present
   (4) 0 degrees
   (3) <10 degrees
   (2) <20 degrees
   (1) >20 degrees

9. VALGUS ANGLE
   When the tibia is
   stressed laterally
   (4) 0–10 degrees
   (3) <20 degrees
   (2) <30 degrees
   (1) >30 degrees

10. VARUS ANGLE
   When the tibia is
   stressed medially
   (5) 0 degrees
   (4) <10 degrees
   (3) <20 degrees
   (2) <30 degrees
   (1) >30 degrees

11. ABILITY TO GET OUT OF CHAIR
   (4) With ease
   (3) With difficulty
   (2) Only by using arms
   (1) Unable

12. ABILITY TO CLIMB STAIRS
   (4) Normal
   (3) One step at a time
   (2) Only with a bannister, stick or both
   (1) Unable or only by bizarre method

APPENDIX

STATE OF OTHER JOINTS
SLIGHTLY AFFECTED
   Infrequent pain
   Minor stiffness – no functional deficit
   Walking minimally affected. No support required

MODERATELY AFFECTED
   Moderate pain
   Joint stiffness producing some function deficit
   Walking interrupted and support required

SEVERELY AFFECTED
   Severe pain
   Stiffness with marked functional disability
   Unable to walk or walking with difficulty using
   a major support

Figure 21-A.2 Knee function assessment chart. Reprinted from Aichroth *et al.* (1978).

Patient Name _____   Surgeon _____

Date of Exam: Mo._____ Day _____ Year _____   Height _____ ' _____ " Weight _____ (lbs.)

Time of Examination (circle one):

    Preoperative.   Postoperative: 3 6 12 18 months,   2 3 4 5 years

---

I. PAIN (30 points possible; circle one):
    A. No pain during walking, standing, or stair climbing activities 30
    B. Occasional ache, no compromise of ambulation activities 26
    C. Mild pain following excessive ambulation, may take aspirin 22
    D. Moderate pain with normal ambulation activities. May require pain medicine stronger than aspirin after
        excessive or unusual activities which cause considerable pain 18
    E. Severe pain, but able to ambulate. Serious limitation of activities. May need prolonged medicine
        stronger than aspirin 10
    F. Totally disabled with pain, unable to ambulate 0

II. FUNCTION (25 points possible):
    A. GAIT (5 points possible; circle one)   B. STANDING (5 points possible; circle one)
        1. No limp 5   1. Comfortable standing without support for ¾ hour 5
        2. Mild limp 3   2. Comfortable standing without support for ½ hour 3
        3. Moderate limp 1   3. Comfortable standing without support for ¼ hour 1
        4. Severe limp 0   4. Not able to stand without discomfort 0

    C. WALKING (5 points possible; circle one)   D. STAIRS (5 points possible; circle one)
        1. Unlimited range 5   1. Foot over foot without use of banister 5
        2. Six blocks 4   2. Foot over foot using banister 3
        3. Two or three blocks 3   3. Using stairs with external support and banister 1
        4. Indoors, around the house only . 1   4. Unable to climb stairs 0
        5. Bed to chair, unable to walk . . 0

            E. SUPPORT (5 points possible; circle one)
                1. No external support needed to walk comfortably . . . 5
                2. Single cane needed for long walks 4
                3. Single cane needed most of the time 3
                4. One crutch needed most of the time 2
                5. Two canes needed most of the time 1
                6. Two crutches or walker needed most of the time . . . 0

III. RANGE OF MOTION (15 points possible; circle one)
    A. 121° or complete flexion 15   Specify: _____° to _____°
    B. 91° to 120° 12
    C. 61° to 90° 9
    D. 31° to 60° 6
    E. 10° to 30° 3
    F. Less than 10° 0

IV. DEFORMITY (12 points possible)
    A. ( ) Extensor lag or ( ) flexion   B. Recurvatum (2 points possible; circle one) Specifiy: _____°
        contracture. Specify: _____°   1. 0° to 5° 2
        (2 points possible; circle one)   2. 6° to 10° 1
        1. 5° or less 2   3. Greater than 10° 0
        2. 6° to 10° 1
        3. Greater than 10° 0   D. Patella alignment (2 points possible; circle one)
                        1. Normal 2
    C. ( ) Varus or ( ) Valgus deformity.   2. Alta or infera 1
        Specify _____°   3. Lateral subluxation 0
        (2 points possible; circle one)
        1. 5° or less 2   F. Limb length discrepancy (2 points possible; circle one)
        2. 6° to 10° 1   1. 1.5 cm or less 2
        3. Greater than 15° 0   2. 1.6 cm to 2.5 cm 1
                        3. Greater than 2.5 cm 0
    E. Effusion (2 points possible; circle one)
        1. None 2
        2. Mild 1
        3. Marked 0

Figure 21-A.3 New Jersey Orthopaedic Hospital Knee Evaluation System. Reprinted from Buechel *et al.* (1982).

Patient category
   A. Unilateral or bilateral (opposite knee successfully replaced)
   B. Unilateral, other knee symptomatic
   C. Multiple arthritis or medical infirmity

Pain	Points	Function	Points
None	50	Walking	50
Mild or occasional	45	Unlimited	40
Stairs only	40	>10 blocks	30
Walking & stairs	30	5–10 blocks	20
Moderate		<5 blocks	10
Occasional	20	Housebound	0
Continual	10	Unable	
Severe	0	Stairs	
		Normal up & down	50
Range of motion		Normal up; down with rail	40
Each degree = 1 point	25	Up & down with rail	30
		Up with rail; unable down	15
(maximum movement in any position)		Unable	0
Anteroposterior		Subtotal	—
<5 mm	10		
5–10 mm	5	**Deductions (minus)**	
>10 mm	0	Cane	5
Mediolateral		Two canes	10
<5°	15	Crutches or walker	20
6°–9°	10	Total deductions	—
10°–14°	5	Function score	—
15°	0		
Subtotal	—		

Deductions (minus)
Flexion contracture

5°–10°	2
10°–15°	5
16°–20°	10
>20°	15
Extension lag	
<10°	5
10°–20°	10
>20°	15
Alignment	
5°–10°	0
0°–4°	3 points each degree
11°–15°	3 points each degree
Other	20
Total deductions	—
Knee score	—

(If total is a minus number, score is 0)

Figure 21-A.4 Knee Score. Rationale of American Knee Society (KSS). Reprinted from Insall *et al.* (1989).

KOOS items	Pre-operative Total group n = 142	ACL n = 12	ACL + Men n = 23	Men n = 49	Men + CD n = 27	CD n = 18	P-value
Pain							
P1. How often is your knee painful? What degree of pain have you experienced the last week, when …?	+	+	+	+	+	+	0.12
P2. Twisting/pivoting on your knee	+		+	+	+	+	0.7
P3. Straightening knee fully		+					0.09
P4. Bending knee fully		+		+	+	+	0.3
P5. Walking on flat suface	−		−	−			0.004
P6. Going up or down stairs					+	+	<0.001
P7. At night while in bed	−	−	−	−			<0.001
P8. Sitting or lying	−	−	−	−			<0.001
P9. Standing upright				−	−		0.002
Symptoms							
S1. How severe is your knee stiffness after first wakening in the morning?	−	−		−			0.07
S2. How severe is your knee stiffness after sitting, lying or resting later in the day?				−			0.007
S3. Do you have swelling in your knee?						+	0.03
S4. Do you feel grinding, hear clicking or any other type of noise when your knee moves?	+	+	+	+	+	+	0.07
S5. Does your knee catch or hang up when moving?							0.5
S6. Can you straighten your knee fully?		+					0.4
S7. Can you bend your knee fully?		+		+		+	0.8
Activities of daily living What difficulty have you experienced in the last week …?							
A1. Descending stairs					+		0.01
A2. Ascending stairs							0.11
A3. Rising from sitting		−					0.001
A4. Standing	−		−	−			0.2
A5. Bending to floor/pick up an object							0.11
A6. Walking on flat surface		−		−			0.01
A7. Getting in/out of car			−				0.03
A8. Going shopping		−	−	−		−	0.003
A9. Putting on socks/stockings	−	−	−	−			0.08
A10. Rising from bed	−	−	−	−			<0.001
A11. Taking off socks/stockings	−	−	−	−			0.11
A12. Lying in bed (turning over, maintaining knee position)			−	−		+	<0.001
A13. Getting in/out of bath/shower	−	−	−	−		−	0.17
A14. Sitting	−	−	−	−		−	<0.001
A15. Getting on/off toilet	−	−	−	−		−	<0.001
A16. Heavy domestic duties (shovelling snow, scrubbing floors etc.)			−				0.01
A17. Light domestic duties (cooking, dusting etc.)	−	−	−	−		−	0.02
Sport and recreation function What difficulty have you experienced in the last week …?							
Sp1. Squatting	+	+	+	+	+	+	0.6
Sp2. Running	+	+	+	+	+	+	0.6
Sp3. Jumping	+	+	+	+	+	+	0.16
Sp4. Turning/twisting on your injured knee	+	+	+	+	+	+	0.7
Sp5. Kneeling	+	+	+	+	+	+	0.3
Knee-related quality of life							
Q1. How often are you aware of your knee problems?	+	+	+	+	+	+	0.18
Q2. Have you modified your life style to avoid potentially damaging activities to your knee?	+		+	+	+	+	0.6
Q3. How troubled are you with lack of confidence in your knee?	+	+	+	+	+	+	0.13
Q4. In general, how much difficulty do you have with your knee?	+	+	+	+	+	+	0.4

The mean score can range from 0 to 4. To simplify interpretation the mean scores are categorized into three groups. A mean score of ≥2, indicating on average at least moderate problems with the item, is indicated by (+). A mean score of ≤1, indicating subjects reporting on average at the most mild problems with the item, is marked by (−). Items not marked by (+) or (−), have a mean score of >1 and <2, indicating mild to moderate problems with the item. P-values are given for comparisons of reported scores with the Kruskal-Wallis test across all groups.

Figure 21-A.5 Mean KOOS scores of each single item for the total group, and for the subgroups isolated ACL-injury (ACL), ACL-injury with associated meniscus injury (ACL + Men), isolated meniscus injury (Men), meniscus injury with associated cartilage damage (Men + CD), and isolated cartilage damage (CD). Reprinted from Roos et al. (1998).

Knee Outcome Survey
Activities of Daily Living Scale

Instructions: The following questionnaire is designed to determine the symptoms and limitations that you experience because of your knee while you perform your usual *daily activities*. Please answer each question by *checking the statement that best describes you over the last 1 to 2 days*. For a given question, more than one of the statements may describe you, but please mark ONLY the statement that best describes you during your usual daily activities.

Symptoms:

1. To what degree does pain in your knee affect your daily activity level?
   _5_ I never have pain in my knee.
   _4_ I have pain in my knee, but it does not affect my daily activity.
   _3_ Pain affects my activity slightly.
   _2_ Pain affects my activity moderately.
   _1_ Pain affects my activity severely.
   _0_ Pain in my knee prevents me from performing all daily activities.

2. To what degree does grinding or grating of your knee affect your daily activity level?
   _5_ I never have grinding or grating in my knee.
   _4_ I have grinding or grating in my knee, but it does not affect my daily activity.
   _3_ Grinding or grating affects my activity slightly.
   _2_ Grinding or grating affects my activity moderately.
   _1_ Grinding or grating affects my activity severely.
   _0_ Grinding or grating in my knee prevents me from performing all daily activities.

3. To what degree does stiffness in your knee affect your daily activity level?
   _5_ I never have stiffness in my knee.
   _4_ I have stiffness in my knee, but it does not affect my daily activity.
   _3_ Stiffness affects my activity slightly.
   _2_ Stiffness affects my activity moderately.
   _1_ Stiffness affects my activity severely.
   _0_ Stiffness in my knee prevents me from performing all daily activities.

4. To what degree does swelling in your knee affect your daily activity level?
   _5_ I never have swelling in my knee.
   _4_ I have swelling in my knee, but it does not affect my daily activity.
   _3_ Swelling affects my activity slightly.
   _2_ Swelling affects my activity moderately.
   _1_ Swelling affects my activity severely.
   _0_ Swelling in my knee prevents me from performing all daily activities.

5. To what degree does slipping of your knee affect your daily activity level?
   _5_ I never have slipping of my knee.
   _4_ I have slipping of my knee, but it does not affect my daily activity.
   _3_ Slipping affects my activity slightly.
   _2_ Slipping affects my activity moderately.
   _1_ Slipping affects my activity severely.
   _0_ Slipping of my knee prevents me from performing all daily activities.

6. To what degree does buckling of your knee affect your daily activity level?
   _5_ I never have buckling of my knee.
   _4_ I have buckling of my knee, but it does not affect my daily activity level.
   _3_ Buckling affects my activity slightly.
   _2_ Buckling affects my activity moderately.
   _1_ Buckling affects my activity severely.
   _0_ Buckling of my knee prevents me from performing all daily activities.

7. To what degree does weakness or lack of strength of your leg affect your daily activity level?
   _5_ My leg never feels weak.
   _4_ My leg feels weak, but it does not affect my daily activity.
   _3_ Weakness affects my activity slightly.
   _2_ Weakness affects my activity moderately.
   _1_ Weakness affects my activity severely.
   _0_ Weakness of my leg prevents me from performing all daily activities.

Functional Disability with Activities of Daily Living

8. How does your knee affect your ability to walk?
   _5_ My knee does not affect my ability to walk.
   _4_ I have pain in my knee when walking, but it does not affect my ability to walk.
   _3_ My knee prevents me from walking more than 1 mile.
   _2_ My knee prevents me from walking more than 1/2 mile.
   _1_ My knee prevents me from walking more than 1 block.
   _0_ My knee prevents me from walking.

9. Because of your knee, do you walk with crutches or a cane?
   _3_ I can walk without crutches or a cane.
   _2_ My knee causes me to walk with 1 crutch or a cane.
   _1_ My knee causes me to walk with 2 crutches.
   _0_ Because of my knee, I cannot walk even with crutches.

10. Does your knee cause you to limp when you walk?
   _2_ I can walk without a limp.
   _1_ Sometimes my knee causes me to walk with a limp.
   _0_ Because of my knee, I cannot walk without a limp.

11. How does your knee affect your ability to go *up stairs?*
   _5_ My knee does not affect my ability to go up stairs.
   _4_ I have pain in my knee when going up stairs, but it does not limit my ability to go up stairs.
   _3_ I am able to go up stairs normally, but I need to rely on use of a railing.
   _2_ I am able to go up stairs one step at a time with use of a railing.
   _1_ I have to use crutches or a cane to go up stairs.
   _0_ I cannot go up stairs.

Figure 21-A.6 Knee Outcome Survey: Activities of Daily Living Scale. Reprinted from Irrgang *et al.* (1998).

12. How does your knee affect your ability to go down stairs?
  _5_ My knee does not affect my ability to go down stairs.
  _4_ I have pain in my knee when going down stairs, but it does not limit my ability to go down stairs.
  _3_ I am able to go down stairs normally, but I need to rely on use of a railing.
  _2_ I am able to go down stairs one step at a time with use of a railing.
  _1_ I have to use crutches or a cane to go down stairs.
  _0_ I cannot go down stairs.

13. How does your knee affect your ability to stand?
  _5_ My knee does not affect my ability to stand. I can stand for unlimited amounts of time.
  _4_ I have pain in my knee when standing, but it does not limit my ability to stand.
  _3_ Because of my knee I cannot stand for more than 1 hour.
  _2_ Because of my knee I cannot stand for more than ½ hour.
  _1_ Because of my knee I cannot stand for more than 10 minutes.
  _0_ I cannot stand because of my knee.

14. How does your knee affect your ability to kneel on the front of your knee?
  _5_ My knee does not affect my ability to kneel on the front of my knee. I can kneel for unlimited amounts of time.
  _4_ I have pain when kneeling on the front of my knee, but it does not limit my ability to kneel.
  _3_ I cannot kneel on the front of my knee for more than 1 hour.
  _2_ I cannot kneel on the front of my knee for more than ½ hour.
  _1_ I cannot kneel on the front of my knee for more than 10 minutes.
  _0_ I cannot kneel on the front of my knee.

15. How does your knee affect your ability to squat?
  _5_ My knee does not affect my ability to squat. I can squat all the way down.
  _4_ I have pain when squatting, but I can still squat all the way down.
  _3_ I cannot squat more than 3/4 of the way down.
  _2_ I cannot squat more than 1/2 of the way down.
  _1_ I cannot squat more than 1/4 of the way down.
  _0_ I cannot squat at all.

16. How does your knee affect your ability to sit with your knee bent?
  _5_ My knee does not affect my ability to sit with my knee bent. I can sit for unlimited amounts of time.
  _4_ I have pain when sitting with my knee bent, but it does not limit my ability to sit.
  _3_ I cannot sit with my knee bent for more than 1 hour.
  _2_ I cannot sit with my knee bent for more than ½ hour.
  _1_ I cannot sit with my knee bent for more than 10 minutes.
  _0_ I cannot sit with my knee bent.

17. How does your knee affect your ability to rise from a chair?
  _5_ My knee does not affect my ability to rise from a chair.
  _4_ I have pain when rising from the seated position, but it does not affect my ability to rise from the seated position.
  _2_ Because of my knee I can only rise from a chair if I use my hands and arms to assist.
  _0_ Because of my knee I cannot rise from a chair.

Figure 21-A.6 Knee Outcome Survey: Activities of Daily Living Scale. (From Irrgang *et al.* 1998). – *continued*

Item	Scoring categories
During the past four weeks	
1) How would you describe the pain you usually have from your knee?	1. None 2. Very mild 3. Mild 4. Moderate 5. Severe
2) Have you had any trouble with washing and drying yourself (all over) because of your knee?	1. No trouble at all 2. Very little trouble 3. Moderate trouble 4. Extreme difficulty 5. Impossible to do
3) Have you had any trouble getting in and out of a car or using public transport because of your knee? (whichever you tend to use)	1. No trouble at all 2. Very little trouble 3. Moderate trouble 4. Extreme difficulty 5. Impossible to do
4) For how long have you been able to walk before the pain from your knee becomes severe? (with or without a stick)	1. No pain > 30 min 2. 16 to 30 min 3. 5 to 15 min 4. Around the house only 5. Not at all – severe on walking
5) After a meal (sat at a table), how painful has it been for you to stand up from a chair because of your knee?	1. Not at all painful 2. Slightly painful 3. Moderately painful 4. Very painful 5. Unbearable
6) Have you been limping when walking, because of your knee?	1. Rarely/never 2. Sometimes or just at first 3. Often, not just at first 4. Most of the time 5. All of the time
7) Could you kneel down and get up again afterwards?	1. Yes, easily 2. With little difficulty 3. With moderate difficulty 4. With extreme difficulty 5. No, impossible
8) Have you been troubled by pain from your knee in bed at night?	1. No nights 2. Only 1 or 2 nights 3. Some nights 4. Most nights 5. Every night
9) How much has pain from your knee interfered with your usual work (including housework)?	1. Not at all 2. A little bit 3. Moderately 4. Greatly 5. Mostly
10) Have you felt that your knee might suddenly 'give way' or let you down?	1. Rarely/never 2. Sometimes or just at first 3. Often not just at first 4. Most of the time 5. All of the time
11) Could you do the household shopping on your own?	1. Yes, easily 2. With little difficulty 3. With moderate difficulty 4. With extreme difficulty 5. No, impossible
12) Could you walk down a flight of stairs?	1. Yes, easily 2. With little difficulty 3. With moderate difficulty 4. With extreme difficulty 5. No, impossible

Figure 21-A.7 The 12-Item Oxford Knee Questionnaire. Reprinted from Dawson *et al.* (1998).

Date of Examination _____

Time: Post Injury/Post Surgery _____

A. Patient's Own Evaluation:_____ ☐
    N = Normal   I = Improved
    S = Severe   W = Worse

B. Pain:_____ ☐
    0 = Yes   1 = No
   Swelling: _____ ☐
    0 = Yes   1 = No
   Stairs Difficulty: _____ ☐
    0 = Yes   1 = No
   Clicking-Numbness:_____ ☐
    0 = Yes   1 = No
   Giving Way: 0–4 _____ ☐
    4 = Normal, none
    2 = With stress only
    1 = With stress upon daily activity
    0 = Regularly upon daily activity
   Return to Sports or Work: 0–3 _____ ☐
    3 = Full return
    2 = Return to orign. with limitations
    1 = Return to different
    0 = No return

C. 1) Functional Tests
    Duck Walk: 0,1,2 _____ ☐
    Run in Place: 0,1 _____ ☐
    Jump on One Leg: 0,1,2 _____ ☐
    Half Squat: 0,1 _____ ☐
    Full Squat: 0,1 _____ ☐
    0 = can not perform
    1 = can perform but with discomfort
    2 = can perform

SCORE CHART	
Excellent	= 46–50
Good	= 41–45
Fair+	= 36–40
Fair	= 31–35
Poor	= <30

Physician's Initials: _____

2) Specific Knee Exam
    Tenderness: 0,1 _____ ☐
    Joint Effusion: 0,1 _____ ☐
    Swelling (soft tissue): 0,1 _____ ☐
    Crepitations: 0,1 _____ ☐
    Muscle Power: 0–3 _____ ☐
      3 = normal
      2 = diminished flex. or ext.
      1 = diminished flex. & ext.
      0 = very weak
    Thigh Sizes: 0–2 _____ ☐
      2 = equal
      1 = 1–2 cm difference
      0 = <2 cm different
    Range of Motion: 0–3 _____ ☐
      3 = normal
      2 = limited flex. or ext.
      1 = limited flex. & ext.
      0 = >90 (degree symbol)
   Stability:
   For all stability scores the answer must
   include both number and letter, e.g. 4a.
    LCL: 0–5, (a/b) _____ ☐
      5 = normal
      4 = mild inst. in flex.
      3 = moderate inst. in flex.
      2 = inst. in flex. & ext.
      0 = gross instability
      a = hard end point
      b = soft or no end point
    MCL: 0–5, (a/b) _____ ☐
      5 = normal
      4 = mild inst. in flex.
      3 = moderate inst. in flex.
      2 = inst. in flex. & ext.
      0 = gross instability
      a = hard end point
      b = soft or no end point
    ACL: 0–5, a/b (= opp. leg) _____ ☐
      5 = normal
      4 = slight jog
      3 = moderate jog
      2 = severe in neutral
      0 = severe in neu. & rot.
        (Pivot Shift, Slocum, Jerk Test)
      a = hard end point
      b = soft or no end point
    PCL: 0–5, a/b (= opp. leg) _____ ☐
      5 = normal
      4 = slight jog
      3 = moderate jog
      2 = severe in neutral
      0 = severe in neu & rot.
      a = hard end point
      b = soft or no end point

Total Score: max–50 pts. _____ ☐

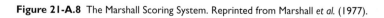

Figure 21-A.8 The Marshall Scoring System. Reprinted from Marshall et al. (1977).

Symptoms (5 points)

Swelling: _____ ☐
- No = 2
- Yes = 0

Locking: _____ ☐
- No = 3
- Yes = 0

Giving Way (20 points)

Severity: _____ ☐
- None = 10
- Transient = 8
- Recovery <1 day = 6
- Recovery <1 week = 2
- Recovery >1 week = 0

Frequency: _____ ☐
- None = 10
- 1 per year = 8
- 2–6 per year = 6
- 1 per month = 4
- 1 per week = 2
- Daily = 0

Function (20 points)

ADL and Work: _____ ☐
- Full return = 4
- Limited, or job change = 2
- Unable due to knee = 0

Sports: _____ ☐
- Full return = 4
- Same but modified = 3
- Different sport = 2
- No return = 0

Ability To: _____ ☐
- Decelerate = 4
- Cut side to side = 4
- Jump = 4

Examination (45 points)

ROM: _____ ☐
- Normal = 3
- Limited flexion or extension = 1
- Both = 0

Effusion: _____ ☐
- No = 4
- Yes = 0

Thigh Circumference: _____ ☐
- Equal to 1 cm difference = 2
- >1 cm difference = 0

Lachman: (note end point) _____ ☐
- Negative = 4
- 1+ (0–5 mm) = 3
- 2+ (5–10 mm) = 2
- 3+ (10–15 mm) = 0

```
SCORE CHART
Excellent 90–100    Fair 70–79
     Good 80–89     Poor <70
```

Examination (45 points)

Anterior Drawer: _____ ☐
- Negative = 2
- 1+ (0–5 mm) = 2
- 2+ (5–10 mm) = 0
- 3+ (10–15 mm) = 0

Posterior Drawer: _____ ☐
- Negative = 5
- 1+ (0–5 mm) = 3
- 2+ (5–10 mm) = 2
- 3+ (10–15 mm) = 0

Pivot Shift: _____ ☐
- Negative (or equal to unaffected side) = 10
- Grind, no movement = 8
- 1+, slight movement = 4
- 2+, definite movement = 2
- 3+, movement and locks = 0

MCL: _____ ☐
- Normal = 5
- 1+ = 3
- 2+ = 2
- 3+ = 0

LCL: _____ ☐
- Normal = 5
- 1+ = 3
- 2+ = 2
- 3+ = 0

Reverse Pivot Shift: _____ ☐
- Negative = 5
- Positive = 0

Functional Exam (10 points)

Standing Forward Jump %
Difference between legs: _____ ☐
- 90–100% = 10
- 75–90% = 7
- 50–75% = 5
- 50% = 0

Score: _____ ☐

Deductions

Derotation Brace: _____ ☐
- Security of mind = 2
- Due to instability = 4

Pain: (if PCL, X3) _____ ☐
- None = 0
- Occasional Aching = 2
- After stressful sports = 5
- After daily activities = 8
- Continuous = 10

Total: _____ ☐

Figure 21-A.9 The Revised Hospital for Special Surgery Knee Ligament Rating Form. Reprinted from Windsor *et al.* (1988).

Limp (5 points)_____ ☐

    None = 5

    Slight or periodical = 3

    Severe and constant = 0

Support (5 points)_____ ☐

    None = 5

    Stick or crutch = 2

    Weight bearing impossible = 0

Locking (15 points)_____ ☐

    No locking and no catching
    sensations = 15

    Catching sensation but no locking = 10

    Locking occasionally = 6

    Frequently = 2

    Locked joint on examination = 0

Instability (25 points)_____ ☐

    Never giving way = 25

    Rarely during athletics or other severe
    exertion = 20

    Frequently during athletics or other
    severe exertion (or incapable of
    participation) = 15

    Occasionally in daily activities = 10

    Often in daily activities = 5

    Every step = 0

Pain (25 points) _____ ☐

    None = 25

    Inconstant and slight during severe
    exertion = 20

    Marked during severe exertion = 15

    Marked on or after walking more than
    2 km = 10

    Marked on or after walking less than
    2 km = 5

    Constant = 0

Swelling (10 points) _____ ☐

    None = 10

    On severe exertion = 6

    On ordinary exertion = 2

    Constant = 0

Stair climbing (10 points) _____ ☐

    No problems = 10

    Slightly impaired = 6

    One step at a time = 2

    Impossible = 0

Squatting (5 points) _____ ☐

    No problems = 5

    Slightly impaired = 4

    Not beyond 90 degrees = 2

    Impossible = 0

TOTAL SCORE _____ ☐

SCORE CHART	
Excellent 95–100	Fair 65–83
Good 84–94	Poor <64

Figure 21-A.10 The Lysholm Knee Scoring Scale. Reprinted from Tegner and Lysholm (1985).

10. Competitive sports
    Soccer-national and international elite

9. Competitive sports
    Soccer, lower divisions
    Ice hockey
    Wrestling
    Gymnastics

8. Competitive sports
    Bandy
    Squash or badminton
    Athletics (jumping, etc.)
    Downhill skiing

7. Competitive sports
    Tennis
    Athletics (running)
    Motorcross, speedway
    Handball
    Basketball

    Recreational sports
    Soccer
    Bandy and ice hockey
    Squash
    Athletics (jumping)
    Cross country track finding
    both recreation and competitive

6. Recreational sports
    Tennis and badminton
    Handball
    Basketball
    Downhill skiing
    Jogging, at least five times per week

5. Work
    Heavy labor (e.g., building, forestry)
    Competitive sports
        Cycling
        Cross-country skiing
    Recreational sports
        Jogging on uneven ground at
        least twice weekly

4. Work
    Moderately heavy labor
    (e.g., truck driving, heavy domestic work)
    Recreational sports
        Cycling
        Cross-country skiing
        Jogging on even ground at least twice weekly

3. Work
    Light labor (e.g., nursing)
    Competitive and recreational sports
        Swimming
    Walking in forest possible

2. Work
    Light labor
    Walking on uneven ground possible but impossible
    to walk in forest

1. Work
    Sedentary work
    Walking on even ground possible

0. Sick leave or disability pension
    because of knee problems

Figure 21-A.11 The Tegner Activity Score. Reprinted from Tegner and Lysholm (1985).

SIDE 1
To be filled out
by patient

A.C.L. FOLLOW-UP FORM
A.O.S.S.M STUDY GROUP

Date: _____

IDENTIFICATION

PLEASE PRINT

Name _____ SS # _____ OFF # _____
(LAST)   (FIRST)   (INITIAL)

Age _____ Sex ☐ M ☐ F   Knee Involved ☐ Right ☐ Left

Phone # _____   Phone # and name ⎫ Name: _____
(AREA CODE)   of someone   ⎬
                                     who can reach you ⎮ Phone #: _____
Sport Causing Injury _____   if you have moved ⎭   (AREA CODE)

Date of Surgery _____ Number of months since surgery: 6   12   18   24   36
(MO)   (DATE)   (YEAR)   (CIRCLE ONE)

POST-OP COURSE

Cast? # weeks in rigid cast _____   # weeks in flexible/hinged cast _____

Brace? ☐ Yes ☐ No   **Current Brace Use?** ☐ All the Time   ☐ Sports Only   ☐ No Longer Use

Physical Therapy? # months in supervised program (Cybex orthotron etc.) _____

Are you still doing a **regular** home program?   ☐ Yes   ☐ No

SYMPTOMS

Knee Pain? [4] None   [3] Mild   [2] Moderate (with activity)   Score
[1] Severe (at rest & preventing activity)   _____

Giving Way? [8] None   [6] Only with Cutting (stop & turn) Sports
[4] Occasional (only with awkward step)   [2] With Normal Daily Activities   _____

Swelling? [4] None   [3] Strenuous Activity   [2] With Moderate Activity
[1] With Any Activity   _____

Stiffness? [4] None   [2] Occasional   [1] Frequent   _____

('x' in appropriate box)   Symptom Summary = Total/4   [_____]

FUNCTION

Activity Level?
[1] No sports   [3] Active, but different sports   [_____]
[2] Sports activities   [4] Same sports, but lower   Function Summary
     significantly limited   performance level   (Activity Level)

Problems with Specific Activities?   [5] Equal performance at same
('x' in appropriate box)   sports as before injury

	NONE	MILD	MODERATE	CAN'T DO
Walking	☐	☐	☐	☐
Running	☐	☐	☐	☐
Turn/Cut	☐	☐	☐	☐
Jumping	☐	☐	☐	☐
Stairs	☐	☐	☐	☐

If your prior injury activity level rates at 10,
what does your current activity level rate? _____

If your normal knee performs 100%, at what %
does your operated knee perform? _____

Figure 21-A.12 The Feagin and Blake Scoring System. The ACL Follow-Up Form. Reprinted from Feagin and Blake (1983).

SIDE 2
To be filled out by physician
(make sure side 1 is complete)

SURGICAL Hx

Type ACL Injury: ☐ Acute (<1 wk) ☐ Sub Acute (1–6 wks) ☐ Chronic (>6 wks) ☐ Acute on Chronic

Associated Injury (acute or chronic): ☐ MCL ☐ PCL ☐ LCL ☐ Med Men ☐ Lat Men

ACL Surgery:
☐ No Repair ☐ Primary Repair Aug with _____
☐ Primary Repair without Augmentation ☐ Reconstruction with _____

Subsequent Injury:
☐ None ☐ Medial Meniscus ☐ Lateral Meniscus
☐ ACL ☐ MCL ☐ LCL ☐ PCL

Subsequent Surgery: ☐ None ☐ Hardware removal ☐ MUA ☐ Meniscectomy ☐ Ligament repair

STABILITY

Ant Draw/Lachmans

R   L

————— 15° —————

————— 90° —————

Sublux (Pivot Shift. Jerk. etc.)

record as 0 tr 1^+ 2^+ 3^+

Varus   **Valgus**   **Varus**

————— 0° —————

————— 30° —————

ROM

R   −10° / 0°

140°   90°   45°

−10° / 0°   L

45°   90°   140°

ADDITIONAL STUDIES

Xray: NONE MILD MOD SEVERE
Med joint DJD ☐ ☐ ☐ ☐
Lat joint DJD ☐ ☐ ☐ ☐
P/F joint DJD ☐ ☐ ☐ ☐
ICN osteophytes ☐ ☐ ☐ ☐

Other (your favorite test):

Cybex/Orthotron (if available)

Strength _____ (rate)   Power _____ (rate)

R   L   R   L

Q   Q

H   H

Thigh Circ
(10 cm ↑ patella)   R _____   L _____

CAPSULE SUMMARY*

Symptoms _____   Function _____   Stability _____

1) The **Symptom** score is the total score/4 of the entire symptom section
2) The **Function** score is the score of the activity level question only
3) The **Stability** score comes from only the Ant Draw/Lach/Sublux portion of the P.E. as follows: 5 = none of the 3 tests > trace; 4 = none of the 3 tests >1^+; 3 = two tests 1^+ one test 2^+; 2 = two tests 2^+ one test 1^+; 1 = all tests ≥2^+.

* The Capsule Summary is intended to give a brief picture of the patient NOT summarise all of the above data.

Figure 21-A.12 The Feagin and Blake Scoring System. The ACL Follow-Up Form. Reprinted from Feagin and Blake (1983). – *continued*

CATEGORIES		DATE:				
A = pain/swelling	B = ROM/strength	___/___/___				
C = stability	D = function	preop. examiner:				
		POINTS: (category)				Total
CRITERION:	NUMBER OF POINTS:	A	B	C	D	
HISTORY						
pain	(5 = no; 3 = rare; 2 = frequ.; 0 = severe)	___				
swelling	(5 = no; 3 = rare; 2 = frequ.; 0 = always)	___				
giving way (true)	(5 = no; 2 = rare; 0 = frequ.)			___		
work	(5 = full; 3 = part.; 1 = change; 0 = unable)				___	
sports	(5 = unlim.; 3 = limit.; 1 = maj.limit.; 0 = unable)				___	
GENERAL FINDINGS AT EXAMINATION						
effusion/swelling	(5 = no; 3 = minim.; 1 = moder.; 0 = severe)	___				
tenderness	(5 = no; 3 = minim.; 1 = moder.; 0 = severe)	___				
diff.circumference thigh	(5 = no; 3 = 2cm; 1 = >2cm)		___			
extension-deficit(pass.)	(5 = no; 3 = 5degr.; 1 = 10degr.; 0 = >10degr.)		___			
flexion (passive)	(5 = free; 3 = >120degr.; 1 = >90degr.; 0 = <90degr.)		___			
INSTABILITY						
anterior	(5 = no; 4 = +; 2 = ++; 0 = +++)			___		
posterior	(5 = no; 4 = +; 2 = ++; 0 = +++)			___		
Lachman	(5 = no; 4 = +; 2 = ++; 0 = +++)			___		
lateral (in 30 degr.Flex)	(5 = no; 4 = +; 2 = ++; 0 = +++)			___		
medial (in 30 degr.Flex)	(5 = no; 4 = +; 2 = ++; 0 = +++)			___		
pivot shift	(5 = no; 3 = uncertain; 0 = pos.)			___		
reversed pivot shift	(5 = neg.; 0 = pos.)			___		
FUNCTIONAL TESTS						
lateral jump on one leg	(5 = free; 3 = difficult; 1 = not possible)				___	
kneeflexion on one leg	(5 = free; 3 = difficult; 1 = not possible)				___	
duck-walking	(5 = free; 3 = difficult; 1 = not possible)				___	
I. MAXIMUM NUMBER OF POINTS IN EACH CATEGORY (+TOTAL)		20	15	40	25	100
II. ACTUAL NUMBER OF POINTS IN EACH CATEGORY (+TOTAL IIA + IIB + IIC + IID)		___	___	___	___	
III. MISSING POINTS IN EACH CATEGORY (IA–IIA; IB–IIB; IC–IIC; ID–IID)		___	___	___	___	
EVALUATION						
EXCELLENT (CATEGORIES: 0–4 missing pts., no parameter 0 pts.		0	0	0	0	
TOTAL: >90 pts. and 'excellent' in all categories)						0
GOOD (CATEGORIES: 5–9 missing pts., no parameter 0 pts.		0	0	0	0	
TOTAL: 81–90 pts. or 'good' in any single category)						0
FAIR (CATEGORIES: 10–14 missing pts. or any parameter 0 pts.		0	0	0	0	
TOTAL: 71–80 pts. or 'fair' in any single category)						0
POOR (CATEGORIES: >14 missing pts.		0	0	0	0	
TOTAL: =<70 pts. or 'poor' in any single category)						0

Figure 21-A.13 Evaluation form of the Swiss Knee Group (OAK). Reprinted from Muller et al. (1988).

Patient Name_____ Date _____ / _____ / _____ Medical Record*_____

Occupation _____ Sport: 1st Choice _____ 2nd Choice _____

Age_____ Sex_____ Ht_____ Wt_____ Involved Knee: ❑ Right ❑ Left Contralateral Normal: ❑Yes ❑ No

Cause of Injury:
❑ ADL ❑ Traffic
❑ Contact ❑ Noncontact

Date of Injury: ___ / ___ / ___

Date of Index Operation: ___ / ___ / ___

Procedure _____

Postop Dx _____

ACTIVITY

	Pre-injury	Pre-Rx	Post-Rx
I. Strenuous Activity jumping, pivoting, hard cutting (football, soccer)			
II. Moderate Activity heavy manual work (skiing, tennis)			
III. Light Activity light manual work (jogging, running)			
IV. Sedentary Activity (housework, ADL)			

Eventual change knee related: ❑ Yes ❑ No

PREVIOUS SURGERY

Arthroscopy: Date (1)_____ (2)_____ (3)_____

Meniscectomy: Dx _____ _____ _____

Stabilization: Procedure _____ _____ _____

MENISCAL STATUS

	N1	1/3	2/3	Total
Med				
Lat				

Morphotype: Lax_____
Normal_____ Tight_____
Knee: Varus_____
Normal _____ Valgus_____

EIGHT GROUPS / FOUR GRADES / *GROUP GRADE

EIGHT GROUPS	A. Normal	B. Nearly Normal	C. Abnormal	D. Sev. Abnorm.	A	B	C	D
1. Patient Subjective Assessment How does your knee function?	❑ 0	❑ 1	❑ 2	❑ 3				
On a scale of 0 to 3, how does your knee affect your activity level?	❑ 0	❑ 1	❑ 2	❑ 3	❑	❑	❑	❑
2. SYMPTOMS (Grade at highest activity level with no significant symptoms. Exclude 0 to slight symptoms.)	I. Strenuous Activity	II. Moderate Activity	III. Light Activity	IV. Sedentary Activity				
Pain	❑	❑	❑	❑				
Swelling	❑	❑	❑	❑				
Partial Giving Way	❑	❑	❑	❑				
Full Giving Way	❑	❑	❑	❑	❑	❑	❑	❑
3. Range of Motion Ext/Flex: Index side: ___ / ___ / ___ Opposite side: ___ / ___ / ___								
Lack of extension (from 0°)	❑ <3°	❑ 3 to 5°	❑ 6 to 10°	❑ >10°				
Δ Lack of flexion	❑ 0 to 5°	❑ 6 to 15°	❑ 16 to 25°	❑ >25°	❑	❑	❑	❑
4. Ligament Evaluation (manual, instrumented, X-ray)								
Δ LACHMAN (25° flex)	❑ −1 to 2mm	❑ 3 to 5mm <−1 to −3 stiff	❑ 6 to 10mm <−3 stiff	❑ >10mm				
Endpoint: firm/soft	❑ firm		❑ soft					
Δ Total A.P. Transl. (70° flex)	❑ 0 to 2mm	❑ 3 to 5mm	❑ 6 to 10mm	❑ >10mm				
Δ Post. sag (70° flex)	❑ 0 to 2mm	❑ 3 to 5mm	❑ 6 to 10mm	❑ >10mm				
Δ Med jt opening (20° flex) (valgus rot)	❑ 0 to 2mm	❑ 3 to 5mm	❑ 6 to 10mm	❑ >10mm				
Δ Lat jt opening (20° flex) (varus rot)	❑ 0 to 2mm	❑ 3 to 5mm	❑ 6 to 10mm	❑ >10mm				
Δ Pivot shift	❑ equal	❑ + (glide)	❑ ++ (clunk)	❑ +++ (gross)				
Δ Reverse pivot shift	❑ equal	❑ glide	❑ marked	❑ gross	❑	❑	❑	❑
5. Compartmental Findings			crepitation with	crepitation with				
Δ Crepitus patellofemoral	❑ none	❑ moderate	❑ mild pain	❑ >mild pain				
Δ Crepitus medial compartment	❑ none	❑ moderate	❑ mild pain	❑ >mild pain				
Δ Crepitus lateral compartment	❑ none	❑ moderate	❑ mild pain	❑ >mild pain				
6. Harvest Sight Pathology	❑ none	❑ mild	❑ moderate	❑ severe				
7. X-Ray Findings								
Med Joint space	❑ none	❑ mild	❑ moderate	❑ severe				
Lat Joint space	❑ none	❑ mild	❑ moderate	❑ severe				
Patellofemoral	❑ none	❑ mild	❑ moderate	❑ severe				
8. Functional Test One leg hop (% of opposite side)	❑ ≥90%	❑ 89% to 76%	❑ 75% to 50%	❑ <50%				
**FINAL EVALUATION					❑	❑	❑	❑

* Group Grade: The lower grade within a group determines the group grade.
** Final Evaluation: The worst group grade determines the final evaluation for acute and subacute patients. For chronic patients compare preoperative and postoperative evaluations. In a final evaluation, only the first 4 groups are evaluated but all groups must be documented.
Δ Difference in involved knee compared to normal or what is assumed to be normal.

Figure 21-A.14 The 1993 International Knee Documentation Committee (IKDC) Knee Ligament Standard Evaluation Form. Reprinted from Hefti et al. (1993).

DIRECTIONS: Using the key below, circle the appropriate boxes on the four scales below which indicate the highest level you can reach WITHOUT having symptoms.

Scale	Description
10	Normal knee, able to do strenuous work/sports with jumping, hard pivoting
8	Able to do moderate work/sports with running, turning and twisting; symptoms with strenuous work/sports
6	Able to do light work/sports with no running, twisting or jumping; symptoms with moderate work/sports
4	Able to do activities of daily living alone; symptoms with light work/sports
2	Moderate symptoms (frequent, limiting) with activities of daily living
0	Severe symptoms (constant, not relieved) with activities of daily living

1. **PAIN**

| 10 | 8 | 6 | 4 | 2 | 0 |

2. **SWELLING** (actual fluid in the knee; obvious puffiness)

| 10 | 8 | 6 | 4 | 2 | 0 |

3. **PARTIAL GIVING-WAY** (partial knee collapse, no fall to the ground)

| 10 | 8 | 6 | 4 | 2 | 0 |

4. **FULL GIVING-WAY** (knee collapse occurs with actual falling to the ground)

| 10 | 8 | 6 | 4 | 2 | 0 |

Patient Grade: Rate the overall condition of your knee at the present time. Circle one number below.

1	2	3	4	5	6	7	8	9	10
	poor		fair		good				normal

poor – I have significant limitations that affect activities of daily living.
fair – I have moderate limitations that affect activities of daily living, no sports possible.
good – I have some limitations with sports but I can participate; I compensate.
normal/excellent – I am able to do whatever I wish (any sport) with no problems.

Sports Activity Scale, Activities of Daily Living Function Scales, Sports Function Scales

Sports Activity Scale

Level I (participates 4–7 days/week)
100	Jumping, hard pivoting, cutting (basketball, volleyball, football, gymnastics, soccer)
95	Running, twisting, turning (tennis, racquetball, handball, ice hockey, field hockey, skiing, wrestling)
90	No running, twisting, jumping (cycling, swimming)

Level II (participates 1–3 days/week)
85	Jumping, hard pivoting, cutting (basketball, volleyball, football, gymnastics, soccer)
80	Running, twisting, turning (tennis, racquetball, handball, ice hockey, field hockey, skiing, wrestling)
75	No running, twisting, jumping (cycling, swimming)

Level III (participates 1–3 times/month)
65	Jumping, hard pivoting, cutting (basketball, volleyball, football, gymnastics, soccer)
60	Running, twisting, turning (tennis, racquetball, handball, ice hockey, field hockey, skiing, wrestling)
55	No running, twisting, jumping (cycling, swimming)

Level IV (no sports)
40	I perform activities of daily living without problems
20	I have moderate problems with activities of daily living
0	I have severe problems with activities of daily living; on crutches, full disability

Figure 21-A.15 The Cincinnati Knee Rating System. (I) Symptom Rating Scales and Patient Perception Scale; (II) Sports Activity Scale, Activities of Daily Living Function Scales, and Sports Function Scales; (III) Occupational Rating Scale; (IV) Overall Rating Scheme; (V) Modifications for Overall Rating Scheme: Symptom and Instability Ratings. Reprinted from Barber-Westin et al. (1999).

Activities of Daily Living Function Scales

1. Walking
check one box:
40 ☐ normal, unlimited
30 ☐ some limitations
20 ☐ only 3–4 blocks possible
0 ☐ less than 1 block; cane, crutch

2. Stairs
check one box:
40 ☐ normal, unlimited
30 ☐ some limitations
20 ☐ only 11–30 steps possible
0 ☐ only 1–10 steps possible

3. Squatting/kneeling
check one box:
40 ☐ normal, unlimited
30 ☐ some limitations
20 ☐ only 6–10 possible
0 ☐ only 0–5 possible

Sports Function Scales

1. Straight running
check one box:
100 ☐ fully competitive
80 ☐ some limitations, guarding
60 ☐ definite limitations, half speed
40 ☐ not able to do

2. Jumping/landing on affected leg
check one box:
100 ☐ fully competitive
80 ☐ some limitations, guarding
60 ☐ definite limitations, half speed
40 ☐ not able to do

3. Hard twists/cuts/pivots
check one box:
100 ☐ fully competitive
80 ☐ some limitations, guarding
60 ☐ definite limitations, half speed
40 ☐ not able to do

Occupational Rating Scale

Check the response which best describes what you actually do at work. Check only one response per column.

Total Points
___ × 2 = ___

Factor 1 sitting	Factor 2 standing/ walking	Factor 3 walking on uneven ground	Factor 4 squatting	Factor 5 climbing	Factor 6 lifting/carrying	Factor 7 pounds carried
0 ☐ 8–10 hrs/day	0 ☐ 0 hr/day	0 ☐ 0 hr/day	0 ☐ 0 times/day	0 ☐ 0 times/day	0 ☐ 0 times/day	0 ☐ 0–5 lbs
1 ☐ 6–7 hrs/day	2 ☐ 1 hr/day	2 ☐ 1 hr/day	1 ☐ 1–5 times/day	2 ☐ 1 flight, 2 times/day	1 ☐ 1–5 times/day	1 ☐ 6–10 lbs
2 ☐ 4–5 hrs/day	4 ☐ 2–3 hrs/day	4 ☐ 2–3 hrs/day	2 ☐ 6–10 times/day	4 ☐ 3 flights, 2 times/day	2 ☐ 6–10 times/day	2 ☐ 11–20 lbs
3 ☐ 2–3 hrs/day	6 ☐ 4–5 hrs/day	6 ☐ 4–5 hrs/day	3 ☐ 11–15 times/day	6 ☐ 10 flights/ ladders	3 ☐ 11–15 times/day	3 ☐ 21–25 lbs
4 ☐ 1 hr/day	8 ☐ 6–7 hrs/day	8 ☐ 6–7 hrs/day	4 ☐ 16–20 times/day	8 ☐ ladders with weight 2–3 days/ week	4 ☐ 16–20 times/day	4 ☐ 26–30 lbs
5 ☐ 0 hr/day	10 ☐ 8–10 hrs/day	10 ☐ 8–10 hrs/day	5 ☐ more than 20 times/ day	10 ☐ ladders daily with weight	5 ☐ more than 20 times/ day	5 ☐ more than 30 lbs

Figure 21-A.15 The Cincinnati Knee Rating System. (I) Symptom Rating Scales and Patient Perception Scale; (II) Sports Activity Scale, Activities of Daily Living Function Scales, and Sports Function Scales; (III) Occupational Rating Scale; (IV) Overall Rating Scheme; (V) Modifications for Overall Rating Scheme: Symptom and Instability Ratings. Reprinted from Barber-Westin *et al.* (1999). – *continued*

Overall Rating Scheme

Subjective: 20 points

- 10 = Normal knee, able to do strenuous work/sports with jumping, hard pivoting
- 8 = Able to do moderate work/sports with running, twisting, turning; symptoms with strenuous work/sports
- 6 = Able to do light work/sports with no running, twisting, jumping; symptoms with moderate work/sports
- 4 = Able to do activities of daily living alone; symptoms with light work/sports
- 2 = Moderate symptoms (frequent, limiting) with ADL
- 0 = Severe symptoms (constant, not relieved) with ADL

*highest level possible with no or rare symptoms

	Levels	Excellent Level	Pts	Good Level	Pts	Fair Level	Pts	Poor Level	Pts
Pain	10 8 6 4 2 0	10	5	8	3	6-4	1	2-0	0
Swelling	10 8 6 4 2 0	10	5	8	3	6-4	1	2-0	0
Partial Giving-Way	10 8 6 4 2 0	10	5	8	3	6-4	1	2-0	0
Full Giving-Way	10 8 6 4 2 0	10	5	8	3	6-4	1	2-0	0

Activity Level: 15 points

	Pts 3	Pts 2	Pts 1	Pts 0		Excellent Pts	Good Pts	Fair Pts	Poor Pts
Walking	Normal, unlimited	Some limitations	Only 3-4 blocks possible	Less than 1 block, cane		3	2	1	0
Stairs	Normal, unlimited	Some limitations	Only 11-30 steps possible	Only 1-10 steps possible	> Score lowest	3	2	1	0
Squatting	Normal, unlimited	Some limitations	Only 6-10 possible	Only 0-5 possible					
Running	Normal, unlimited	Some limitations	Run 1/2 speed	Not able to do		3	2	1-0	
Jumping	Normal, unlimited	Some limitations	Definite limitations, 1/2 speed	Not able to do		3	2	1-0	
Twists/Cuts	Normal, unlimited	Some limitations	Definite limitations, 1/2 speed	Not able to do		3	2	1-0	

Examination: 25 points

	NL	Pts	MILD	Pts	MOD	Pts	SEV	Pts	Excellent Pts	Good Pts	Fair Pts	Poor Pts
Effusion	NL	5	≤25 cc	4	26-60 cc	2	>60 cc	0	5	4	2	0
Lack of Flexion	0-5°	5	6-15°	4	16-30°	2	>30°	0	5	4	2	0
Lack of Extension	0-3°	5	4-5°	4	6-10°	2	>10°	0	5	4	2	0
Tibiofemoral Crepitus	NL	5	Mild		Mod*	2	Sev*	0	5		2	0
Patellofemoral Crepitus	NL	5	Mild		Mod*	2	Sev*	0	5	2	2	0

(*indicates definite fibrillation, cartilage abnormality; moderate 25-50°, severe > 50°)

Instability: 20 points

	<3 mm	Pts	MILD	Pts	MOD	Pts	SEV	Pts	Excellent	Good	Fair	Poor
Anterior (KT-1000)	<3 mm	10	3-5 mm	7	6 mm	4	>6 mm	0	10	7	4	0
Pivot Shift	negative	10	slip	7	definite	4	severe	0	10	7	4	0

Radiographs: 10 points

	4 pts	3 pts	2 pts	0 pt	
Medial Tibiofemoral	NL	Mild	Mod	Sev	narrowing <1/2 joint space
Lateral Tibiofemoral	NL	Mild	Mod	Sev	narrowing >1/2 joint space
Patellofemoral	NL	Mild	Mod	Sev	

Convert sum   Sum points:___

Excellent	Good	Fair	Poor
x-ray pts: 12 x-ray pts = 10 final pts	11-9 x-ray pts = 7 final pts	8-6 x-ray pts = 4 final pts	5-0 x-ray pts = 0 final pts

Function Testing: 10 points

Use any two

- One-Legged Hop, 1 hop for distance ___ % limb symmetry
- One-Legged Hop, 3 hops for distance ___ % limb symmetry
- One-Legged Hop, timed hop over 6 meters ___ % limb symmetry
- One-Legged Hop, cross-over for distance ___ % limb symmetry

___ average % limb symmetry

	Excellent Symmetry	Pts	Good Symmetry	Pts	Fair Symmetry	Pts	Poor Symmetry	Pts
	100-85	10	84-75	7	74-65	4	<65	0

Final Rating Chronic Injury Studies: Point Sum _____

Final Rating Acute Injury Studies: Category
Excellent: all in 'excellent' (may have one in 'good'); Good: all in 'excellent' and 'good'
Fair: any one in 'fair'; Poor: any one in 'poor'

Modifications for Overall Rating Scheme: Symptom and Instability Ratings

Subjective: 20 points

6 = Able to do light/moderate/strenuous work/sports without symptoms
4 = Able to do activities of daily living alone; symptoms with light/moderate strenuous work/sports
2 = Moderate symptoms (frequent, limiting) with ADL
0 = Severe symptoms (constant, not relieved) with ADL

				Excellent		Good		Fair		Poor	
				Level	Pts.	Level	Pts.	Level	Pts.	Level	Pts.
Pain	6	4	2	0	6	5	4	3	2	1	0	0
Swelling	6	4	2	0	6	5	4	3	2	1	0	0
Partial Giving-Way	6	4	2	0	6	5	4	3	2	1	0	0
Full Giving-Way	6	4	2	0	6	5	4	3	2	1	0	0

Instability*: 20 points

		Pts.		Pts.		Pts.	Excellent Pts.	Good Pts.	Fair	Poor Pts.
ACL	<3 mm	5	3–5.5 mm	3	≥6 mm	0	5	3		0
PCL	<3 mm	5	3–5.5 mm	3	≥6 mm	0	5	3		0
MCL	<3 mm	5	3–5 mm	3	≥6 mm	0	5	3		0
LCL/PL complex	<3 mm & <5° ER	5	3–5 mm or 6–10° ER	3	>5 mm or > 10° ER	0	5	3		0

*ACL: use knee arthrometer test total AP displacement 20°, 134 N, involved-noninvolved limb
PCL: use knee arthrometer test (70°, 89 N) or stress radiographs (70°, 89 N)
MCL: use valgus stress test, 25
LCL/PL complex: use varus stress test 25°, external tibial rotation test 30° & 90°, varus recurvatum test

Figure 21-A.15 The Cincinnati Knee Rating System. (I) Symptom Rating Scales and Patient Perception Scale; (II) Sports Activity Scale, Activities of Daily Living Function Scales, and Sports Function Scales; (III) Occupational Rating Scale; (IV) Overall Rating Scheme; (V) Modifications for Overall Rating Scheme: Symptom and Instability Ratings. Reprinted from Barber-Westin et al. (1999). – continued

KNEE DISORDERS SUBJECTIVE HISTORY

NAME _____

CHART _____ DATE _____ SIDE: L R

INSTRUCTIONS:

For each question, shade in a box between the two descriptions which you think describes your knee **relative** to the two extremes. Please complete both sides of this form.

1. How often does your knee hurt?
   never — daily even at rest

2. How bad is the pain at its worst?
   none — severe, requiring pain pills every few hours

3. Do you have swelling in your knee?
   never — daily, even at rest

4. Does your knee give way or buckle?
   never — I must gaurd my knee to prevent giving way even with normal everyday activity

5. Does your knee lock up so you are unable to straighten it?
   never — I must gaurd my knee to prevent locking even with normal everyday activity

6. Does your knee catch or hang up when moving?
   never — I must gaurd my knee to prevent catching even with normal everyday activity

7. Is your knee stiff?
   none — I can barely move my knee because of stiffness

8. Are you able to walk on level groud?
   no problem — unable

9. Are you able to walk on rough ground, inclines, or negotiate curves?
   no problem — unable

10. Do you need crutches, cane, or walker to walk?
    never — always

11. Do you feel grinding when your knee moves?
    none — severe

12. Do you have problems twisting or pivoting on your injured knee?
    none — unable

13. Do you have problems carrying heavy objects because of your knee?
    none — unable ☐ not attempted

14. Do you have problems climbing stairs?
    none — unable ☐ not attempted

15. Do you have problems going down stairs?
    none — unable ☐ not attempted

16. Do you have problems running?
    none — unable ☐ not attempted

17. Do you have problems decelerating (slowing down) after running or jogging?
    none — unable ☐ not attempted

18. Do you have problems cutting (changing directions while running by pivoting on affected knee)?
    none — unable ☐ not attempted

19. Do you have problems jumping?
    none — unable ☐ not attempted

20. Do you have problems taking part in competitive sports?
    none — unable ☐ not attempted

21. Do you have night pain?
    none — severe

22. Do you have problems kneeling?
    no problem — unable ☐ not attempted

23. Do you have problems squatting?
    no problem — unable ☐ not attempted

24. Do you have problems getting in and out of a car?
    no problem — unable

25. Does your knee ache while you are sitting?
    never — always

26. Do you have problems getting in or out of a chair?
    no problem — unable

27. Do you have stiffness or discomfort when you first start to walk?
    none — always

28. Do you have problems turning over in bed?
    none — unable

HUGHSTON SPORTS MEDICINE FOUNDATION, INC.

Figure 21-A.16 Visual analogue scales for assessing subjective knee complaints. Reprinted from Flandry et al. (1991).

Symptoms and Physical Complaints

1. With respect to your overall knee function. How troubled are you by giving way episodes? (Make a slash at the extreme right, i.e., 100, if you are experiencing no giving way episodes in your knee. Please note that this question has two parts. It is concerned with both the severity (1a) and frequency (1b) of the giving way episodes.)

1a 0 _____ 100
   Major giving way   Minor giving way
      episodes   episodes

1b 0 _____ 100
   Constantly   Never
   giving way   giving way

2. With any kind of prolonged activity (i.e., greater than half an hour) how much pain or discomfort do you get in your knee?

   0 _____ 100
   Severe   No pain
   pain   at all

3. With respect to your overall knee function, how much are you troubled by stiffness or loss of motion in your knee?

   0 _____ 100
   Severely   Not troubled
   troubled   at all

4. Consider the overall function of your knee and how it relates to the strength of your muscles: How *weak* is your knee?

   0 _____ 100
   Extremely   Not weak
   weak   at all

Work-Related Concerns

The following questions are being asked with respect to your job or vocation. The questions are concerned with your ability to function at work and how your knee has affected your current work situation, i.e., your work-related concerns. If you are a full-time student or home maker consider this and any part-time work together. Consider the last three months.

If you are currently not employed for *reasons other than your knee* then place a check on this line._____

5. How much trouble do you have, because of your knee, with turning or pivoting motions at work? (Make a slash at the extreme left, i.e., 0, if you are unable to work because of the knee.)

   0 _____ 100
   Severely   No trouble
   troubled   at all

6. How much trouble do you have, because of your knee, with squatting motions at work? (Make a slash at the extreme left, i.e., 0, if you are unable to work because of the knee.)

   0 _____ 100
   Severely   No trouble
   troubled   at all

7. How much of a concern is it for you to miss days from work due to problems or reinjury to your knee? (Make a slash at the extreme left, i.e., 0, if you are unable to work because of the knee.)

   0 _____ 100
   An extremely   No concern
   significant concern   at all

8. How much of a concern is it for you to lose time from 'school' or work because of the treatment of your ACL-deficient knee?

   0 _____ 100
   An extremely   No concern
   significant concern   at all

Recreational Activities and Sport Participation or Competition

The following questions are concerned with your ability to function and participate in these activities as they relate to your ACL-deficient knee. Consider the last three months.

9. How much limitation do you have with sudden twisting and pivoting movements or changes in direction?

   0 _____ 100
   Totally   No
   limited   limitations

10. How much of a concern is it for you that your sporting or recreational activities may result in the status of your knee worsening?

    0 _____ 100
    An extremely   No concern
    significant concern   at all

11. How does your current level of athletic or recreational performance compare with your preinjury level?

    0 _____ 100
    Totally   No
    limited   limitations

12. With respect to the activities or sports that you currently desire to be involved with, how much have your expectations changed because of the status of your knee?

    0 _____ 100
    Expectations totally   Expectations
    lowered   not lowered at all

13. Do you have to play your recreation or sport under caution? (Make a slash at the extreme left, i.e., 0, if you are unable to play your recreation or sport because of your knee.)

    0 _____ 100
    Always play   Never play
    under caution   under caution

14. How fearful are you of your knee giving way when playing recreation or sport? (Make a slash at the extreme left, i.e., 0, if you are unable to play recreation or sport because of your knee.)

    0 _____ 100
    Extremely   No fear
    fearful   at all

Figure 21-A.17 Quality of Life Assessment in anterior cruciate ligament (ACL) deficiency. Note: on the actual form, the lines are 100 mm long. Reprinted from Mohtadi (1998).

15. Are you concerned about environmental conditions such as a wet playing field, a hard court, or the type of gym floor when involved in your recreation or sport? (Make a slash at the extreme left, i.e., 0, if you are unable to play recreation or sport because of your knee.)

0 _____ 100
Extremely   Not concerned
concerned   at all

16. Do you find it frustrating to have to consider your knee with respect to your recreation or sport?

0 _____ 100
Extremely   Not frustrated
frustrated   at all

17. How difficult is it for you to 'go full out' at your recreation or sport? (Make a slash at the extreme left, i.e., 0, if you are unable to play recreation or sport because of your knee.)

0 _____ 100
Extremely   Not difficult
difficult   at all

18. Are you fearful of playing contact sports? (Circle the 'N/A' at the right of the scale if you do not play contact sport for reasons other than the knee.)

0 _____ 100 N/A
Extremely   No fear
fearful   at all

The following questions are specifically asking about the two most important sports or recreational activities that you do or that you wish to do. Please write them in order.

1._____
2._____

19. How limited are you in playing the number "1" sport or activity? (Make a slash at the extreme left, i.e., 0, if you are unable to play the recreation or sport because of your knee.)

0 _____ 100
Extremely   Not limited
limited   at all

20. How limited are you in playing the number '2' sport or activity? (Make a slash at the extreme left, i.e., 0, if you are unable to play the recreation or sport because of your knee.)

0 _____ 100
Extremely   Not limited
limited   at all

Life Style

The following questions are concerned with your life style in general and should be considered outside of your work and recreational or sport activities as they relate to your ACL-deficient knee.

21. Do you have to concern yourself with general safety issues (e.g., carrying small children, working in the yard) with respect to your ACL-deficient knee?

0 _____ 100
Extremely   No concern
concerned   at all

22. How much has your ability to exercise and maintain fitness been limited by your knee problem?

0 _____ 100
Totally   Not limited
limited   at all

23. How much has your enjoyment of life been limited by your knee problem?

0 _____ 100
Totally limited   Not limited at all

24. How often are you aware of your knee problem?

0 _____ 100
All of   None of
the time   the time

25. Are you concerned about your knee with respect to life style activities that you and your family do together?

0 _____ 100
Extremely   No concern
concerned   at all

26. Have you modified your life style to avoid potentially damaging activities to your knee?

0 _____ 100
Totally   No
modified   modifications

Social and Emotional

The following questions are about your attitudes and feelings as they relate to your ACL-deficient knee.

27. Does it concern you that your competitive needs are no longer being met because of your knee problem? (Make a slash at the extreme right, i.e., 100, if your competitive needs are being met.)

0 _____ 100
Extremely   Not concerned
concerned   at all

28. Have you had difficulty being able to psychologically 'come to grips' with your knee problem?

0 _____ 100
Extremely   Not difficult
difficult   at all

29. How often are you apprehensive about your knee?

0 _____ 100
All of   None of
the time   the time

30. How much are you troubled with lack of confidence in your knee?

0 _____ 100
Severely   No trouble
troubled   at all

31. How fearful are you of reinjuring your knee?

0 _____ 100
Extremely   No fear
fearful   at all

Figure 21-A.17 Quality of Life Assessment in anterior cruciate ligament (ACL) deficiency. Note: on the actual form, the lines are 100 mm long. Reprinted from Mohtadi (1998). – *continued*

Knee instability scale modified for evaluation of patellofemoral pain and instability

Pain/instability	No. of available points
Limp	
None	10
Slight	5
Severe	0
Support	
Full	10
Cane or crutch necessary at times	3
Weightbearing impossible	0
Stair climbing	
No problem	10
Slightly impaired	6
One step at a time	2
Unable	0
Squatting	
No problem	5
Slightly impaired	4
Not past 90° of knee flexion	2
Unable	0
Instability	
Never gives way	10
With vigorous activity	5
Occasionally in daily activities	5
Often in daily activities	3
Every day	0
Pain	
None	45
Slight during vigorous exercise only	40
Moderate with vigorous exercise	35
Severe after vigorous exercise	25
Severe after walking 1 mile	20
Severe after walking less than ½ mile	10
Constant and severe	2
Swelling	
None	10
With giving way	7
On severe exertion	5
On mild exertion	2
Constant	0

Scoring of overall surgical result	
95–100	Excellent
90–94	Very good
80–89	Good
70–79	Fair
<70	Poor

Figure 21-A.18 The Fulkerson modification of the Lysholm score for assessing the outcome of anterior knee pain. Reprinted from Fulkerson *et al.* (1990).

ANTERIOR KNEE PAIN (Sheet code: _____)
Name: _____ Date: _____
Age: _____
Knee: L/R
Duration of symptoms: ____ years ____ months
For each question, circle the latest choice (letter) which corresponds to your knee symptoms.

1. Limp
   (a) None (5)
   (b) Slight or periodical (3)
   (c) Constant (0)
2. Support
   (a) Full support without pain (5)
   (b) Painful (3)
   (c) Weight bearing impossible (0)
3. Walking
   (a) Unlimited (5)
   (b) More than 2 km (3)
   (c) 1–2 km (2)
   (d) Unable (0)
4. Stairs
   (a) No difficulty (10)
   (b) Slight pain when descending (8)
   (c) Pain both when descending and ascending (5)
   (d) Unable (0)
5. Squatting
   (a) No difficulty (5)
   (b) Repeated squatting painful (4)
   (c) Painful each time (3)
   (d) Possible with partial weight bearing (2)
   (e) Unable (0)
6. Running
   (a) No difficulty (10)
   (b) Pain after more than 2 km (8)
   (c) Slight pain from start (6)
   (d) Severe pain (3)
   (e) Unable (0)

7. Jumping
   (a) No difficulty (10)
   (b) Slight difficulty (7)
   (c) Constant pain (2)
   (d) Unable (0)
8. Prolonged sitting with the knees flexed
   (a) No difficulty (10)
   (b) Pain after exercise (8)
   (c) Constant pain (6)
   (d) Pain forces to extend knees temporarily (4)
   (e) Unable (0)
9. Pain
   (a) None (10)
   (b) Slight and occasional (8)
   (c) Interferes with sleep (6)
   (d) Occasionally severe (3)
   (e) Constant and severe (0)
10. Swelling
   (a) None (10)
   (b) After severe exertion (8)
   (c) After daily activities (6)
   (d) Every evening (4)
   (e) Constant (0)
11. Abnormal painful kneecap (patellar) movements (subluxations)
   (a) None (10)
   (b) Occasionally in sports activities (6)
   (c) Occasionally in daily activities (4)
   (d) At least one documented dislocation (2)
   (e) More than two dislocations (0)
12. Atrophy of thigh
   (a) None (5)
   (b) Slight (3)
   (c) Severe (0)
13. Flexion deficiency
   (a) None (5)
   (b) Slight (3)
   (c) Severe (0)

Figure 21-A.19 The Kujala scoring system for anterior knee pain, and its evaluation form. Reprinted from Kujala *et al.* (1993).

The following grading system was used:

1. *Excellent*: The patient had no symptoms and no disability related to his knee;

2. *Good:* The patient had minimum symptoms, such as aching or weakness after heavy use or effusion after heavy exertion, but there was essentially no disability;

3. *Fair*: The patient had symptoms, such as trouble kneeling or climbing stairs; weakness, pain, or discomfort had became enough of a problem to interfere some-what with everyday activities and the patient thought he had some disability; and he was active but could not participate in vigorous sports (such as skiing, tennis, football, and so forth);

4. *Poor*: The symptoms were severe and included all of those listed under *fair* as well as the presence of pain at rest, limited motion, and locking. The patient was clearly disabled, and his activities, including walking, were definitely limited because of his knee.

Figure 21-A.20 Grading system related to meniscal disorders. Reprinted from Tapper and Hoover (1969).

	Points	Acceptable		Unacceptable	
		Excellent	Good	Fair	Poor
A. Subjective complaints					
a. Pain					
No pain	6				
Occasional ache, bad weather pain	5				
Stabbing pain in certain positions	4	5	4	2	0
Afternoon pain, intense, constant pain around the knee after activity	2				
Night pain at rest	0				
b. Walking capacity					
Normal walking capacity (in relation to age)	6				
Walking outdoors at least one hour	4	6	4	2	1
Short walks outdoors >15 minutes	2				
Walking indoors only	1				
Wheel-chair/bedridden	0				
B. Clinical signs					
a. Extension					
Normal	6				
Lack of extension (0 to 10 degrees)	4	6	4	2	2
Lack of extension >10 degrees	2				
b. Total range of motion					
At least 140	6				
At least 120	5				
At least 90	4	5	4	2	1
At least 60	2				
At least 30	1				
0	0				
c. Stability					
Normal stability in extension and 20 degrees of flexion	6				
Abnormal instability 20 degrees of flexion	5	5	4	2	2
Instability in extension <10 degrees	4				
Instability in extension >10 degrees	2				
Sum (minimum)		27	20	10	6

Figure 21-A.21 Evaluation of treatment for tibial condylar fractures: the Rasmussen criteria. Reprinted from Rasmussen (1973).

22

The ankle and hindfoot

Mark L. Herron and Michael M. Stephens

INTRODUCTION

The factors to measure in assessing outcome of the ankle and hindfoot comprise either signs, symptoms, complications or investigations (Pynsent 2001), and these are most often variously combined within a scoring system. 'Signs' by definition are objective, and these most commonly encompass ranges of movement, quantification of deformity and stability. Although historically there has been a tendency towards placing more credence in these objective criteria, this approach is changing as it is becoming fairly well recognized that the measurement of some objective criteria are open to significant error (Dawson and Carr 2001) and the measures themselves may be non-validated and poorly reproducible (Drake *et al.* 1994; Conboy *et al.* 1996). There is little doubt that both the range of movement and alignment at the ankle and hindfoot may be affected by both pathology and treatment. The exact relationship of this to function and correlation with outcome is however less well defined. If these are assessed it is important to define the reference landmarks for clinical measurements of movement or deformity, as this may significantly effect the results (Bohannon *et al.* 1989), though this is almost universally ignored. The singular lack of inter-observer agreement in clinical measurements at both ankle and subtalar joints is documented (Elveru *et al.* 1988), though intra-observer agreement can be within acceptable limits, as can radiographic measurement of movement (Backer and Kofoed 1989). Clinical measurements of ankle and subtalar movement, once made, should probably be compared with a contralateral normal side – if this exists – given the recognized wide variation in documented normal ranges (Oatis 1988). In addition, it has been demonstrated that the clinical measurement of subtalar movement is poorly reproducible (Leicht and Kofoed 1992). Despite these well-recognized sources of error, most of the scoring systems in usage avoid addressing these issues all together. It is increasingly appreciated that a patient's subjective assessment of outcome such as pain, functional ability and satisfaction may fulfil the criteria of being valid, reliable and sensitive to change if gathered by a correctly designed and tested patient-centred questionnaire (Dawson and Carr 2001). The WOMAC score for osteoarthritis of the hip and knee is one such instrument (Bellamy *et al.* 1988), but there exists no comparable fully validated disease-specific measure for the ankle and hindfoot. The Foot Function Index (Budiman-Mak *et al.* 1991) is the only fully validated regional scoring system, but this has only been used in a rheumatoid arthritis population, excluding operated cases and those with fixed deformities. It has however seen wider usage (Skalley *et al.* 1994; Coester *et al.* 2001) which should be regarded with some caution. There has been a move towards the use of patient-based generic scores of health, in particular the SF-36 (Ware and Sherbourne 1992), in conjunction with more traditional outcome scores of ankle and hindfoot. Generally, its elements have been used either as a yardstick against which to regard a non-validated score (Heffernan *et al.* 2000), or to provide a more holistic view of the patient's response to intervention (Egol *et al.* 2000).

This chapter is not intended as a treatise on what ideal measures should encompass, but rather as a critical and practical review of the better and more commonly used tools – imperfect as they are – which are at present available to the researcher in the field. Outcome measures used in clinical research should be demonstrated to be valid, reliable and sensitive to change (Pynsent 2001). With a few exceptions, the specific outcome measures in common usage for the ankle and hindfoot are unlikely to have been demonstrated to fulfil all – if any – of these criteria. Attention has therefore been drawn, where appropriate, to reports where several independent measures have been used and an attempt made at correlation, for example the use of an outcome score as well an assessment of patient satisfaction. Such information is not validation and must be treated with circumspect. As has been pointed out (Dawson and Carr 2001), the reason for a disparity between the patient's satisfaction level and other measures may simply be explained by inappropriately informed patient expectations. Additionally, the most commonly used scores are reviewed, invariably those with a number of features to recommend them and with which there is well-established clinical experience. In general, outcome scores with a high proportion of subjective fields have been emphasized given the recognized limitations of objective measurements. This also reflects the way in which current research is moving. The natural history of many of the commonly encountered conditions and their longer-term response to interventions is not unequivocally known. In addition, a number of procedures may have good short- and intermediate-term results (e.g. triple arthrodesis) but result in long-term sequelae (Saltzman et al. 1999). Both of these factors mean that the most appropriate time (or times) when to measure outcome must be considered. The following conditions and procedures discussed should be regarded as representative rather than complete. They encompass the areas most commonly encountered or where useful developments have been made.

regarded as the absolute arbiter of outcome. There may be poor agreement between the presence of joint incongruency (Bauer et al. 1985) or even non-union (Angus and Cowell 1986) and clinical outcome. A poor correlation between clinical outcome and radiographic changes is not infrequent in the case of osteoarthritis (Southwell and Sherman 1981; Lindsjo et al. 1985; Pell et al. 2000). This could be inferred from the fact that only rarely are radiographs included directly with other measures in a score. Nevertheless, there would be little contention that the presence of osteoarthritis or a non-union could be regarded as a measure of outcome in the ankle and hindfoot. However, the issue of at what stage a measurement of radiographic alignment may come to be regarded as an outcome measure is less clear, and will rely upon an identified and strong correlation between the variable and end result. Given the less than full understanding of the natural history of many of the pathologies, this is often not known. In terms of osteoarthritis, the two main features which have been used radiographically to define and quantify it are: (i) the presence and extent of osteophytes; and (ii) the degree of reduction in joint space. Both are included in the classification systems of Kellgren and Moore (1952) and Mazur et al. (1979), although the relevance of osteophytes is questionable (Croft 1990). Other scales such as that of Olerud and Molander (1984) rely simply upon the extent of reduction in joint space. In both cases, however, validity and reliability data are either lacking or not complementary to the scores. Scales for osteoarthritis of the ankle joint have also been suggested (Mazur et al. 1979; Olerud and Molander 1984; Takakura et al. 1998a; Pell et al. 2000) and also for the subtalar joint (Morrey and Wiedeman 1980; Paley and Hall 1993). However, there is little scientific advice available to help recommend one scale over another, and which to use – if any.

RADIOGRAPHIC OUTCOME

The role of radiographs in the measurement of outcome may be categorized into the assessment of extra-articular alignment and joint congruency, and the assessment of union and detection of osteoarthritis. The information yielded by radiographs cannot be

ACHILLES TENDON DISORDERS

This is an area where debate continues between operative or conservative treatment for acute rupture. Evidence either way is certainly hampered by the lack of agreed outcome measures (Maffulli 1999).

It is generally accepted that the re-rupture rate following operative repair is usually lower (Kellam *et al.* 1985). Such complete failure however is an infrequent result, and various scores for measuring subtler outcomes are worth considering.

Two scores in particular merit attention. The first is that of Leppilahti *et al.* (1998) (Table 22.1), which was designed to measure the outcome for operatively treated tendon ruptures. Seven criteria were assessed, and all given equal weighting, with subjective measures comprising five of these. The criteria were pain, stiffness, subjective calf weakness, footwear restrictions, and patient satisfaction as well as difference in the range of movement between ankles and the isokinetic muscle strength. Of note is the fact that one criterion included is the subjective result, the four categories of which allow a direct comparison with the overall score, which is also subdivided into four classes. Of the 101 patients reported, there appeared to be a good agreement between the patients' subjective assessment and the overall score in terms of the numbers and proportions in each of the outcome classes: very satisfied, satisfied with minor reservations; satisfied with major reservations; or dissatisfied correlating with excellent (90–100 points), good (75–85 points), fair (60–70 points) or poor (<50 points).

The quantification of muscle function using isokinetic torque measurements with a dynamometer in this score is not without contention. As pointed out by Maffulli (1999), the technique is expensive, time-consuming and not widely available. In addition, there may be an issue with its sensitivity. Haggmark *et al.* (1986) found that the system did not discriminate any difference between operatively and non-operatively treated tendon ruptures, in contradistinction to a single heel rise fatigability test which did so clearly. However, other authors have not noted any problem with its discriminative ability (Wapner *et al.* 1993; Gallant *et al.* 1995).

The VISA-A (Victorian Institute of Sports Assessment-Achilles) outcome score (Robinson *et al.* 2001) (Table 22.2) offers hope that it may provide a means of standardizing the assessment of the injured or degenerate tendoachilles and the results of treatment. This system comprises eight questions, each weighted with 10 points on a visual analogue scale. It is purely subjective and covers the three most relevant areas of pain, function in daily living, and sporting activity, all of which were chosen as a result of clinician and patient input. Designed as an 'instrument to measure the severity of Achilles tendonopathy', this system is based on an already accepted and proven score used for the assessment of the patella tendinitis, the VISA score (Visentini *et al.* 1998). Its validity and reliability have been tested and demonstrated in terms of its 'ability to differentiate' between degrees of Achilles' tendinopathy and normal tendons. There is no evidence yet to demonstrate the sensitivity of the VISA-A to detect change with intervention over time; neither has it been used in any study other than that in which it was initially reported.

Table 22.1: Achilles tendon repair score. Reprinted from Leppilahti *et al.* (1998)

Clinical factors	Scores (points)
Pain	
None	15
Mild, no limited recreational activities	10
Moderate, limited recreational, but not daily activities	5
Severe, limited recreational and daily activities	0
Stiffness	
None	15
Mild, occasional, no limited recreational activities	10
Moderate, limited recreational but not daily activities	5
Severe, limited recreational and daily activities	0

Table 22.1: Achilles tendon repair score. Reprinted from Leppilahti *et al.* (1998) – *continued*

Clinical factors	Scores (points)
Calf muscle weakness (subjective)	
None	15
Mild, no limited recreational activities	10
Moderate, limited recreational but not daily activities	5
Severe, limited recreational and daily activities	0
Footwear restrictions	
None	10
Mild, most shoes tolerated	5
Moderate, unable to tolerate fashionable shoes, modified shoes tolerated	0
Active range of motion difference between ankles	
Normal ($\leqslant 5°$)	15
Mildly limited (6–10°)	10
Moderately limited (11–15°)	5
Severely limited ($\geqslant 16°$)	0
Subjective result	
Very satisfied	15
Satisfied with minor reservations	10
Satisfied with major reservations	5
Dissatisfied	0
Isokinetic muscle strength (score)	
Excellent	15
Good	10
Fair	5
Poor	0
Overall results	
Excellent	90–100
Good	75–85
Fair	60–70
Poor	$\leqslant 55$

Table 22.2: The VISA-A Questionnaire. Reprinted from Robinson *et al.* (2001): The VISA-A questionnaire, *Br J Sports Med*, **35**, 335–41, with permission from the BMJ Publishing Group

1. For how many minutes do you have stiffness in the Achilles region on first getting up?

100 min	0	1	2	3	4	5	6	7	8	9	10	0 min	POINTS

2. Once you are warmed up for the day, do you have pain when stretching the Achilles tendon fully over the edge of a step? (keeping knee straight)

Strong Severe Pain	0	1	2	3	4	5	6	7	8	9	10	No pain	POINTS

Table 22.2: The VISA-A Questionnaire. Reprinted from Robinson *et al.* (2001): The VISA-A questionnaire, *Br J Sports Med*, **35**, 335–41, with permission from the BMJ Publishing Group – *continued*

3. After walking on flat ground for 30 minutes, do you have pain within the next 2 hours? (if unable to walk on flat ground for 30 minutes because of pain, score 0 for this question).

Strong Severe Pain | 0 | 1 | 2 | 3 | 4 | 5 | 6 | 7 | 8 | 9 | 10 | No pain   POINTS [ ]

4. Do you have pain on walking downstairs with normal gait cycle?

Strong Severe Pain | 0 | 1 | 2 | 3 | 4 | 5 | 6 | 7 | 8 | 9 | 10 | No pain   POINTS [ ]

5. Do you have pain during or immediately after doing 10 (single leg) heel raises from a flat surface?

Strong Severe Pain | 0 | 1 | 2 | 3 | 4 | 5 | 6 | 7 | 8 | 9 | 10 | No pain   POINTS [ ]

6. How many single leg hops can you do without pain?

0 | 0 | 1 | 2 | 3 | 4 | 5 | 6 | 7 | 8 | 9 | 10 | 10   POINTS [ ]

7. Are you currently undertaking sport or other physical activity?

0 [ ] Not at all

4 [ ] Modified training ± modified competition

7 [ ] Full training ± but not at same level as when symptoms began

10 [ ] Competing at the same or higher level as when symptoms began

POINTS [ ]

8. Please complete EITHER A, B, C in this question.

A. If you have no pain while undertaking Achilles tendon loading sports, for how long can you train/practise?

NIL	1–10 min	11–20 min	21–30 min	>30 min	POINTS
[ ]	[ ]	[ ]	[ ]	[ ]	[ ]
0	7	14	21	30	

OR

B. If you have some pain while undertaking Achilles tendon loading sports, but it does not stop you from completing your training/practice, for how long can you train/practise?

NIL	1–10 min	11–20 min	21–30 min	>30 min	POINTS
[ ]	[ ]	[ ]	[ ]	[ ]	[ ]
0	7	14	21	30	

Table 22.2: The VISA-A Questionnaire. Reprinted from Robinson *et al.* (2001): The VISA-A questionnaire, *Br J Sports Med*, **35**, 335–41, with permission from the BMJ Publishing Group – *continued*

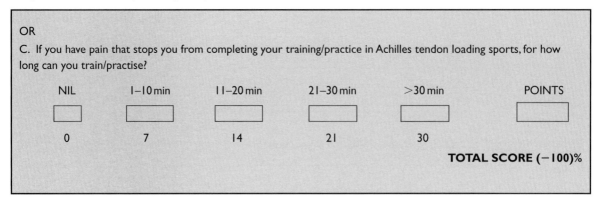

LATERAL LIGAMENT COMPLEX

The only score for which any attempt has been made to demonstrate validity and reliability is that of Kaikkonen *et al.* (1994) (Table 22.3). This is worthy of description – flawed though its methodology is in parts. A maximum 100 points are awarded – 40 for subjective symptoms and assessment of function, and 60 points for four objective tests of function (one for balance, one for functional stability, two for muscle strength), assessment of antero-posterior (AP) laxity and range of movement. The objective tests were selected from a larger group following side-to-side comparison testing. The reproducibility of the objective measures has been tested and appears high, but may be artificially so as figures quoted are Pearson's correlation coefficients rather than intra-class correlation coefficients. In addition, the discriminatory ability between 100 normal and 148 operatively treated lateral ligament injuries for each of the test fields was demonstrated. The validity of the score was assessed by correlating the total scores achieved with isokinetic strength measurements and subjective functional assessment. The former produced a low correlation, whereas the latter correlated strongly with the score. Issue could be taken for using this functional assessment as the

'gold standard' with which to compare the scores. No longitudinal data were supplied, and so it is not possible to comment upon the sensitivity to change of the score. Other scores worthy of mention are those of Karlsson and Peterson (1991) (Table 22.4) and St. Pierre *et al.* (1982) and Good *et al.* (1975). Of these scores, that of Karlsson and Peterson has probably been the most widely used. A purely subjective score 45 of the 100 points are given to instability and pain. Results with this score have corresponded well with a simplified version by Nimon *et al.* (2001) which just comprised four categories of pain and four of subjective instability. It is interesting to note from this study that whilst only 65 per cent of patients experienced no pain or instability, this correlated with an 86 per cent satisfaction rate and with 97.7 per cent of patients willing to opt for the operation again given the same circumstances. The difficulty with the heterogeneity of scoring systems used in this area is emphasized in a meta-analysis by Pijnenburg *et al.* (2000). In examining data from randomized controlled trials between 1966 and 1998 for the treatment of lateral ligament injury, these authors were only able to extrapolate and analyse three common measures of outcome for analysis, which were simply the time off work, residual pain and giving way.

Table 22.3: A scoring scale for subjective and functional follow-up evaluation.[1] Reprinted from Kaikkonen *et al.* (1994): A performance test protocol and scoring scale for the evaluation of ankle injuries. *Am J Sports Med*, **22**, 462–9

I	Subjective assessment of the injured ankle	
	No symptoms of any kind[2]	15
	Mild symptoms	10
	Moderate symptoms	5
	Severe symptoms	0
II	Can you walk normally?	
	Yes	15
	No	0
III	Can you run normally?	
	Yes	10
	No	0
IV	Climbing down stairs[3]	
	Under 18 seconds	10
	18–20 seconds	5
	Over 20 seconds	0
V	Rising on heels with injured leg	
	Over 40 times	10
	30–39 times	5
	Under 30 times	0
VI	Rising on toes with injured leg	
	Over 40 times	10
	30–39 times	5
	Under 30 times	0
VII	Single-limbed stance with injured leg	
	Over 55 seconds	10
	50–55 seconds	5
	Under 50 seconds	0
VIII	Laxity of ankle joint (ADS)	
	Stable ($\leqslant 5$ mm)	10
	Moderate instability (6–10 mm)	5
	Severe instability (>10 mm)	0
IX	Dorsiflexion range of motion, injured leg	
	$\geqslant 10°$	10
	5–9°	5
	<5°	0

[1] Total: Excellent, 85–100; good, 70–80; fair, 55–65; poor, $\leqslant 50$.
[2] Pain, swelling, stiffness, tenderness, or giving way during activity (mild, only 1 of these symptoms is present; moderate, 2 to 3 of these symptoms are present; severe, 4 or more of these symptoms are present).
[3] Two levels of staircase (length, 12 m) with 44 steps (height, 18 cm; depth, 22 cm).

Table 22.4: Scoring scale for assessment of functional results.[1] Reprinted from Karlsson and Peterson (1991)

Instability	
None	25
1 or 2 times per year (during exercise)	20
1 or 2 times per month (during exercise)	15
Walking on uneven ground	10
Walking on even ground	5
Constant (severe), using ankle support	0
Pain	
None	20
During exercise	15
Walking on uneven surface	10
Walking on even surface	5
Constant (severe)	0
Swelling	
None	10
After exercise	5
Constant	0
Stiffness	
None	5
Moderate (morning after exercise)	2
Marked (constant, severe)	0
Work, sport activities and activities of daily living	
Same as pre-injury	15
Same work, less sport, normal leisure activities	10
Impaired working capacity, no sports, normal leisure activities	5
Severely impaired working capacity, decreased leisure activities	0
Stair climbing	
No problems	10
Impaired (instability)	5
Impossible	0
Running	
No problems	10
Impaired	5
Impossible	0
Support	
None	5
Ankle support during exercise	2
Ankle support during daily activities	0

[1] The maximum score is 100 points.

Table 22.5: Summary of abridged ankle scores

	AOFAS	Mazur	Takakura	Kofoed
Pain	40	50	40	50
Function				
Limitations	10			
Walk distance	5	6	20	
Walk surface	5			
Gait	8	6	4	
Hills		6		
Stairs		6	8	6
Support		6		6
Running		5		
Single leg stand			4	6
Sitting			4	
Heel rise		5		3
Heel walk				3
Footwear				6
Ankle movement	8	10	20	10
Hindfoot movement	6			6
Alignment	10			4
Stability	8			
TOTAL POINTS	100	100	100	100

ANKLE ARTHRODESIS AND ARTHROPLASTY

The four most commonly used scores are compared in Table 22.5 and discussed specifically below. Generally, they have all been applied for the assessment of both ankle arthrodesis and arthroplasty and at present probably represent the best scores available, though there are few significant differences between them. All need to share the criticism that they are entirely non-validated. The choice of which system is to be used remains based imperfectly on factors such as the proportion of subjective to object-ive measurements included, a personal assessment of the factors most specifically affected by the procedure or disease under investigation or which scores have been most commonly adopted by the previous authors with whom one may be comparing results.

Mazur score

The Mazur score (Mazur *et al.* 1979) was 'designed' to assess ankle arthrodesis, and originally reported on 12 patients. Its authors attribute its inspiration to be the Harris hip score. As can be seen by comparison with subsequent ankle outcome scores, the basic template and weighting have seen little change, though the specific variables may have done. Of the 100 points available, 50 are assigned to pain, 40 to function, and 10 to range of movement. Some 78 of these points are allocated to subjective assessments, and only 22 to objective. One could take issue with the illogical weighting between the categories of pain, or with the weighting in general. Other points worth noting are the use of absolute values in the assessment of ankle movement and the number of single heel rises performable being used as an objective test of stability (which is rather non-specific and obviously subject to other pathologies not related to stability). Their combined effect however on the score is low. A grading scheme, though arbitrary (excellent 80–90 points; good 70–79; fair 60–69; poor <60), does stand up to common-sense scrutiny.

Takakura score

The Takakura scoring system (Takakura *et al.* 1990) was originally developed for the assessment of total ankle replacements, and then subsequently applied by the same authors to ankle arthrodesis (Takakura *et al.* 1998b) and supramalleolar osteotomies (Takakura *et al.* 1998a). Again, there are a total of 100 points: 40 for pain, 20 for range of movement, and 40 for function (including the ability to sit cross-legged 'Japanese style'). Objective measurements comprise just 20 points, and the remaining 80 points subjective measurements. Again, the range of movement is assessed in absolute terms and is restricted to ankle saggital movements.

The American Foot and Ankle Society score

This score (Kitaoka *et al.* 1994) is deserving of detailed mention if, for no other reason, it has been widely adopted as the standard measure in much of the American and European literature. It remains non-validated for all of its postulated indications (namely ankle, talar and hindfoot fractures, ankle instability, ankle and hindfoot arthrodesis and arthroplasty). Its scoring is subdivided into 40 points for pain, 50 points for function, and 10 points for alignment. In all, the subjective part of the score constitutes 60 points and the objective portion 40 points. The score is not classified into arbitrary divisions of excellent, good, etc., although subsequent authors have assigned their own categories (Mann *et al.* 1998). A minor point is that its use of 'blocks' to quantify walking distance does not immediately translate into any recognized European

or British measure. Again, one could take issue with some aspects of the weighting – for example, the subjective assessment of function accounting for just 20 points. This compares with 30 points for objective assessment of movement, stability and gait. However, in terms of the assessment of movement this is the only one of the scores to use comparative rather than absolute measurements. The equal weighting of all aspects of the score, irrespective of the different conditions or procedures assessed, needs to be considered carefully before application to particular investigations. For example, it has been used to assess lateral ligament reconstruction and found to yield inappropriately good results when compared with more specific measures (Nimon *et al.* 2001).

Kofoed score

The Kofoed score (Kofoed 1995) was designed for the assessment of outcomes following total ankle arthroplasty. Again, it essentially adheres to the blueprint of Mazur's score and has a very similar overall breakdown to the AOFAS score, with a total of 100 points: 50 for pain, 20 for range of movement, and 30 for function. The total allocated to subjective evaluation is potentially 74 points, and to objective 26. Range of movement is assessed in absolute terms and includes subtalar motion. As with other scores, weighting can seem arbitrary. Any score below 70 is deemed 'not acceptable'; this may describe a patient with only occasional pain, an inability to heel or tip-toe walk, but otherwise a normal functional score and mid to low ranges of movement.

More recent developments are the movement towards assessment of patients with the use of the SF-36, in tandem with these scores (Marsh *et al.* 1997).

ANKLE OSTEOARTHRITIS AND ANTERIOR IMPINGEMENT

The syndrome of chronic anterior ankle pain and restriction of dorsiflexion secondary to osteophytic tibial spurring (with or without reciprocal talar neck

Table 22.6: Scoring system used to assess results in five categories for anterior ankle impingement. Reprinted from Ogilvie-Harris et al. (1993)

	1 Poor	2 Fair	3 Good	4 Excellent
Pain	Severe	Moderate	Mild	None
Swelling	Moderate/severe	Mild with ADL	With exercise	None/minimal
Stiffness	Minimal motion	Painful deficit	Mild deficit	None/minimal
Limping	Severe (cane/crutch)	Moderate	Slight	None
Activity	Limited ADL	Moderate limits	Minor limits	No limits

ADL = Activities of Daily Living

changes) is well recognized. It may arise in an otherwise radiographically normal ankle or with varying degrees of degenerative change. Arthroscopic débridement with osteophyte removal has become the mainstay of surgical treatment in the salvageable joint.

One of the most commonly used scoring systems is that of Ogilvie-Harris (Ogilvie-Harris et al. 1993) (Table 22.6), which is purely subjective and allows one of four responses to each of the criteria of pain, swelling, stiffness, limping, and activity. Both the original author as well as subsequent ones (Tol et al. 2001) have noted a lack of correlation between patient satisfaction (excellent or good in 53%) and the scores yielded (similar gradings in only 29%). In context, this was only in ankles with associated established arthritic changes. Those with none or early changes however showed a high level of agreement between the score and patient satisfaction judged with the same four categories (Tol et al. 2001).

OSTEOCHONDRAL LESIONS OF THE TALAR DOME

The aetiology of these lesions is frequently, though not exclusively, post-traumatic. There are a proportion of cases with no history of trauma (Campbell and Ranawat 1966), and various hypotheses have been suggested including spontaneous osteonecrosis or ossification defects (Hepple et al. 1999). The investigator is not spoilt for choice of outcome measures in this field. The phenomenon of talar dome osteochondral lesions was first tackled substantively during the late 1950s (Berndt and Harty, 1959). Both the clinical outcome grading as well as the radiographic classification, based on the degree of displacement, described by the original authors saw wide (though not unqualified) acceptance. In particular, the value of their preoperative radiographic classification is being increasingly questioned in the light of magnetic resonance imaging (MRI) (Hepple et al. 1999) and arthroscopic (Kumai et al. 1999; Tol et al. 2000) findings. Likewise, their outcome score continues to be used (Pritisch et al. 1986; Kumai et al. 1999), and has in its favour that it is simple and subjective but potentially has low discriminatory power given the presence of only three categories. A good result corresponds to occasional symptoms but no disabling pain; a fair result to a decrease in symptoms but still some disabling pain; and a poor result to no decrease in symptoms. Other scores with a mixture of subjective and objective criteria and a greater detail have also been used. Examples are: (i) the Hannover score (Hangody et al. 1997; Gautier et al. 2002) (Table 22.7), which encompasses 68 points for subjective and 36 for objective outcomes; and (ii) the AOFAS (Kitaoka et al. 1994). These have been shown to correlate well statistically with each other, but are no more validated than the score of Berndt and Harty (1959).

Table 22.7: Hannover Scoring System. Reprinted from Shereff (1993)

	Excellent	Good	Satisfactory	Poor	Points
Subjective					
Pain	None	On exertion	Moderate	Constant	12/9/6/3
Swelling	None	With sports	With daily exertion	Constant	8/6/4/2
Deficit in ROM	None	Moderate	Considerable	Stiff	8/6/4/2
Postop. improvement	Normal function	Considerable	Moderate	None/worse	8/6/4/2
Limping	None	After strenuous exercise	Intermittent	Constant	4/3/2/1
Locking	None	Causing no limitations	Causing intermittent limitations	Considerable limitations	8/6/4/2
Giving way	None	With exercise	Intermittent, uneven ground	Regularly	8/6/4/2
Objective					
Function	Normal	<10° deficit pf/df	11–15° deficit pf/df	>15° deficit pf/df	16/12/8/4
Instability	None	1+	1–2+	2+	4/3/2/1
Arthritis	No signs	1°	2°	3°	8/6/4/2
Perception disorders	None	Temporary, <2	Month, >2	Month persistent	8/6/4/2

* ROM, range of motion; Postop., postoperative; pf, plantarflexion; df, dorsiflexion.

Activity score (points) pain with rest, 2; light work, pain with daily activities, rest required, no sports, 4; normal work, pain only after light sports (bicycling, jogging on even ground), 6; heavy work, normal sports (jogging on uneven ground, team sports), 8; competitive sports, 10; high-performance sports, 12.

Result: poor, <34; satisfactory, 64–35; good, 84–65; excellent, 100–85; points total, maximum 100; professional sport activity without complaints, 104–100.

HINDFOOT ARTHRODESES (SUBTALAR, TRIPLE, PANTALAR AND TIBIOCALCANEAL)

The range of pathological conditions to which each of these operations may be applied is wide, united simply by a combination of pain and deformity. It may be important to bear the case mix in mind when comparing the results of patients or series with these often very diverse pathologies. For example, subtalar arthrodesis may be an appropriate procedure at stages in the surgical management of calcaneal fractures, tarsal coalition, pes planus due to tibialis posterior dysfunction and talpies equinovarus (Mann *et al.* 1998; Trnka *et al.* 2001). For the subtalar joint,

the most common outcome score in usage is the AOFAS, modified appropriately by removal of the six points usually allocated for the subtalar movement which has been ablated surgically (Mann *et al.* 1998; Chandler *et al.* 1999; Easley *et al.* 2000; Trnka *et al.* 2001). Other authors (Marti *et al.* 1999) have adopted scores developed for the original pathology, such as that of Paley (Paley and Hall 1993) for subtalar fusion following calcaneal trauma. For triple arthrodesis, the AOFAS has again been widely adopted with appropriate modification for the loss of subtalar motion, and has been shown to agree well with patient satisfaction (Pell *et al.* 2000). The simpler subjective system of Angus and Cowell (1986) has also been used (Saltzman *et al.* 1999).

Table 22.8: Modified American Orthopaedic Foot and Ankle Society Clinical Rating Scale. Reprinted from Kitaoka *et al.* (1994). © 1997 by the American Orthopaedic Foot and Ankle Society, originally published in Foot and Ankle International, reproduced here with permission

	POINTS
Pain (40 points)	
Severe (Always present)	0
Moderate (Daily)	20
Mild (Occasional)	30
None	40
Function (40 points)	
Dependent, Wheelchair	
Housebound, Supports	0
Partially Dependent, Supports	5
Household Ambulator	
Walk <15 minutes, Single Support	10
Community Ambulator	
Walk 15–30 minutes, Cane	20
Perform Activities of Daily	30
Living, No support	
Recreational Activities	
Walk 30+ minutes	40
Shoe wear (10 points)	
Modified shoes, with pain	0
Modified shoes, without pain	5
Regular shoes, without pain	10
Alignment (10 points)	
Poor (Severe deformity)	0
Fair (Mild/moderate deformity)	5
Good (Plantigrade foot, well aligned)	10

Tibiocalcaneal and pantalar fusions self-evidently will result in the loss of all true hindfoot movement. In addition, a successful result is likely to result in significant functional impairment, and is often performed in patients with very poor function. Any scoring system with a fair proportion of weighting given to range of movement and emphasis upon function such as the AOFAS will be inappropriate in these circumstances. A modified version lacking the measurement of movement and with more appropriate functional parameters has been suggested (Acosta *et al.* 2000) (Table 22.8). A simpler and purely subjective score with appropriate levels of functional attainment for tibiocalcaneal fusion also exists (Kitaoka and Patzer 1998).

FRACTURES

Ankle fractures

Various non-specific scores have been adopted to assess the outcome of ankle fractures including the AOFAS and Mazur's score as well as the SF-36, individually and in combination. The specific outcome measure most commonly applied is that of Olerud and Molander (1984) (Table 22.9). This is a purely subjective score with a total of 100 points, broken down into 25 for pain, 20 for stiffness and swelling, and 55 for function. One could take issue with the exact weighting of some aspects of the score and an illogical allocation of points within categories, in particular pain. The authors did attempt validation by correlating the scores obtained for 90 operated ankles with four other independent measurements of outcome, including a linear analogue scale of ankle function with which it correlated well. Some authors (Makwana *et al.* 2001) have found however that a significant difference in the Olerud and Molander score between groups with ankle fractures has not been associated with any significant difference either in visual analogue scores or general satisfaction levels.

Calcaneal fractures

The question of whether or not to fix displaced intra-articular calcaneal fractures still excites debate. There is general acceptance that providing robust evidence for either side of the argument is hampered by the lack of an accepted, validated scoring system. The outcome scores commonly used fall into four categories:

- The AOFAS scores (Park *et al.* 2000);

- The specialized calcaneal fracture scores comprising a mixture of subjective and objective criteria; examples include the Maryland foot score (Sanders *et al.* 1993), the Creighton-Nebraska score (Crosby and

Table 22.9: The scoring system of Olerud and Molander (1984). Reproduced by permission of Springer-Verlag

Parameter	Degree	Score
I. Pain	None	25
	While walking on uneven surface	20
	While walking on even surface outdoors	10
	While walking indoors	5
	Constant and severe	0
II. Stiffness	None	10
	Stiffness	0
III. Swelling	None	10
	Only evenings	5
	Constant	0
IV. Stair-climbing	No problem	10
	Impaired	5
	Impossible	0
V. Running	Possible	5
	Impossible	0
VI. Jumping	Possible	5
	Impossible	0
VII. Squatting	No problems	5
	Impossible	0
VIII. Supports	None	10
	Taping, wrapping	5
	Stick or crutch	0
IX. Work, activities of daily life	Same as before injury	20
	Loss of tempo	15
	Change to a simpler job/part-time work	10
	Severely impaired work capacity	0

Table 22.10: Maryland foot score. Reprinted from Sanders *et al.* (1993)

I. Pain		
	None: including sports	45
	Slight: no change in ADLs	40
	Mild: minimal change in ADLs	35
	Moderate: significant decrease in ADLs	30
	Marked: during minimal ADLs (e.g. bathroom, simple housework. Stronger, frequent analgesics)	10
	Disabled: unable to work or shop	5
2. Function		
Gait		
	Distance walked	
	Unlimited	10
	Slight limitation	8
	Moderate (2–3 blocks)	5
	Severe limitation (1 block)	2
	Indoors only	0
Stability		
	Normal	4
	Weak feeling – no true giving way	3
	Occasional giving way (1–2 months)	2
	Frequent giving way	1
	Orthotic device used	0
Support		
	None	4
	Cane	3
	Crutches	1
	Wheelchair	0
Limp		
	None	4
	Slight	3
	Moderate	2
	Severe	1
	Unable to walk	0
Shoes		
	Any type	10
	Minor concessions	9
	Flat, laced	7
	With orthotics	5
	Space shoes	2
	Unable to wear shoes	0
Stairs		
	Normally	4
	With bannister	3

Fitzgibbons 1990), and Paley's score (Paley and Hall 1993);

- a specialized subjective score (Kerr *et al.* 1996); and

- the SF-36 (Heffernan *et al.* 2000).

Probably the most widely used system is the Maryland foot score (Table 22.10) which awards 45 points for pain and 55 for function. However, few investigations have been conducted on validation,

Table 22.10: Maryland foot score. Reprinted from Sanders *et al.* (1993) – *continued*

	Any method	2
	Unable	0
Terrain		
	No problem, any surface	4
	Problems on stones, hills	2
	Problems on flat surfaces	0
Cosmesis		
	Normal	10
	Mild deformity	8
	Moderate	6
	Severe	0
	Multiple deformities	0
Motion (ankle, subtalar, mid-foot, metatarsophalangeal)		
	Normal	5
	Slightly decreased	4
	Markedly decreased	2
	Ankylosed	0

Table 22.11: Calcaneal fracture scoring system. Maximum score = 100 points. Reprinted from Kerr *et al.* (1996)

1. Pain (36 points)

At rest		On activity	
None	18	None	18
Slight	12	Slight	12
Moderate	6	Moderate	6
Severe	0	Severe	0

2. Work (25 points)

No change in job	25
Modification of job	16
Enforced change of job	8
Unable to work	0

3. Walking (25 points)

No change in walking ability	25
Minimal restriction	16
Moderate restriction	8
Severe restriction	0

4. Walking aids (14 points)

None	14
Occasional stick	10
Constant stick	6
2 sticks	3
Crutches	0

with the exception of a study by Heffernan *et al.* (2000). This compared the results yielded by the pain and functional components of the SF-36 with the Maryland score, separated into its equivalent parts, for internally fixed calcaneal fractures. Correlation coefficients were calculated to be 0.78 for pain and 0.64 for function ($P < 0.001$). A useful contribution has also been made by Kerr *et al.* (1996) (Table 22.11), who performed a regression analysis of six such scores upon their variables, having been first applied to a 'diverse' group of intra-articular fractures. There was considerable overlap between the different scores, with a total of 17 different components examined. In the final analysis, four components accounted for 98 per cent of the variation, all of which were subjective. These variables were pain, work capacity, walking ability and the use of walking aids. They were selected for a new scoring system, and their weighting was based on that in the original scores. The resulting score was not subjected to validity or reliability testing, but is based on a sound premise, and has seen some – albeit limited – acceptance amongst researchers (Squires *et al.* 2001; Mishra *et al.* 2002).

USE OF THE SF-36 IN HINDFOOT AND ANKLE

The SF-36 is a patient-based, subjective, validated outcome score which has been shown to provide reliable information on the general health – both psychological and physical – of a patient group (Ware and Sherbourne 1992). It assesses eight areas, these being physical functioning, role limitations due to physical factors, role limitations due to emotional problems, pain, general health perceptions, vitality, social functioning and general mental health. The score yields numerical outcomes in each of these categories, which are not combined and may be used for comparison with age-matched control figures as well as pre- and post-treatment figures. As can be appreciated from these broad fields, the SF-36 is an instrument which may be affected by many factors extraneous to the procedure or condition under review. A number of examples of its application have already been discussed. It has been used to provide an additional measure of the health status of a patient group and as such has proved useful. For example, in a small study of ankle arthrodeses (following pilon fractures), Marsh *et al.* (1997) found – despite a preponderance of excellent and good results measured on the score of Mazur *et al.* (1979) – that all SF-36 results were lower than age-matched controls, in particular for physical function, role limitations and pain. Others (Egol *et al.* 2000) again used both the SF-36 and Mazur's score in a study comparing casting and bracing for ankle fractures. Here, the SF-36 identified differences between the groups at 12 months post injury (though just in vitality and general health perceptions), whereas the ankle score detected none.

CONCLUSION

Since publication of the first edition of this book, a move has occurred in the scientific literature towards patient-centred, subjective measures of outcome. With this shift away from 'traditional', predominantly objective, measures there has been an evolution of the scoring systems in use. For the ankle and hindfoot there is as yet none which fulfils all the requirements of being valid, reliable and sensitive to change, though some, such as the VISA-A, come close. In their absence, some have adopted the SF-36 as a 'gold standard', but this has clear limitations. Much work remains to be done, both with the validation of newer scores as well as the scientific development and testing of alternative scores where needs exist, though progress is clearly being made.

ACKNOWLEDGEMENTS

The authors wish to acknowledge the assistance of Mrs Judy Dawson in the preparation of this manuscript.

REFERENCES

Acosta, R., Ushiba, J., and Cracchiolo, A. (2000): The results of primary and staged pantalar arthrodesis and tibiotalocalcaneal arthrodesis in adult patients. *Foot Ankle Int* **21**, 182–94.

Angus, P. D., and Cowell, H. R. (1986): Triple arthrodesis a critical long term review. *J Bone Joint Surg* **68B**, 260–5.

Backer, M., and Kofoed, H. (1989): Passive ankle mobility. Clinical measurement compared with radiography. *J Bone Joint Surg* **71B**, 696–8.

Bauer, M., Jonsson, K., and Nilsson, B. (1985): 30 year follow-up of ankle fractures. *Acta Orthop Scand* **56**, 103–6.

Bellamy, N., Buchanan, W. W., Goldsmith, C. H., Campbell, J., and Stitt, L. W. (1988): Validation study of WOMAC a health status instrument for measuring clinically important patient relevant outcomes to anti-rheumatic drug therapy in patients with osteoarthritis of the hip or knee. *Rheumatology* **15**, 1833–40.

Berndt, A. L., and Harty, M. (1959): Transchondral fractures of the talus. *J Bone Joint Surg* **41A**, 988–1020.

Bohannon, R. W., Tiberio, D., and Zito, M. (1989): Selected measures of ankle dorsiflexion range of motion: differences and inter-correlations. *Foot Ankle* **10**, 99–103.

Budiman-Mak, E., Conrad, K. J., and Roach, K. E. (1991): The foot function index: a measure of foot pain and disability. *Clin Epidemiol* **44**, 561–70.

Campbell, C. J., and Ranawat, C. S. (1966): Osteochondritis dissecans: the question of etiology. *J Trauma* **6**, 201–21.

Chandler, J. T., Bonar, S. K., Anderson, R. B., and Davis, W. (1999): Results of in situ subtalar arthrodesis for late sequelae of calcaneus fractures. *Foot Ankle Int* **20**, 18–24.

Coester, L. M., Saltzman, C. L., Leupold, J., and Pontarelli, W. (2001): Long term results following ankle arthrodesis for post-traumatic arthritis. *J Bone Joint Surg* **83A**, 219–28.

Conboy, V. B., Morris, R. W., Kiss, J., and Karr, A. J. (1996): An evaluation of the Constant-Murley shoulder assessment. *J Bone Joint Surg Br* **78B**, 229–32.

Croft, P. (1990): Review of UK data on the rheumatic diseases. 3. Osteoarthritis. *Br J Rheumatol* **29**, 391–5.

Crosby, L. A., and S Fitzgibbons, T. (1990): Computerised tomography scanning of acute intra-articular fractures of the calcaneus. *J Bone Joint Surg* **72A**, 852–9.

Dawson, J., and Carr, A. (2001): Outcomes evaluation in orthopaedics. *J Bone Joint Surg* **83B**, 313–15.

Drake, B. G., Callahan, C. M., Dittus, R. S., and Wright, J. G. (1994): Global rating systems used in assessing knee arthroplasty outcomes. *Arthroplasty* **9**, 409–17.

Easley, M. E., Trnka, H., Schon, L. C., and Myerson, M. S. (2000): Isolated subtalar arthrodesis. *J Bone Joint Surg* **82A**, 613–24.

Egol, K. A., Dolan, R., and Koval, K. J. (2000): Functional outcome of surgery for fractures of the ankle. *J Bone Joint Surg* **82B**, 246–9.

Elveru, R. A., Rothstein, J. M., and Lamb, R. L. (1988): Goniometric reliability in a clinical setting. Subtalar and ankle joint measurements. *Phys Ther* **68**, 672–7.

Gallant, G., Massie, C., and Turco, V. (1995): Assessment of eversion and plantarflexion strength after repair of Achilles' tendon rupture using peroneus brevis tendon transfer. *Am J Orthop* **24**, 257–61.

Gautier, E., Kolker, D., and Jakob, R. P. (2002): Treatment of cartilage of the talus by autologous osteochondral grafts. *J Bone Joint Surg* **84B**, 237–44.

Good, C., Jones, M., and Livingstone, B. M. (1975): Reconstruction of the lateral ligament of the ankle. *Injury* **7**, 63–5.

Haggmark, T., Liedberg, H., Eriksson, E., and Wredmark, T. (1986): Calf muscle atrophy and muscle function after non-operative vs. operative treatment of Achilles' tendon ruptures. *Orthopaedics* **9**, 160–4.

Hangody, L., Kish, G., Karpati, Z., Szerb, I., and Eberhardt, R. (1997): Treatment of osteochondritis dissecans of the talus: use of the mosaicplasty technique – a preliminary report. *Foot Ankle Int* **18**, 628–34.

Heffernan, G., Khan, F., Awan, N., O'Riordain, C., and Corrigan, J. (2000): A comparison of outcomes scores in oscalcis fractures. *Irish J Med Sci* **169**, 127–8.

Hepple, S., Winson, I. G., and Gew, D. (1999): Osteochondral lesions of the talus: a revised classification. *Foot Ankle Int* **20**, 789–93.

Kaikkonen, A., Kannus, P., and Javinen, M. (1994): A performance test protocol and scoring scale for the evaluation of ankle injuries. *Am J Sports Med* **22**, 462–9.

Karlsson, J., and Peterson, L. (1991): Evaluation of ankle joint function; the use of a scoring scale. *Foot* **1**, 15–19.

Kellam, J. F., Huner, G. A., and McElwein, J. P. (1985): Review of the operative treatment of Achilles' tendon rupture. *Clin Orthop* **201**, 80–3.

Kellgren, J. H., and Moore, R. (1952): Generalised oestoarthrosis and Heberden's nodes. *Br Med J* **1**, 181–7.

Kerr, P. S., Prothero, D. L., and Atkins, R. M. (1996): Assessing outcome following calcaneal fracture: a rational scoring system. *Injury* **27**, 35–8.

Kitaoka, H. B., and Patzer, G. L. (1998): Arthrodesis for the treatment of arthrosis of the ankle and osteonecrosis of the talus. *J Bone Joint Surg* **80A**, 370–9.

Kitaoka, H. B., Alexander, I. J., Adellar, R. S., Nunley, J. A., Myerson, M. S., and Sanders, M. (1994): Clinical rating systems for the ankle-hindfoot midfoot hallux and lesser toes. *Foot Ankle Int* **15**, 349–53.

Kofoed, H. (1995): Cylindrical cemented ankle arthroplasty: a prospective series with long term follow-up. *Foot Ankle Int* **16**, 474–9.

Kumai, T., Takakura, Y., Higashiyama, I., and Tamai, S. (1999): Arthroscopic drilling for treatment of oesteochondral lesions of the talus. *J Bone Joint Surg* **81A**, 1229–35.

Leicht, P., and Kofoed, H. (1992): Subtalar arthrosis following ankle arthrodesis. *Foot* **II**, 89–92.

Leppilahti, J., Forsman, K., Peranem, J., and Orava, S. (1998): Outcome and prognostic factors of achilles rupture repair using a new scoring method. *Clin Orthop Rel Res* **346**, 152–61.

Lindsjo, U., Danckwardt-Lilliest, R. O. M. G., and Sahlstedt, B. (1985): Measurement in the motion range in the loaded ankle. *Clin Orthop Rel Res* **199**, 68–71.

Maffulli, N. (1999): Rupture of the Achilles tendon. *J Bone Joint Surg* **81A**, 1019–36.

Makwana, N. K., Bhowal, B., Harper, W. M., and Hui, A. W. (2001): Comparative versus operative for displaced ankle fractures in patients over 55 years of age. *J Bone Joint Surg* **83B**, 525–9.

Mann, R. A., Beaman, D. N., and Horton, G. A. (1998): Isolated subtalar arthrodesis. *Foot Ankle Int* **19**, 511–19.

Marsh, J. L., Ratty, R. E., and Dulaney, T. (1997): Results of ankle arthrodesis for treatment of supramalleolar non-union and ankle arthrosis. *Foot Ankle Int* **18**, 138–43.

Marti, R. K., de Heus, J. A., Roolker, W., Poolman, R. W., and Besselarr, P. P. (1999): Subtalar arthrodesis with correction of deformity after fractures of the os calcis. *J Bone Joint Surg* **81B**, 611–16.

Mazur, J. M., Schwartz, E., and Simon, S. R. (1979): Ankle arthrodesis long term follow-up with gait analysis. *J Bone Joint Surg* **61A**, 964–75.

Mishra, V., Umedi, U., Durkin, P., and Marsh, D. R. (2002): Outcome analysis in displaced 2 part intra-articular fractures of the os calcis. *J Bone Joint Surg* **84B** (Suppl. 1), 5–6.

Morrey, B. F., and Wiedeman, G. P. (1980): Complications and long term results of ankle arthrodeses following trauma. *J Bone Joint Surg* **62A**, 777–84.

Nimon, G. A., Dobson, P. J., Angel, K. R., Lewis, P. L., and Stevenson, T. M. (2001): A long term review of a modified Evans procedure. *J Bone Joint Surg* **83B**, 14–18.

Oatis, C. A. (1988): Biomechanics of the foot and ankle under static conditions. *Physiotherapy* **68**, 815–21.

Ogilvie-Harris, D. J., Mahomed, N., and Demaziere, A. (1993): Anterior impingement of the ankle treated arthroscopic removable of boney spurs. *J Bone Joint Surg* **75B**, 437–40.

Olerud, C., and Molander, H. (1984): A scoring scale for symptom evaluation after ankle fracture. *Arch Orthop Trauma Surg* **103**, 190–4.

Paley, D., and Hall, H. (1993): Intra-articular fractures of the calcaneus. *J Bone Joint Surg* **75A**, 342–54.

Park, I.-H., Song, K.-W., Shin, S.-I., Lee, J.-Y., Kim, T.-G., and Park, R.-S. (2000): Displaced intra-articular calcaneal fracture treated surgically with limited posterior incision. *Foot Ankle Int* **21**, 195–205.

Pell, R. F., Myerson, M. S., and Schon, L. C. (2000): Clinical outcome after primary triple arthrodesis. *J Bone Joint Surg* **82A**, 47–57.

Pijnenberg, C. M., Van Dijk, C. N., Bossuyt, P. M., and Marti, R. K. (2000): Treatment of ruptures of the lateral ankle ligaments: a meta-analysis. *J Bone Joint Surg* **82A**, 761–73.

Pritisch, M., Horoshovski, H., and Farine, B. (1986): Arthroscopic treatment of osteochrondral lesions of the talus. *J Bone Joint Surg* **68A**, 862–5.

Pynsent, P. B. (2001): Choosing an outcome measure. *J Bone Joint Surg* **83B**, 792–4.

Robinson, J., Cook, J., Purdam, C., et al. (2001): The VISA-A questionnaire: a valid and reliable index of the clinical severity of achilles tendonopathy. *Br J Sports Med* **35**, 335–41.

Saltzman, C. L., Fehrle, M. J., Cooper, R. R., Spencer, E. C., and Ponseti, I. V. (1999): Triple arthrodesis 25 and 44 year average follow-up of the same patients. *J Bone Joint Surg* **81A**, 1391–402.

Sanders, R., Fortin, P., Dipasquale, T., and Walling, A. (1993): Operative treatment in 120 displaced intra-articular calcaneal fractures. Results using a prognostic. *Clin Orthop* **290**, 87–95.

Shereff, M. J. (1993): *Atlas of Foot and Ankle Surgery*. W. B. Saunders, Philadelphia.

Skalley, T. C., Schon, L. C., Hinton, R. Y., and Myerson, M. S. (1994): Clinical results following revision tibial nerve release. *Foot Ankle Int* **15**, 360–7.

Southwell, R. B., and Sherman, F. C. (1981): Triple arthrodesis: a long term study with force plate analysis. *Foot Ankle* **2**, 15–24.

Squires, B., Allen, P. E., Livingstone, J., and Atkins, R. M. (2001): Fractures of the tuberocity of the calcaneus. *J Bone Joint Surg* **83B**, 55–61.

St. Pierre, R., Allman, F., Bassett, F., *et al.* (1982): A review of lateral ankle ligamentous reconstructions. *Foot Ankle* 3, 114–23.

Takakura, Y., Tanaka, Y., Sugimoto, K., Tamai, S., and Masuhara, K. (1990): Ankle arthroplasty: a comparative study of cemented metal and uncemented ceramic prostheses. *Clin Orthop Rel Res* 252, 209–16.

Takakura, Y., Takaoka, T., Tanaka, Y., Yajima, H., and Tamai, S. (1998a): Results of opening – wedge osteotomy for the treatment of a post-traumatic varus deformity of the ankle. *J Bone Joint Surg* 80A, 213–18.

Takakura, Y., Tanaka, Y., Sugimoto, K., Akiyama, K., and Tamai, S. (1998b): Long term results of arthrodesis for osteoarthritis of the ankle. *Clin Orthop Rel Res* 361, 178–85.

Tol, J. L., Struijs, P. A., Bossuyt, P. M., Verhagen, R. A., and van Dijk, C. N. (2000): Treatment strategies in oesteochondral defects of the talar dome: a systematic review. *Foot Ankle Int* 21, 119–26.

Tol, J. L., Verheyen, C. P., and Van Dijk, C. N. (2001): Arthroscopic treatment of anterior impingement in the ankle. *J Bone Joint Surg* 83B, 9–13.

Trnka, H. J., Easley, M. E., Lam, P. W., Anderson, C. D., Schon, L. C., and Myerson, M. S. (2001): Subtalar distraction bone block arthrodesis. *J Bone Joint Surg* 83B, 849–54.

Visentini, P., Khan, K., Cook, J., *et al.* (1998): The VISA score an index of the severity of jumper's knee (patellar tendinosis). *J Sci Med Sport* 1, 22–8.

Wapner, K., Pavlock, G., Hecht, P., *et al.* (1993): Repair of chronic Achilles tendon rupture with flexor hallucis longus transfer. *Foot Ankle* 14, 443–9.

Ware, J. E., and Sherbourne, C. D. (1992): The MOS 36 item short form health survey (SF36). I. Conceptual framework and item selection. *Med Care* 30, 473–83.

23

The foot

Roger M. Atkins

INTRODUCTION

Some 20 per cent of orthopaedic practice relates to the foot (Mann and Plattner 1990), outcome measurements are poorly developed. An outcome instrument must determine the extent of residual disability and the degree of correction of the abnormality addressed by the index treatment. With respect to the foot there are several particular difficulties.

There is no satisfactory definition of normality, with wide variation in both shape (Steel *et al.* 1980; Staheli *et al.* 1987; Perlman *et al.* 1989; Welton 1992), range of joint motion (Oatis 1988; Lundberg *et al.* 1989a–d) and gait (Katoh *et al.* 1983), which is also influenced by sex and age (Roass and Andersson 1982; Nigg *et al.* 1992). Jahss (1984) has suggested that surgery should aim to produce a flexible plantigrade foot with painless metatarsal head weight-bearing rather than an arbitrary normality.

The anatomy and biomechanics of the foot are complex, and heretofore poorly understood. The advent of computed tomography (CT), foot pressure analysis and automated gait analysis has allowed an accurate understanding of foot function. Indeed, until the use of CT scanning, the correct analysis of common problems such as calcaneal fracture was not possible (Eastwood *et al.* 1993; Langdon *et al.* 1994).

In the past, there has been a nihilistic attitude to foot function after injury. It has even been suggested that satisfactory function occurs despite severe residual derangement (Pozo *et al.* 1984). This supposition has been reinforced by the minimization of symptoms using orthotics, as well as a natural tendency to make the most of residual function. Nevertheless, the re-establishment of normal anatomy may not be necessary for a return of apparently normal function following injury (Aitken 1963).

Outcome may be assessed by two different, overlapping methods:

- *Clinical outcomes*: these measure such variables as range of joint movement, foot pressures or radiographic indices. These are readily seen to be relevant to the index intervention, but may have little effect on the patient's perception of efficacy of treatment. Furthermore, the measurements may be unreproducible and therefore of poor scientific validity.

- *Functional outcomes*: these measure the patient's overall ability to perform within their social environment. With respect to isolated foot problems they may be insensitive, since the majority are directed at systemic disease. However, even after severe generalized body trauma, foot injury can be the major determinant of the ultimate level of function (Turchin *et al.* 1999; Stiegelmar *et al.* 2001).

Some outcome measures aim to combine the two categories of assessment, usually with specific reference to a particular region of the foot or disease (Kitaoka *et al.* 1994); however, scientific validation of these may be wanting. An increasing emphasis is being placed on functional rather than clinical outcomes (Saltzman 2001) but this must not obscure the researcher from his or her primary goal – the investigation and validation of intervention.

For the foot, bilateral disease is a potential, severe confounding variable. This is because it is almost impossible to separate individual foot contributions from functional disability and because it is more reliable to compare radiographic outcomes with the contralateral side rather than with a normal range. Where possible – for example in calcaneal fracture – it is probably better to exclude bilateral cases.

CLINICAL MEASUREMENTS

Range of movement

Movement ranges are an acceptable clinical technique for evaluating disability (Boone and Azen 1979), and represent a measure of return to normality after injury. Foot movements are described as occurring around theoretical axes perpendicular to the cardinal planes, sagittal (median), coronal (frontal) and transverse (horizontal) occur, and are respectively described as dorsiflexion/plantarflexion, eversion/inversion and abduction/adduction (Kirkup et al. 1988; Alexander 1990). Combinations of plantarflexion, adduction and inversion produce supination, whereas dorsiflexion, eversion and abduction produce pronation. The true axes of joint movement do not coincide with the theoretical and vary with joint position (Oatis 1988; Lundberg et al. 1989a–d). It is usually assumed that joint motion is uniplanar, but this approximation may be a source of error in the presence of gross mal-alignment. Measurement reliability varies with the joint (Low 1976) and is reduced for smaller bones and with increasing complexity of movement (Gadjosik and Bohannon 1987). All studies report similarity between the two sides in any subject, so for unilateral pathology comparison against the opposite limb is valid.

The metatarsophalangeal joints move in the sagittal and transverse planes, whereas the interphalangeal joints move only in the sagittal plane. Reported normal ranges vary, with significant differences between techniques and no reproducible data are available (Boone and Azen 1979; Roass and Andersson 1982; Norkin and White 1985; Backer and Kofoed 1987 1989; Oatis 1988; Alexander 1990).

The anatomical complexity and the number of articulations in the midfoot mean that movements can be only grossly assessed (Alexander 1990). No clinical method has been described to measure the motion of these joints discretely, although others (Lundberg et al. 1989a–c) have studied the joints using stereophotogrammetric techniques. In the absence of objective data, attempted quantification is inadvisable.

METHOD OF MEASUREMENT

Visual assessment is insufficiently reliable (Hellebrandt et al. 1949), while goniometric measurement is superior (Low 1976), though even the latter technique is inaccurate for small ranges of movement. The use of different goniometers does not seem to affect reliability, as long as the instruments are of appropriate size for the joint examined (Rothstein et al. 1983; Stratford et al. 1984). The reliability of goniometric measurement varies from joint to joint, being least acceptable in small joints, such as those of the foot, where it is difficult to accurately identify the centre of motion, the axes of movement, and consistent surface landmarks. Reliability may be improved by moving only one goniometer arm (Stratford et al. 1984). Electronic and pendulum goniometers are not an improvement on simple measurement (Clapper and Wolf 1988; Whittle 1991). With consistent positioning, the most accurate method of measuring joint motion is radiographic, although radiation dosage limits the use of this technique (Backer and Kofoed 1989; Bohannon et al. 1989).

Reliability is increased by the standardization of examination method (Ekstrand et al. 1982) and use of the neutral zero position (the normal anatomical position of the body) as the optimal starting point for measurements (American Academy of Orthopaedic Surgeons 1965; Debrunner 1982; Stratford et al. 1984).

GUIDELINES

Although the measurement of joint range of motion in the foot is unreliable, loss of mobility in the foot is a common complaint after injury or surgery. Hence, quantification may be useful, either as a direct outcome measure or for prognostic purposes. Intra-observer reliability is consistently higher than inter-observer reliability. Thus, in serial studies the same investigator should perform all the measurements using the same technique, which should be documented with its reproducibility. This also implies caution in direct comparison of data from different studies (Boone and Azen 1979; Stratford *et al.* 1984; Gadjosik and Bohannon 1987; Elveru *et al.* 1988). Comparisons to the unaffected limb are more valid than the use of 'normal ranges' (Boone and Azen 1979; Backer and Kofoed 1989).

Measuring deformity

CLINICAL EXAMINATION

Qualitative observational assessment of clinical deformity is simple, although quantification is all but impossible. Fixed deformity must be measured with the foot unloaded in order to avoid compensatory actions of unaffected joints (Oatis 1988).

RADIOGRAPHIC EXAMINATION

Routine projections include antero-posterior (AP), lateral, internal oblique and external oblique views. Non-weight-bearing views are adequate for assessing structural anatomy, including common normal variants. Weight-bearing studies are important for reproducible serial measurements, particularly where the radiographic angle may be susceptible to changes in axis and where the stress of weight bearing may alter the measurement, such as in hallux valgus or in tibialis posterior insufficiency. It is essential to employ standardized techniques both for radiographic examination and measurement (Schneider and Knahr 1998). Radiographic appearances vary widely in the normal, asymptomatic foot and some common radiographic measurements have unacceptably narrow reference ranges or are inaccurate (Steel *et al.* 1980). For angular measurements in hallux valgus, scientific studies of reproducibility have been undertaken and show good reproducibility for the hallux valgus angle and the 1–2 metatarsal angle (Smith *et al.* 1984; Coughlin *et al.* 2002). However the inter-observer reliability of the distal metatarsal articular angle is poor, as is the ability to discriminate joint congruency (Coughlin 2001).

These data imply caution in the use of radiographic outcome measures. However, in many disorders of the foot – for example, hallux valgus – the clinically perceived abnormalities are mirrored by radiographic parameters, and success or failure in radiographic correction provides a useful outcome measure to supplement clinical or functional assessment. Serial measurements or comparison with a contralateral normal are probably more meaningful than reference to a normal range. Common measurements and normal ranges are provided in Table 23.1.

Osteoarthritis

The development of osteoarthritis is a common outcome measure particularly following trauma (Olerud and Molander 1984; Heim 1989), and minimization of late degeneration is one argument for the anatomic operative fixation of fractures (Wright 1990), though exact reduction may not be necessary (Bauer *et al.* 1985).

The relationship between arthritic symptoms and severity of radiographic change is inconsistent (Bagge *et al.* 1991; Hart *et al.* 1991), in part due to the radiographic assessment methods. The Kellgren and Lawrence scale (Kellgren and Lawrence 1957) is the most widely used, but it places significant weight on the presence of osteophytes (Kellgren *et al.* 1963; Mazur *et al.* 1979; Hattrup and Johnson 1988; Heim 1989; Merchant and Dietz 1989), which may be inappropriate (Croft 1990). It is also insensitive to early or mild disease, and if comparisons between studies are to be undertaken then standardized radiographs must be employed.

At the knee joint, scales based predominantly upon loss of joint space are more reproducible than those based on osteophytes (Dacre *et al.* 1988; Cooper *et al.* 1990), but although this type of scale has been used (Olerud and Molander 1984; Ahl *et al.* 1989) it has not been formally evaluated for the foot. The only joint in the foot where the width has been analysed is the ankle (Jonsson *et al.* 1984). Reliability data for radiographic scales of osteoarthritis are scant. Both Wright and Acheson (1970) and Kellgren

Table 23.1: Radiographic measurements from plain radiographs, with normal values

Measurement	Normal range (°)
Measurements on antero-posterior radiograph	
Hallux-interphalangeal angle	6–24
Hallux valgus (Hallux-metatarsophalangeal) angle	0–20
First intertarsal angle	<9
Metatarsal break angle (angle formed by line drawn tangential to first and second metatarsal heads plus line tangential to second and fifth metatarsal heads)	140
First to fifth intertarsal angle	14–35
Talar-second metatarsal angle	6–42
Talocalcaneal angle	30–50 under 5 years old 15–30 over 5 years
Measurements on lateral radiograph	
Lateral talocalcaneal angle	25–30
Fifth metatarsal base height	2.3–3.8
Calcaneal pitch angle	10–30
Bohler's angle	22–48
Tibiocalcanean angle	60–90
Talar-first metatarsal angle	−4 to +4

and Lawrence (1957) reported relatively poor intra- and inter-observer reliability but did not provide data for the measurement of joint width alone. Hattrup and Johnson (1988) presented a scale for the assessment of the severity of osteoarthritis of the first metatarsophalangeal joint in hallux rigidus, but without scientific validation (Table 23.2).

Gait analysis

Normal human gait consists of a series of complex coordinated movements, which are measured systematically and quantified by gait analysis. Gait analysis can be visual, or it can be achieved by monitoring force and pressure measurements at the foot–ground interface, by measuring muscle action potentials (electromyography), or by the

Table 23.2: Grading of hallux rigidus. Reprinted from Hattrup and Johnson (1988)

Grade 1: Mild to moderate osteophyte formation but good joint space preservation

Grade 2: Moderate osteophyte formation with joint space narrowing and subchondral cyst formation

Grade 3: Marked osteophyte formation and loss of the visible joint space, with or without subchondral cyst formation

measurement of energy expenditure during locomotion (Whittle 1991).

VISUALIZATION

The visual inspection of gait is unsystematic, subjective and observer skill-dependent (Whittle 1991). Even skilled observers miss subtle abnormalities and have difficulty quantifying simple parameters such as cadence, stride length and velocity (Saleh and Murdoch 1985). Gait laboratory analysis provides a more stringent assessment of function than do either subjective analysis or clinical examination. However, notwithstanding improved instrumentation and measurement techniques, it has not gained widespread clinical use except in the management of cerebral palsy, and is more suitable for the evaluation of movement in large joints than in the foot and ankle.

ELECTROMYOGRAPHY

Electromyography is primarily useful to determine the timing of muscle contraction during the gait cycle, but it may be difficult to obtain satisfactory recordings from a walking subject. It is useful in planning tendon transfers in cerebral palsy (Perry and Hoffer 1977), but has little place in outcome assessment in the foot.

ENERGY CONSUMPTION

Abnormalities of gait increase the energy required for walking. Energy consumption can be measured by whole body calorimetry, and this methodology has been applied mainly as a research tool for the investigation of abnormalities of gait associated with large joint disease such as osteoarthritis of the hip. It has not been used for the analysis of foot function.

FOOT–GROUND INTERFACE

The amount and direction of ground-to-foot reaction forces can be measured using force plates. This allows calculation of joint moments and forces. In clinical practice it is more useful to measure the pressure distribution beneath the foot (Lord 1981) if a convenient system which provides accurate, reproducible, clinically relevant and reliable data in an understandable form is available (Duckworth et al. 1988).

Three types of device are available:

- the Harris mat;

- the force plate (Dhanendran et al. 1978); and
- the pedobarograph (Duckworth et al. 1982).

In a comparative study (Hughes et al. 1987), the force plate was found to be the most precise method, though spatial resolution and reliability were poor [Coefficient of variation (CV) 18.3–23.3%], and it was also the most expensive to operate. The Harris mat, which is cheap and easy to use, could be quantitated only with difficulty, though its reliability was similar to that of the pedobarograph (CV 12%). The pedobarograph was less accurate but more reliable (CV 10.9%), the resolution was markedly better, and the print-out clearly showed pressure distribution.

Advances in computing and sensor technology have allowed major developments in pedobarography. Data are collected and analysed using a portable computer. Here, two modern systems will be described as examples, namely the Musgrave Footprint™ pressure plate (Preston Communications, Ltd., Dublin, Ireland) and the GAITRite system (CIR Systems, Inc., East Darby Road, Havertown, PA, USA).

The Musgrave Footprint™

This is a flush-mounted, platform-based, vertical pressure measurement system. Force is measured by an array of 2048 high-quality force-sensitive resistor (FSR) sensors, which are sampled at approximately 60 Hz. Since each sensor is 5 mm × 5 mm (0.25 cm^2), pressure (force per unit area) may be quantified. Pressure magnitudes can be recorded from 0 to 15 kg/cm^2. Plantar pressures <3 kg/cm^2 during posture and <11 kg/cm^2 during normal walking are pathological.

The GAITRite system

This system measures not only spatial gait parameters but, by using a longer walkway, temporal parameters between footfalls are also assessed and recorded on a computer. The standard GAITRite electronic walkway contains six sensor pads encapsulated in a roll-up carpet to produce an active area which is 61 cm (24 inches) wide and 366 cm (144 inches) long. In this arrangement, the active area is a grid of 48 × 288 sensors placed on 1.27-cm (0.5-inch) centres, totalling 13 824 sensors.

In addition to the visual representation of the foot-step and cadence, a number of quantifiable functions may be derived. The centre of pressure curve is comprised of the centroids of the vertical pressures exerted upon the foot at each instant sampled throughout stance phase. The centre of pressure is also the origin of the three-dimensional ground reaction force vector of the entire body. The centre of pressure excursion index (CPEI) describes the lateral deviation of the centre of pressure from the centre of pressure reference line (CPRL, i.e. the line connecting the initial and the final centre of pressures values) in the region of the metatarsal conic curve (i.e. the anterior one third trisection of the foot). In a pronated foot, the concavity of the centre of pressure line will be decreased and a smaller CPEI value will be observed. The primary value of the CPEI measurement is objectively to document dynamic foot function (e.g. excessive pronation) during gait.

The GAITRite system places great weight on the Functional Ambulatory Performance (FAP) score, the basis for which is a linear relationship of Step Length/Leg Length ratio to step time when the velocity is 'normalized' to Leg Length in healthy adults (Grieve and Gear 1966; Al-Obaidi 1991; Leiper and Craik 1991).

In choosing between these devices, the trade-off is between the increased accuracy of the Musgrave Footprint (0.25 cm² area for each sensor compared with 1.61 cm² for the GAITRite) against the ability of the GAITRite system to analyse multiple footfalls.

An alternative approach is the Pedar™ insole system (Novel GmbH, Munich, Germany), which consists of an in-shoe array of capacitive sensors embedded in a 2.6-cm flexible shoe insert (Graf 1993). This is probably more applicable to shoe-wear and insole design.

As computing power and sensor technology develop, these techniques will continue to become more readily and cheaply available, and are likely to allow increasingly sophisticated insights into foot function. At present, the correlation between individual measurements and their changes and patient symptoms is incomplete. However, it seems probable that these types of analysis will in the future become essential for research and clinical applications.

FUNCTIONAL ASSESSMENTS

A number of functional assessment instruments exist which may be applied to patients with foot disease. These consist of a series of questions that are either self-administered or (less desirably) require a trained operator. The questions are designed to represent the patient's function in different aspects of their life (Guyatt et al. 1992). The five most widely used scoring systems which have been validated for musculoskeletal disease are:

- the Short Form 36 (SF-36) (Ware 1992);
- the Sickness Impact Profile (SIP) (Bergner et al. 1981);
- the Nottingham Health Profile (NHP) (McEwen 1983);
- the Quality of Wellbeing Scale (QWS) (Williams 1991), upon which the Quality of Life Years (QALYs) are based; and
- the Musculoskeletal Functional Assessment (MFA) (Engelberg et al. 1996), together with its shortened form (Swiontkowski et al. 1999).

In use, the SIP is lengthy, while the QWS and NHP require professional administration; hence, the SF-36 and MFA are the preferred outcome measures. The MFA is probably more reliable for foot disability, particularly if the general effects are minor. However, the SF-36 has been more widely used.

As an alternative, Rowan (2001) has developed and validated a multi-dimensional measure of chronic pain specifically aimed at the foot (the Rowan Foot Pain Assessment Questionnaire; ROF-PAQ). The final scale demonstrates better than standard readability, and has both a short completion time and a simple scoring method. This is a potentially exciting approach, which is as yet incompletely explored.

Where the major functional limitation is pain, a visual analogue scale may be valuable (Huskisson 1974).

THE AMERICAN ORTHOPAEDIC FOOT AND ANKLE SOCIETY (AOFAS) SCORING SYSTEMS

Kitaoka *et al.* (1994) (Tables 23.3–23.5) described a series of instruments aimed specifically at disability in various parts of the foot and ankle. These are hybrid-scoring systems because they combine elements of functional outcome with clinical evaluation. Although it is tempting to employ scoring systems which have been developed specifically for the foot, these systems have not been subjected to rigorous statistical analysis (Kerr *et al.* 1996), and preliminary analysis suggests that they may not behave in a statistically reliable fashion (Guyton 2001). Hence, the scores may not be susceptible to analysis, at least using parametric methods. Retrospective use of these scoring systems is unreliable (Toolan *et al.* 2001). The increasing use of these systems is providing a spurious validity, but it is imperative that a full analysis be performed before they are accepted scientifically.

GENERAL CONSIDERATIONS

The following should always be reported where relevant. Wound healing, chronic sepsis, fracture or osteotomy healing, non-union, revision surgeries, failures, recovery times, nerve or vessel damage associated with the index procedure, and any other significant complication (Chen *et al.* 2001).

RECOMMENDATIONS

Where the outcome of injury is being investigated, reports should include at least two years of follow-up. In other surgical interventions, one year is probably usually adequate, though the outcome of replacement arthroplasty will require long-term results.

Functional assessment should be made with the SF-36 or MFA, while the AOFAS scores should be

Table 23.3: American Orthopaedic Foot and Ankle Society Grading for the midfoot. Reprinted from Kitaoka *et al.* (1994)

Pain (40 points)	
None	40
Mild, occasional	30
Moderate, daily	20
Severe, almost always present	0
Function (45 points)	
Activity limitations, support	
No limitations, no support	10
No limitations of daily activities, limitation of recreational activities, no support	7
Limited daily and recreational activities, cane	4
Severe limitation of daily and recreational activities, walker, crutches, wheelchair	0
Footwear requirements	
Fashionable, conventional shoes, no insert required	5
Comfort footwear, shoe insert	3
Modified shoes or brace	0
Maximum walking distance in blocks	
>6	10
4–6	7
1–3	4
<1	0
Walking surfaces	
No difficulty on any surface	10
Some difficulty on uneven terrain, stairs, inclines, ladders	5
Severe difficulty on uneven terrain, stairs, inclines, ladders	0
Gait abnormality	
None, slight	10
Obvious	5
Marked	0
Alignment (15 points)	
Good, plantigrade foot, midfoot well-aligned	15
Fair, plantigrade foot, some degree of mid-foot mal-alignment observed, no symptoms	8
Poor, non-plantigrade foot, severe mal-alignment, symptoms	0

Table 23.4: American Orthopaedic Foot and Ankle Society Grading for the hallux metatarsophalangeal joint. Reprinted from Kitaoka *et al.* (1994)

Pain (40 points)	
None	40
Mild, occasional	30
Moderate, daily	20
Severe, almost always present	0
Function (45 points)	
Activity limitations	
No limitations	10
No limitations of daily activities, limitation of recreational activities	7
Limited daily and recreational activities	4
Severe limitation of daily and recreational activities	0
Footwear requirements	
Fashionable, conventional shoes, no insert required	10
Comfort footwear, shoe insert	5
Modified shoes or brace	0
MTPJ motion (dorsiflexion plus plantarflexion)	
Normal or mild restriction ($\geq 75°$)	10
Moderate restriction (30–74°)	5
Severe restriction ($< 30°$)	0
IP joint motion (plantarflexion)	
No restriction	5
Severe restriction	0
MTP-IP stability (all directions)	
Stable	5
Unstable	0
Callus related to hallux mtp-ip joints	
No callus or asymptomatic	5
Symptomatic	0
Alignment (15 points)	
Good, hallux well-aligned	15
Fair, some degree of hallux mal-alignment, no symptoms	8
Poor, obvious symptomatic mal-alignment	0

Table 23.5: American Orthopaedic Foot and Ankle Society Grading for the lesser metatarsophalangeal-interphalangeal joints. Reprinted from Kitaoka *et al.* (1994)

Pain (40 points)	
None	40
Mild, occasional	30
Moderate, daily	20
Severe, almost always present	0
Function (45 points)	
Activity limitations	
No limitations	10
No limitations of daily activities, limitation of recreational activities	7
Limited daily and recreational activities	4
Severe limitation of daily and recreational activities	0
Footwear requirements	
Fashionable, conventional shoes, no insert required	10
Comfort footwear, shoe insert	5
Modified shoes or brace	0
MTPJ motion (dorsiflexion plus plantarflexion)	
Normal or mild restriction ($\geq 75°$)	10
Moderate restriction (30–74°)	5
Severe restriction ($< 30°$)	0
IP joint motion (plantarflexion)	
No restriction	5
Severe restriction	0
MTP-IP stability (all directions)	
Stable	5
Unstable	0
Callus related to lesser mtp-ip joints	
No callus or asymptomatic	5
Symptomatic	0
Alignment (15 points)	
Good, lesser toes well-aligned	15
Fair, some degree of lesser toe mal-alignment, no symptoms	8
Poor, obvious symptomatic mal-alignment	0

employed with great reservation and not used in isolation.

Radiographic outcome should include relevant measurements compared to the contralateral side and, where possible, compared to the pre-intervention situation (Okuda *et al.* 2001). The presence of arthritis should be reported simply.

Clinical outcomes should include a form of pedobarography (Metaxiotis *et al.* 2000), combined with relevant ranges of movement compared with the contralateral side and the situation prior to intervention.

REFERENCES

Ahl, T., Dalen, N., and Selvik, G. (1989): Ankle fractures. *Clin Orthop Rel Res* **245**, 246–55.

Aitken, A. P. (1963): Fractures of the os calcis – treatment by closed reduction. *Clin Orthop Rel Res* **30**, 67–75.

Al-Obaidi, S. (1991): *The Relationship of Anticipated and Experienced Chronic Knee Pain to Kinematic and Proficiency of Walking in Adults*. Ph.D. Thesis, Dept. of Physical Therapy, New York University.

Alexander, I. A. (1990): *The Foot: Examination and diagnosis*. Churchill Livingstone, New York.

American Academy of Orthopaedic Surgeons (1965): *Joint Motion: Method of measuring and recording*. American Academy of Orthopaedic Surgeons, Chicago.

Backer, M., and Kofoed, H. (1987): Weightbearing and non-weightbearing ankle joint mobility. *Med Sci Res* **15**, 1309–10.

Backer, M., and Kofoed, H. (1989): Passive ankle mobility: clinical measurement compared with radiography. *J Bone Joint Surg* **71-B**, 696–8.

Bagge, E., Bjelle, A., Eden, S., and Svanborg, A. (1991): Osteoarthritis in the elderly: clinical and radiological findings in 79 and 85 year olds. *Ann Rheum Dis* **50**, 535–9.

Bauer, M., Jonsson, K., and Nilsson, B. (1985): Thirty-year follow up of ankle fractures. *Acta Orthop Scand* **56**, 103–6.

Bergner, M., Bobbitt, R. A., and Carter, W. B. (1981): The Sickness Impact Profile: development and final revision of a health status measure. *Med Care* **19**, 787–805.

Bohannon, R. W., Tiberio, D., and Zito, M. (1989): Selected measures of ankle dorsiflexion range of motion: differences and intercorrelations. *Foot Ankle* **10**, 99–103.

Boone, D. C., and Azen, S. P. (1979): Normal ranges of motion of joints in male subjects. *J Bone Joint Surg* **61-A**, 756–9.

Chen, C.-H., Huang, P.-J., Chen, T.-B., Cheng, Y.-M., Lin, S.-Y., Chiang, H.-C., and Chen, L.-C. (2001): Isolated talonavicular arthrodesis for talonavicular arthritis. *Foot Ankle Int* **22**, 633–41.

Clapper, M. P., and Wolf, S. L. (1988): Comparison of the reliability of the Orthoranger and the standard goniometer for assessing active lower extremity range of motion. *Phys Ther* **68**, 214–18.

Cooper, C., Cushnaghan, J., Kirwan, J., Rogers, J., McAlindon, T., McCrae, F., and Dieppe, P. A. (1990): Radiographic assessment of the knee joint in osteoarthritis. *Br J Rheumatol* **29** (Suppl. 1), 19–26.

Coughlin, M. J. (2001): The reliability of angular measurement in hallux valgus deformities. *Foot Ankle Int* **22**, 369–79.

Coughlin, M. J., Saltzman, C. L., and Nunley, J. A. (2002): Angular measurements in the evaluation of hallux valgus deformities: a report of the Ad Hoc committee of the American Orthopaedic Foot and Ankle Society on angular measurements. *Foot Ankle Int* **23**, 68–74.

Croft, P. (1990): Review of UK data on the rheumatic diseases. 3: Osteoarthritis. *Br J Rheumatol* **29**, 391–5.

Dacre, J. E., Herbert, K. E., Perret, D., and Huskisson, E. (1988): The use of digital image analysis for the assessment of radiographs in osteoarthritis. *Br J Rheumatol* **27** (Suppl. 1), 46.

Debrunner, H. U. (1982): *Orthopaedic Diagnosis*. Georg Thieme Verlag, Stuttgart.

Dhanendran, M., Hutton, W., and Paker, Y. (1978): The distribution of force under the human foot: an on-line measuring system. *Meas Control* **11**, 261–4.

Duckworth, T., Betts, R. P., Franks, C. I., and Burke, J. (1982): The measurement of pressures under the foot. *Foot Ankle* **3**, 130–41.

Duckworth, T., Helal, B., and Wilson, D. (1988): Pedobarography. In: *The Foot*. Churchill Livingstone, Edinburgh, pp. 108–30.

Eastwood, D. M., Gregg, P., and Atkins, R. M. (1993): Calcaneal fractures: pathological anatomy and classification. *J Bone Joint Surg Br* **75-B**, 183–9.

Ekstrand, J., Witkorsson, M., Oberg, B., and Gillquist, J. (1982): Lower extremity goniometry measurements: a study to determine their reliability. *Arch Phys Med Rehabil* **63**, 171–5.

Elveru, R. A., Rothstein, J. M., and Lamb, R. L. (1988): Goniometric reliability in a clinical setting: subtalar and ankle joint measurements. *Phys Ther* **68**, 672–7.

Engelberg, R., Martin, D. P., Agel, J., Obremsky, W., Coronado, G., and Swiontkowski, M. F. (1996): Musculoskeletal function assessment instrument: criterion and construct validity. *J Orthop Res Mar* **14**, 182–92.

Gadjosik, R. L., and Bohannon, R. W. (1987): Clinical measurement of range of motion: review of goniometry emphasising reliability and validity. *Phys Ther* **67**, 1867–72.

Graf, P. M. (1993): The EMED system of foot pressure analysis. *Clin Podiatr Surg* **10**, 445–54.

Grieve, D., and Gear, R. (1966): The relationships between length of stride, step frequency, time of swing, and speed of walking for children and adults. *Ergonomics* **5**, 379.

Guyatt, G. H., Kirshner, B., and Jaeschke, R. (1992): Measuring health status: what are the necessary measurement properties? *J Clin Epidemiol* **118**, 622–9.

Guyton, P. G. (2001): Theoretical limitations of the AOFAS scoring systems: an analysis using Monte Carlo modelling. *Foot Ankle Int* **22**, 779–87.

Hart, D. J., Spector, T. D., Brown, P., Wilson, P., Doyle, D. V., and Silman, A. J. (1991): Clinical signs of early osteoarthritis: reproducibility and relation to X-ray changes in 541 women in the general population. *Ann Rheum Dis* **50**, 467–70.

Hattrup, S. J., and Johnson, K. A. (1988): Subjective results of hallux rigidus following treatment with cheilectomy. *Clin Orthop Rel Res* **226**, 182–91.

Heim, U. F. A. (1989): Trimalleolar fractures: late results after fixation of the posterior fragment. *Orthopaedics* **12**, 1053–9.

Hellebrandt, F. A., Duvall, E. N., and Moore, M. L. (1949): The measurement of joint motion: Part III. Reliability of goniometry. *Phys Ther Rev* **29**, 302–7.

Hughes, J., Kriss, S., and Klenerman, L. (1987): A clinician's view of foot pressure: a comparison of three different methods of measurement. *Foot Ankle* **7**, 277–84.

Huskisson, E. C. (1974): Measurement of pain. *Lancet* **2**, 1127–31.

Jahss, M. H. (1984): Editorial. *Foot Ankle* **4**, 227–8.

Jonsson, K., Fredin, H. O., Cederlund, C. G., and Bauer, M. (1984): Width of the normal ankle joint. *Acta Radiol Diag* **25**, 147–9.

Katoh, V., Chao, E. Y. S., Laughman, R. K., Schneider, E., and Morrey, B. F. (1983): Biomechanical analysis of foot function during gait and clinical applications. *Clin Orthop Rel Res* **177**, 23–33.

Kellgren, J. H., and Lawrence, J. S. (1957): Radiological assessment of osteoarthritis. *Ann Rheum Dis* **16**, 494–502.

Kellgren, J. H., Jeffrey, M., and Ball, J. (1963): *The Epidemiology of Chronic Rheumatism. Volume 2. Atlas of Standard Radiographs.* Blackwell Scientific, Oxford.

Kerr, P. S., Prothero, D., and Atkins, R. M. (1996): Assessing outcome after calcaneal fracture: a rational scoring system. *Injury* **27**, 35–9.

Kirkup, J., Helal, B., and Wilson, D. (1988): Terminology. In: *The Foot*. Churchill Livingstone, Edinburgh, pp. 202–10.

Kitaoka, H., Alexander, I. J., Adelaar, R. S., Nunley, J. A., Myerson, M. S., and Sanders, M. (1994): Clinical rating systems for the ankle-hindfoot, midfoot, hallux and lesser toes. *Foot Ankle Int* **15**, 349–53.

Langdon, I., Kerr, P., and Atkins, R. M. (1994): Pathologic anatomy of intra-articular fractures of the calcaneum. The anterolateral fragment. *J Bone Joint Surg Br* **76-B**, 303–5.

Leiper, C., and Craik, R. (1991): Relationships between physical activity and temporal-distance characteristics of walking in elderly women. *Phys Ther* **71**, 791.

Lord, M. (1981): Foot pressure measurement: a review of methodology. *J Biomed Eng* **3**, 91–9.

Low, J. (1976): Reliability of joint measurements. *Physiotherapy* **62**, 227–9.

Lundberg, A., Goldie, I., Kalin, B., and Selvik, G. (1989a): Kinematics of the ankle/foot complex: plantarflexion and dorsiflexion. *Foot Ankle* **9**, 194–200.

Lundberg, A., Svensson, O. K., Bylund, C., Goldie, I., and Selvik, G. (1989b): Kinematics of the ankle/foot complex. Part 2: pronation and supination. *Foot Ankle* **9**, 248–53.

Lundberg, A., Svensson, O. K., Bylund, C., and Selvik, G. (1989c): Kinematics of the ankle/foot complex. Part 3: influence of leg rotation. *Foot Ankle* **9**, 304–9.

Lundberg, A., Svensson, O. K., Nemeth, G., and Selvik, G. (1989d): The axis of rotation of the ankle joint. *J Bone Joint Surg* **71-B**, 94–9.

Mann, R. A., and Plattner, P. F. (1990): Ankle and foot: editorial overview. *Curr Opin Orthop* **1**, 111–12.

Mazur, J. M., Schwartz, E., and Simon, S. R. (1979): Ankle arthrodesis: long-term follow-up with gait analysis. *J Bone Joint Surg* **61-A**, 964–75.

McEwen, J. (1983): The Nottingham Health Profile. A measure of perceived health, In Teeling-Smith, G. (ed.), *Measuring the Social Benefits of Medicine*. Office of Health Economics, London, pp. 75–84.

Merchant, T. C., and Dietz, F. R. (1989): Long-term follow-up after fractures of the tibial and fibular shafts. *J Bone Joint Surg* **71-A**, 599–606.

Metaxiotis, D., Accles, W., Pappas, A., and Doederlein, L. (2000): Dynamic pedobarography (DPB) in the management of cavovarus foot deformity. *Foot Ankle Int* **21**, 935–47.

Nigg, B. M., Fisher, V., Allinger, T. L., Ronsky, J. R., and Engsberg, J. R. (1992): Range of motion of the foot as a function of age. *Foot Ankle* **13**, 336–44.

Norkin, C. C., and White, D. J. (1985): *Measurement of Joint Motion: A Guide to Goniometry*. F. A. Davis, Philadelphia.

Oatis, C. A. (1988): Biomechanics of the foot and ankle under static conditions. *Phys Ther* **68**, 1815–21.

Okuda, R., Kinoshita, M., Morikawa, J., Jotoku, T., and Abe, M. (2001): Surgical treatment for hallux valgus with painful plantar callosities. *Foot Ankle Int* **22**, 203–8.

Olerud, C., and Molander, H. (1984): A scoring scale for symptom evaluation after ankle fracture. *Arch Othop Trauma Surg* **103**, 190–4.

Perlman, M. D., Leveille, D., and Gale, B. (1989): Traumatic classifications of the foot and ankle. *J Foot Surg* **28**, 551–85.

Perry, J., and Hoffer, M. M. (1977): Preoperative and postoperative dynamic electromyography as an aid in planning tendon transfers in children with cerebral palsy. *J Bone Joint Surg* **59-A**, 531–7.

Pozo, J. L., Kirwan, E. O. G., and Jackson, A. M. (1984): The long-term results of conservative management of severely displaced fractures of the calcaneus. *J Bone Joint Surg* **66-B**, 386–90.

Roass, A., and Andersson, G. B. J. (1982): Normal range of motion of the hip, knee and ankle joints in male subjects, 30–40 years of age. *Acta Orthop Scand* **53**, 205–8.

Rothstein, J. M., Miller, P. J., and Roettger, R. F. (1983): Goniometric reliability in a clinical setting: elbow and knee measurements. *Phys Ther* **63**, 1611–15.

Rowan, K. J. (2001): Development and validation of a multi-dimensional measure of chronic foot pain: the Rowan Foot Pain Assessment Questionnaire (ROFPAQ). *Foot Ankle Int* **22**, 795–809.

Saleh, M., and Murdoch, G. (1985): In defence of gait analysis. *J Bone Joint Surg* **67-B**, 237–41.

Saltzman, C. L. (2001): Why outcomes research? (Editorial). *Foot Ankle Int* **22**, 773–4.

Schneider, W., and Knahr, K. (1998): Metatarsophalangeal and intermetatarsal angle: different values and interpretation of post-operative results dependent on the technique of measurement. *Foot Ankle Int* **19**, 532–6.

Smith, R. W., Reynolds, J. C., and Steward, M. J. (1984): Hallux valgus assessment: report of research committee of American Foot and Ankle Society. *Foot Ankle* **5**, 92–103.

Staheli, L. T., Chew, D. E., and Corbett, M. (1987): The longitudinal arch: a survey of eight hundred and eighty two feet in normal children and adults. *J Bone Joint Surg Am* **69A**, 426–8.

Steel, M. W., Johnson, K. A., DeWitz, M. A., and Ilstrup, D. M. (1980): Radiographic measurements of the normal adult foot. *Foot Ankle* **1**, 151–8.

Stiegelmar, R., McKee, M. D., Waddell, J. P., and Schemitsch, E. H. (2001): Outcome of foot injuries in multiply injured patients. *Orthop Clin North Am* **32**, 193–204.

Stratford, P., Agostino, V., Brazeau, C., and Gowitzke, B. A. (1984): Reliability of joint angle measurement: a discussion of methodology issues. *Physiotherapy Canada* **36**, 5–9.

Swiontkowski, M. F., Engelberg, R., Martin, D. P., and Agel, J. (1999): Short musculoskeletal function assessment questionnaire: validity, reliability, and responsiveness. *J Bone Joint Surg Am* **81**, 1245–60.

Toolan, B. C., Wright Quinones, V. J., Cunningham, B. J., and Brage, M. E. (2001): An evaluation of the use of retrospectively acquired preoperative AOFAS clinical rating scores to assess surgical outcome after elective foot and ankle surgery. *Foot Ankle Int* **22**, 775–87.

Turchin, D. C. J., Schemitsch, E. H., McKee, M. D., and Waddell, J. P. (1999): Do foot injuries significantly affect the functional outcome of multiply injured patients? *J Orthop Trauma* **13**, 1–4.

Ware, J. E. (1992): The MOS 36 short-form health survey (SF-36). *Med Care* **30**, 473–83.

Welton, E. A. (1992): The Harris and Beath footprint: interpretation and clinical value. *Foot Ankle* **13**, 462–8.

Whittle, M. (1991): *Gait Analysis: An Introduction.* Butterworth-Heinemann Ltd., Oxford.

Williams, A. (1991): Setting priorities in healthcare: an economist's view. *J Bone Joint Surg* **73-B**, 365–7.

Wright, E. C., and Acheson, R. M. (1970): New Haven survey of joint diseases. XI: Observer variability in the assessment of x-rays for osteoarthrosis of the hands. *Am J Epidemiol* **91**, 378–92.

Wright, V. (1990): Post-traumatic osteoarthritis – a medico-legal minefield. *Br J Rheumatol* **29**, 474–8.

Index